Margarita Sordo, Sachin Vaidya and Lakhmi C. Jain (Eds.)

Advanced Computational Intelligence Paradigms in Healthcare - 3

Studies in Computational Intelligence, Volume 107

Editor-in-chief
Prof. Janusz Kacprzyk
Systems Research Institute
Polish Academy of Sciences
ul. Newelska 6
01-447 Warsaw
Poland
E-mail: kacprzyk@ibspan.waw.pl

Further volumes of this series can be found on our homepage: springer.com

Vol. 84. Marek R. Ogiela and Ryszard Tadeusiewicz
Modern Computational Intelligence Methods for the Interpretation of Medical Images, 2008
ISBN 978-3-540-75399-5

Vol. 85. Arpad Kelemen, Ajith Abraham and Yulan Liang (Eds.)
Computational Intelligence in Medical Informatics, 2008
ISBN 978-3-540-75766-5

Vol. 86. Zbigniew Les and Mogdalena Les
Shape Understanding Systems, 2008
ISBN 978-3-540-75768-9

Vol. 87. Yuri Avramenko and Andrzej Kraslawski
Case Based Design, 2008
ISBN 978-3-540-75705-4

Vol. 88. Tina Yu, David Davis, Cem Baydar and Rajkumar Roy (Eds.)
Evolutionary Computation in Practice, 2008
ISBN 978-3-540-75770-2

Vol. 89. Ito Takayuki, Hattori Hiromitsu, Zhang Minjie and Matsuo Tokuro (Eds.)
Rational, Robust, Secure, 2008
ISBN 978-3-540-76281-2

Vol. 90. Simone Marinai and Hiromichi Fujisawa (Eds.)
Machine Learning in Document Analysis and Recognition, 2008
ISBN 978-3-540-76279-9

Vol. 91. Horst Bunke, Kandel Abraham and Last Mark (Eds.)
Applied Pattern Recognition, 2008
ISBN 978-3-540-76830-2

Vol. 92. Ang Yang, Yin Shan and Lam Thu Bui (Eds.)
Success in Evolutionary Computation, 2008
ISBN 978-3-540-76285-0

Vol. 93. Manolis Wallace, Marios Angelides and Phivos Mylonas (Eds.)
Advances in Semantic Media Adaptation and Personalization, 2008
ISBN 978-3-540-76359-8

Vol. 94. Arpad Kelemen, Ajith Abraham and Yuehui Chen (Eds.)
Computational Intelligence in Bioinformatics, 2008
ISBN 978-3-540-76802-9

Vol. 95. Radu Dogaru
Systematic Design for Emergence in Cellular Nonlinear Networks, 2008
ISBN 978-3-540-76800-5

Vol. 96. Aboul-Ella Hassanien, Ajith Abraham and Janusz Kacprzyk (Eds.)
Computational Intelligence in Multimedia Processing: Recent Advances, 2008
ISBN 978-3-540-76826-5

Vol. 97. Gloria Phillips-Wren, Nikhil Ichalkaranje and Lakhmi C. Jain (Eds.)
Intelligent Decision Making: An AI-Based Approach, 2008
ISBN 978-3-540-76829-9

Vol. 98. Ashish Ghosh, Satchidananda Dehuri and Susmita Ghosh (Eds.)
Multi-Objective Evolutionary Algorithms for Knowledge Discovery from Databases, 2008
ISBN 978-3-540-77466-2

Vol. 99. George Meghabghab and Abraham Kandel
Search Engines, Link Analysis, and User's Web Behavior, 2008
ISBN 978-3-540-77468-6

Vol. 100. Anthony Brabazon and Michael O'Neill (Eds.)
Natural Computing in Computational Finance, 2008
ISBN 978-3-540-77476-1

Vol. 101. Michael Granitzer, Mathias Lux and Marc Spaniol (Eds.)
Multimedia Semantics - The Role of Metadata, 2008
ISBN 978-3-540-77472-3

Vol. 102. Carlos Cotta, Simeon Reich, Robert Schaefer and Antoni Ligeza (Eds.)
Knowledge-Driven Computing, 2008
ISBN 978-3-540-77474-7

Vol. 103. Devendra K. Chaturvedi
Soft Computing Techniques and its Applications in Electrical Engineering, 2008
ISBN 978-3-540-77480-8

Vol. 104. Maria Virvou and Lakhmi C. Jain (Eds.)
Intelligent Interactive Systems in Knowledge-Based Environment, 2008
ISBN 978-3-540-77470-9

Vol. 105. Wolfgang Guenthner
Enhancing Cognitive Assistance Systems with Inertial Measurement Units, 2008
ISBN 978-3-540-76996-5

Vol. 106. Jacqueline Jarvis, Dennis Jarvis, Ralph Rönnquist and Lakhmi C. Jain (Eds.)
Holonic Execution: A BDI Approach, 2008
ISBN 978-3-540-77478-5

Vol. 107. Margarita Sordo, Sachin Vaidya and Lakhmi C. Jain (Eds.)
Advanced Computational Intelligence Paradigms in Healthcare - 3, 2008
ISBN 978-3-540-77661-1

Margarita Sordo
Sachin Vaidya
Lakhmi C. Jain (Eds.)

Advanced Computational Intelligence Paradigms in Healthcare - 3

With 90 Figures and 14 Tables

Springer

Dr. Margarita Sordo
Decision Systems Group
Harvard Medical School
900 Commonwealth Ave, 3rd Floor
Boston MA 02215
USA

Dr. Sachin Vaidya
Adelaide
Australia

Prof. Lakhmi C. Jain
University of South Australia
School of Electrical &
Information Engineering
KES Centre
Mawson Lakes Campus
Adelaide SA 5095
Australia

ISBN 978-3-540-77661-1 e-ISBN 978-3-540-77662-8

Studies in Computational Intelligence ISSN 1860-949X

Library of Congress Control Number: 2008921396

Cover design: Deblik, Berlin, Germany

Printed on acid-free paper

9 8 7 6 5 4 3 2 1

springer.com

Foreword

Advances in computational intelligence have created powerful tools for manipulating vast amounts of patient data and transform it into valuable information from which expert knowledge can be extracted. The significance of this statement is understood best if one considers the large amounts of data healthcare applications most often need to handle in order to provide the key information for early detection, diagnosis and decision support – all critical aspects of healthcare.

This book shows the wide role computational intelligence can play in the development of healthcare applications. It introduces the core concepts of computational intelligence and demonstrates their usability in healthcare. After introducing the basic concepts, the book's subsequent chapters cover the development of various applications ranging from cancer detection in optical spectroscopy, image interpretation, optimized medication regimens and diagnostic support, to ubiquitous computing, computational tools to assist disabled people, and ethical systems.

As a whole, the book is a major reference for practitioners and researchers alike, interested in both computational intelligence and healthcare. I believe this is an excellent resource and I hope it will encourage readers to immerse in this fascinating field and further explore the challenges that lay ahead.

Gabriela Ochoa, PhD
School of Computer Science
University of Nottingham, UK

Preface

Computational Intelligence rises to the imperative challenge of implementing robust computer applications to process the vast amount of information captured by computers and to extract meaningful knowledge from it. This is particularly true in healthcare where the most compelling reasons for developing computational intelligence applications are to foster safety, quality and efficacy in all aspects of patient care.

This book is an attempt to cover the latest applications of Computational Intelligence in Healthcare. It includes ten chapters covering all the aspects of healthcare ranging from cancer detection in optical spectroscopy and imaging, optimized medication regimens, and diagnostic support, to ubiquitous computing, computational tools to assist disabled people, and ethical systems in healthcare.

A summary of the book layout is as follows: Chapter one introduces the concept of computational intelligence from a healthcare point of view. Artificial intelligence techniques are explored in chapter two to detect and diagnose cancer based on optical imaging and spectra. The authors have presented a review on applications of AI paradigms in optical spectroscopy for cancer detection and diagnosis. A case study on oral cancer diagnosis using polarized light spectra is presented.

Chapter three is on decision making for ranking medicine effectiveness. Fuzzy decision making models are used to mimic physician judgment and medication effectiveness. Chapter four is on cognitive categorization for image analysis in medical information systems. The computational efficient algorithms of this system make it exceptionally useful for semantic interpretation of medical images.

Chapter five is on intelligent pervasive healthcare systems. It presents pervasive healthcare systems in controlled environments and/or in sites where immediate health support is not possible. Chapter six is on agent middleware for ubiquitous computing in healthcare. The authors have implemented an agent-based ubiquitous computing environment for enhancing medical activities. Chapter seven is on detection and classification of microcalcification clusters in mammograms using evolutionary neural networks. It is shown by the authors that the present approach offers improvement in overall accuracy compared to other reported methods in the literature.

Chapter eight reports the use of a Bayesian constrained spectral method for segmentation of noisy medical images. It is shown that the proposed method is applicable to a number of clinical applications. Chapter nine is on the application of computational intelligence paradigms for processing music for blind people, music teachers, students, hobbyists and musicians. The final chapter is on ethical healthcare agents. The system advises human beings as to the ethically correct action related to the healthcare issues.

We certainly appreciate the vast and varied opportunities for developing novel computational intelligence approaches with the potential to revolutionize healthcare in the coming years. We are grateful to the authors and reviewers for their vision and wonderful contributions. We also like to thank Sridevi Ravi for her valuable assistance in preparing the final manuscript. We hope that the latest advances of Computational Intelligence in Healthcare presented in this book will encourage readers to immerse in this field and further explore the exciting opportunities that this field presents to us.

Editors

Contents

1

An Introduction to Computational Intelligence in Healthcare: New Directions

M. Sordo[1], S. Vaidya[2], and L.C. Jain[3]

[1] Decision Systems Group, Brigham & Women's Hospital, Harvard Medical School
[2] Adelaide South Australia
[3] School of Electrical & Information Engineering, University of South Australia

Summary. Computational intelligence paradigms offer tremendous advantages in many areas including healthcare, engineering, science and management. This chapter presents a brief introduction to computational intelligence in healthcare.

1.1 Introduction

Computers are seamlessly integrated in all realms of our daily lives and the amount of information they capture is staggering. This poses tremendous challenges to our ability to not only store data, but more importantly, to process such vast information to extract meaningful knowledge. This is particularly true in healthcare where computers have been used to obtain patient information, and assist physicians in making difficult clinical decisions.

Computational Intelligence rises to the imperative challenge of implementing robust computer applications to foster healthcare safety, quality and efficacy. An emerging discipline, Computational Intelligence (CI) comprises computational models and theories that draw inspiration from neurocognitive and biological functions. Unlike traditional Artificial Intelligence (AI) which mainly focuses on high-cognition formalisms and reasoning about symbolic representations, CI focuses on low-level cognitive functions such as perception and control [1].

In this chapter we seek to provide the reader with an introduction to the three core disciplines of Computational Intelligence, namely Neural Networks, Genetic Algorithms and Fuzzy Logic. We devote a section to the discussion of a series of Computational Intelligence applications developed over the past several years to aid the healthcare community in various aspects of prevention, diagnosis, treatment, and management of illnesses. We conclude this chapter with a summary of the latest advances of Computational Intelligence in Healthcare, as presented in this book. We hope that the work presented in this book will encourage readers to immerse in this field and further explore the possibilities that lay ahead.

M. Sordo et al.: *An Introduction to Computational Intelligence in Healthcare: New Directions*, Studies in Computational Intelligence (SCI) **107**, 1–26 (2008)
www.springerlink.com

1.2 Computational Intelligence

An emerging discipline, Computational Intelligence (CI) comprises computational models and theories that draw inspiration from neurocognitive and biological functions. Unlike traditional Artificial Intelligence (AI) which mainly focuses on high-cognition formalisms and reasoning about symbolic representations, CI focuses on low-level cognitive functions such as perception and control [1].

According to the IEEE Computational Intelligence Society, the field of Computational Intelligence comprises three core disciplines and their applications:

- Neural Networks are computational paradigms based on mathematical models with strong pattern recognition capabilities;
- Fuzzy Logic is an extension of traditional propositional logic. It deals with approximate reasoning by extending the binary membership {0,1} of a conventional set into a continuous membership in the interval [0,1];
- Evolutionary Computation refers to computer-based methods inspired by biological mechanisms of natural evolution.

These three core disciplines are highly complementary, and they can be synergistically applied to tackle complex problems – like those encountered in real life.

Given the fact that CI is a relatively new, evolving discipline, a more modern definition of CI may comprise any computational, non-algorithmic approach capable of handling 'raw' numerical sensory data directly [2, 3]. Hence, under this wider *umbrella* we may consider, among others, intelligent agents, belief networks, and swarm intelligence, parts of CI. In either case, the goal is not to simulate human intelligence but rather to understand the underlying mechanisms of natural or artificial intelligent systems, and to some extent be able to incorporate such mechanisms into intelligent systems capable of performing tasks we deem as *intelligent*.

The following sections briefly describe the three core disciplines of CI, namely Neural Networks, Fuzzy Logic and Genetic Algorithms – the most widely used Evolutionary Computation technique.

1.2.1 Neural Networks

Artificial Neural Networks or Neural Networks (NN) for short are computational paradigms based on mathematical models that unlike traditional computing have a structure and operation that resembles that of the mammal brain. Neural networks are also called connectionist systems, parallel distributed systems or adaptive systems, because they are comprised by a series of interconnected processing elements that operate in parallel. Neural networks lack centralized control in the classical sense, since all the interconnected processing elements change or "adapt" simultaneously with the flow of information and adaptive rules.

One of the original aims of Neural Networks was to understand and shape the functional characteristics and computational properties of the brain when it performs cognitive processes such as sensorial perception, concept categorization, concept association and learning. However, today a great deal of effort is focused on the development of Neural Networks for applications such as pattern recognition and classification, data compression and optimization.

Model for a Neural Network

An artificial neural network can be defined as a computational system consisting of a set of highly interconnected processing elements, called *neurons*, which process information as a response to external stimuli. An artificial neuron is a simplistic representation that emulates the signal integration and threshold firing behavior of biological neurons by means of mathematical equations. Like their biological counterpart, artificial neurons are bound together by connections that determine the flow of information between peer neurons. Stimuli are transmitted from one processing element to another via *synapses* or interconnections, which can be excitatory or inhibitory. If the input to a neuron is excitatory, it is more likely that this neuron will transmit an excitatory signal to the other neurons connected to it. Whereas an inhibitory input will most likely be propagated as inhibitory.

The inputs received by a single processing element (Figure 1.1) can be represented as an input vector $A = (a_1, a_2, \ldots, a_n)$, where a_i is the signal from the ith input. A weight is associated with each connected pair of neurons. Weights connected to the jth neuron can be represented as a weight vector of the form $Wj = (w_{1j}, w_{2j}, \ldots, w_{nj})$, where w_{ij} represents the weight associated with the connection between the processing element a_i, and the processing element a_j with i != j. A neuron contains a threshold value that regulates its action potential. While action potential of a neuron is determined by the

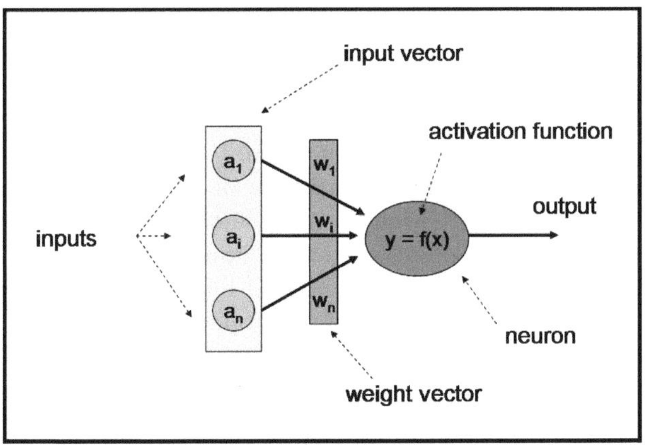

Fig. 1.1. Basic model of a single neuron

weights associated with the neuron inputs (Eq. 1.1), a threshold modulates the response of a neuron to a particular stimulus confining such response to a pre-defined range of values. Equation 1.2 defines the output y of a neuron as an activation function f of the weighted sum of $n+1$ inputs. These $n+1$ inputs correspond to the n incoming signals and a threshold value. The threshold value is incorporated into the equation as an extra incoming weight denoted by $-\mathrm{w}_0$.

$$SUM = \sum_{i=1}^{n} x_i w_i \tag{1.1}$$

$$y = f\left(\sum_{i=0}^{n} x_i w_i\right) \tag{1.2}$$

Activation functions are generally chosen to be continuous, non-monotonic and differentiable; the most commonly used being the step or saturation (Eq. 1.3), sigmoid (Eq. 1.4) and hyperbolic tangent or tanh (Eq. 1.5) functions [4].

$$f(x) = \left\{\begin{matrix} 1 & if & \sum_{i=1}^{n} x_i w_i > 0 \\ 0 & if & \sum_{i=1}^{n} x_i w_i \leq 0 \end{matrix}\right\} \tag{1.3}$$

$$f(x) = \frac{1}{1+e^{-x}} \tag{1.4}$$

$$f(x) = \frac{e^{x} - e^{-x}}{e^{x} + e^{-x}} \tag{1.5}$$

Multilayer Feedforward Networks

A multilayer feedforward network can be defined as an array of processing elements arranged in layers. Information flows through each element in an input-output manner. In other words, each element receives an input signal, manipulates it and forwards an output signal to the other connected elements in the following layer. A common example of such a network is the *Multilayer Perceptron* (MLP) [5] (Figure 1.2). Multilayer networks normally have three layers of processing elements with only one hidden layer, but there is no restriction on the number of hidden layers. The only task of the input layer is to receive the external stimuli and to propagate it to the next layer. The hidden layer receives the weighted sum of incoming signals sent by the input units (Eq. 1.1) and processes it by means of an activation function. The hidden units in turn send an output signal towards the neurons in the next layer. This adjacent layer could be either another hidden layer of arranged processing elements or the output layer. The units in the output layer receive the

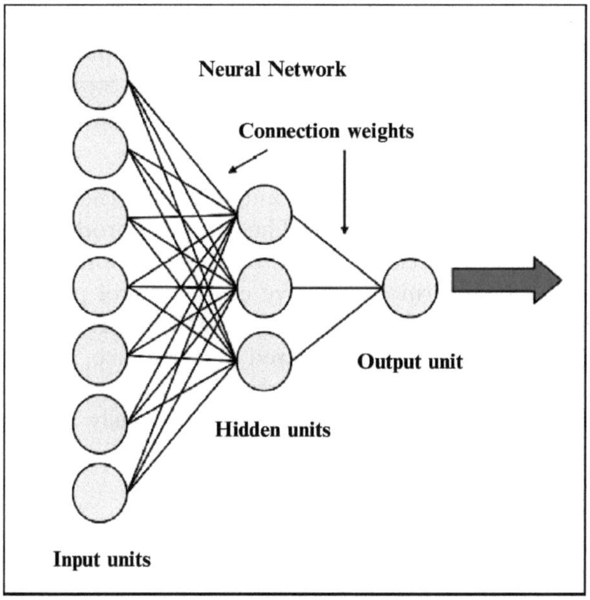

Fig. 1.2. Multilayered Feedforward Network

weighted sum of incoming signals and process it using an activation function. Information is propagated *forwards* until the network produces an output.

Based on the input-output relationship, Neural Networks can be of two types: If the desired output is different from the input, it is said that the network is hetero-associative, because it establishes a link or mapping between different signals; while in an auto-associative network, the desired output is equal to the input.

A Neural Network operates in two different modes: learning and testing. The learning stage is the process in which the network modifies the weights of each connection in order to respond to a presented input. At the testing stage, the network processes an input signal and produces an output. If the network has correctly learnt, the outputs produced at this stage should be almost as good as the ones produced in the learning stage for similar inputs. There are three main learning modes:

Supervised learning. The network receives an input and the desired output. After each trial the network compares the actual output with the desired output and corrects any difference by adjusting all the weights in the net until the output produced is similar enough to the desired output or the network cannot improve its performance any further. Pattern classification is one of the typical tasks of this learning mode.

Unsupervised learning. The network receives an input signal but not the target output. Instead, the network organizes itself internally with each processing element responding to a particular stimulus or a group of similar stimuli. This set of inputs forms clusters in the input space. Each cluster represents a set of elements of the real world with some common features. Clustering, filtering and estimation are common tasks normally carried out by unsupervised learning.

Reinforcement learning. At each point in time t the network receives an input signal and generates an output. The response produced by the network is evaluated by a cost function c_t. The aim of this function is to minimize some measure of a long-term cumulative cost. Control problems, games and sequential learning are examples of applications using reinforcement learning. Once the network has reached the desired performance, the learning stage is over and the associated weights are frozen. The final state of the network is preserved and it can be used to classify new, previously unseen inputs.

Backpropagation Learning Algorithm

During the learning stage weights in a network are adapted to optimize the network response to a presented input. The way in which these weights are adapted is specified by the learning rule. The most common rules are generalizations of the Least Mean Square Error (LMS) rule, being the generalized delta rule or Backpropagation the most used for supervised learning in feed-forward networks [6, 7].

As described before, the supervised learning procedure consists of presenting the network with pairs of input-output examples. The network produces an output in response to the presented input. An error E is calculated as the difference between the current o_p and desired t_p output. Weights are changed to minimize the overall output error (Eq. 1.6).

$$E = \frac{1}{2} \sum_j (t_{pj} - o_{pj})^2 \tag{1.6}$$

The error is propagated backwards and appropriate adjustments in the weights are made. A summarized mathematical description of the Backpropagation learning algorithm extracted from Rumelhart et al. [7] and Aleksander and Morton [8] is presented as follows:

1. Present the input-output pair p and produce the current output o_p.
2. Calculate the error δ_{pj} for each output unit j for that particular input-output pair p. The error is the difference between the desired t_{pj} and the current output o_{pj} times the derivative of the activation function $f_j(net_{pj})$ which maps the total input to an output value (Eq. 1.7).

$$\delta_{pj} = (t_{pj} - o_{pj})\, f_j\,(net_{pj}) \tag{1.7}$$

3. Calculate the error by the recursive computation of δ for each of the hidden units j in the current layer. Where w_{kj} are the weights in the k

output connections of the hidden unit j, δ_{pk} are the error signals from the k units in the next layer and $f_j(net_{pj})$ is the derivative of the activation function (Eq. 1.8). Propagate *backwards* the error signal through all the hidden layers until the input layer is reached.

$$\delta_{pj} = \sum_k \delta_{pk} w_{kj} f_j(net_{pj}) \tag{1.8}$$

This section introduced the basic concepts of Neural Networks from structure to learning modes. Probably the most used supervised learning algorithm is the Backpropagation algorithm. It is mainly used to train multilayered feed-forward neural networks. There are, however, several more types of networks and learning algorithms equally powerful. We encourage the reader to consult the following excellent sources [4, 8–11].

1.2.2 Fuzzy Logic

Proposed by Lotfi A. Zadeh in 1965 [12], Fuzzy Logic is an extension of one of the fundamental underlying concepts of Classic Propositional Logic: dichotomization. In propositional logic, truth values are binary. For example, under this dichotomous assumption, we should be able to unequivocally determine, based on the characteristics of an object, whether it belongs to a set or not. In other words, an object x is either a member of a set A or not (Eq. 1.9).

$$A(x) = \begin{cases} 1 & if \quad x \in A \\ 0 & if \quad x \notin A \end{cases} \tag{1.9}$$

However powerful this concept may be, the condition defining the boundaries of a set is very rigid. Fuzzy sets extend the binary membership {0,1} of a conventional set into a continuous one in the interval [0,1], where the membership values express the degree of compatibility of an object with the properties or characteristics distinctive of the collection it belongs to. The membership value can range from 0 (complete exclusion) to 1 (complete membership). Thus, a fuzzy set A is a set of ordered pairs defined by [3]:

$$A = \{(x, \mu_A(x)) : x \in X\} \tag{1.10}$$

where x is any object of a universal set X and $\mu_A(x)$ is the degree of membership of the element x in A. Let us define the following example in a clinical context. Let us say we want to develop a monitoring system using fuzzy logic to keep track of the resting heart rate of adult patients at risk of developing some complications. So, let X be the universal set of RESTING HEART RATE (RHR) measurements for adults where an element x in X could have any value in the range $[0, 250]$ beats per minute. We may also want to define three fuzzy sets to classify our patients, e.g. LOW, NORMAL, HIGH. We may even want to define some sort of alarms to warn us when a patient heart rate deviates from normal. All possible heart rates in the interval [0, 250] are members of each fuzzy set, though with different membership values in the interval [0, 1]. For example, a RHR = 70 is a member of all three sets, but the membership functions $\mu_{LOW}(70)$, $\mu_{NORMAL}(70)$ $\mu_{HIGH}(70)$ will have very different membership values for the same heart rate (see Figure 1.3).

In fuzzy systems, membership functions can be continuous, and expand over a continuous spectrum of values (Figure 1.3), or discrete, sampling values at regular intervals over the whole range of possible values (Figure 1.4).

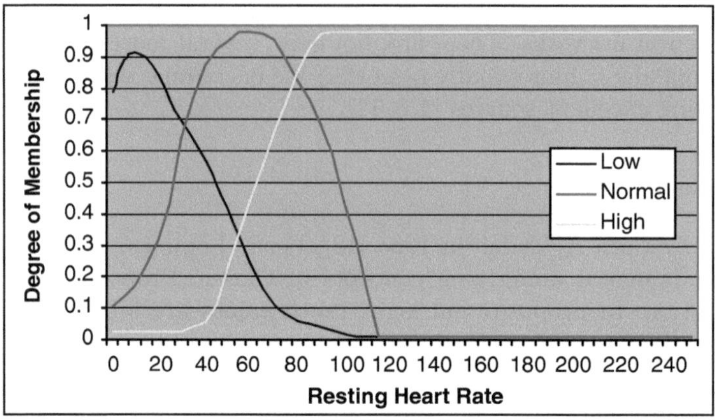

Fig. 1.3. Membership curves for the fuzzy sets Low, Normal and High. The x-axis denotes the resting heart rate for adults. The y-axis denotes the degree of membership of the given fuzzy sets at different heart rates

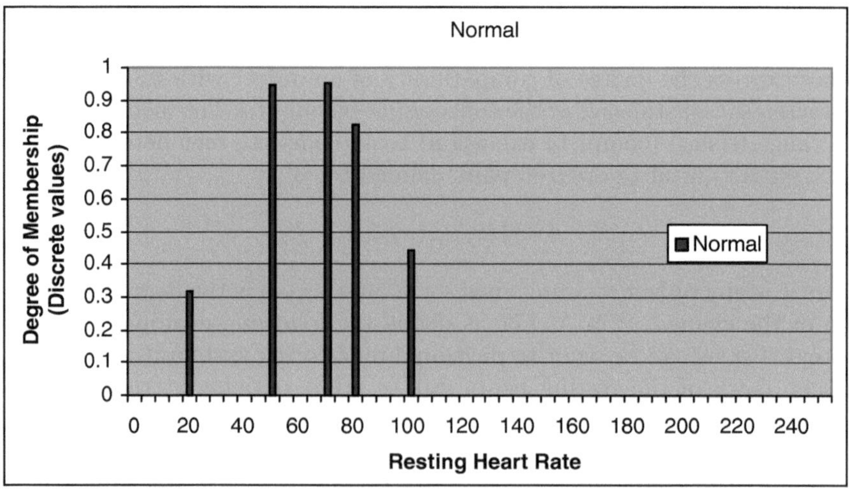

Fig. 1.4. Non-uniform sampling of discrete resting heart rate values at non-uniform intervals for the Normal fuzzy set

Membership Functions

Although any continuous function of the form $A : X \to [0,1]$ can be used as membership function of a fuzzy set, the most commonly used are:

- **Triangular membership function** or bell-shaped function determines the degree of membership by comparing a given value x against an upper and lower values a, b and a modal value m as shown in Eq. 1.11. The graphic representation of this type of function is depicted in Figure 1.5a.

$$A(x) = \begin{cases} 0 & if \quad x \leq a \\ \dfrac{x-a}{m-a} & if \quad x \in [a,m] \\ \dfrac{b-x}{b-m} & if \quad x \in [m,b] \\ 0 & if \quad x \geq b \end{cases} \tag{1.11}$$

- **Trapezoidal membership function** is typically used to represent the fuzzy linguistic conditions *neither so high nor so low* [3]. In our heart rate example, we could use this function to express that a given heart rate is *neither too high nor too low*, for those values between the threshold boundaries determined by m, n, calculated by Eq. 1.12. See Figure 1.5b.

$$A(x) = \begin{cases} 0 & if \quad x < a \\ \dfrac{x-a}{m-a} & if \quad x \in [a,m] \\ 1 & if \quad x \in [m,n] \\ \dfrac{b-x}{b-n} & if \quad x \in [n,b] \\ 0 & if \quad x > b \end{cases} \tag{1.12}$$

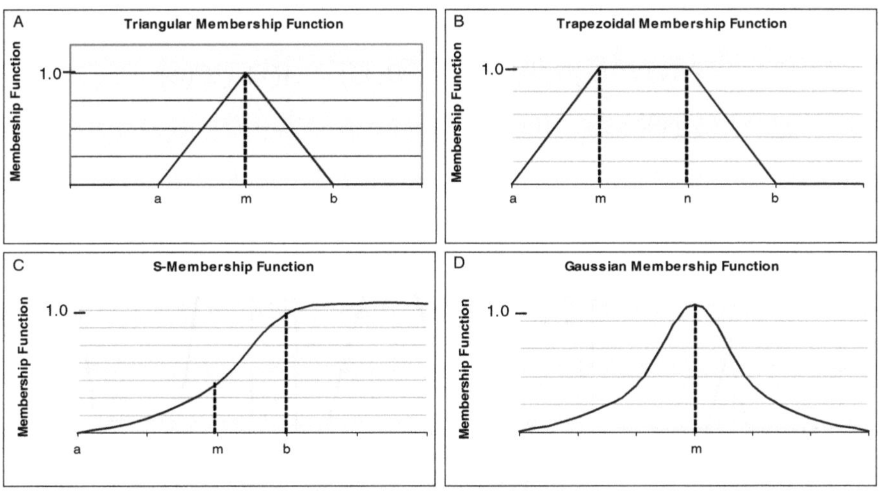

Fig. 1.5. Typical Membership functions: A) Triangular; B) Trapezoidal; C) S-Membership; and D) Gaussian

- **S-Membership function** has a smoother slope. In our example, we could use it to calculate the membership for the fuzzy set HIGH. One typical form of the S-Function is depicted in Figure 1.5c, and the curve is calculated by Eq. 1.13 as follows:

$$A(x) = \begin{cases} 0 & if \quad x \leq a \\ 2\left(\dfrac{x-a}{b-a}\right)^2 & if \quad x \in [a,m] \\ 1-2\left(\dfrac{x-b}{b-a}\right)^2 & if \quad x \in [m,b] \\ 1 & if \quad x > b \end{cases} \tag{1.13}$$

- Gaussian membership function has a wide application on fuzzy sets. In our example, this function could be used to calculate the membership for the fuzzy set NORMAL, with mean value of e.g. 60. To shape the curve we can experiment with different values for the variance; the smaller the value, the higher and sharper the curve around the mean value. A typical Gaussian curve is depicted in Figure 1.5d, and it is calculated by Eq. 1.14.

$$A(x) = e^{-k(x-m)^2} \quad where \quad k > 0 \tag{1.14}$$

Fuzzy Set Operations

Fuzzy sets support the same operations as *crisp* conventional set theory: Union, Intersection and Negation. In [12] L.A. Zadeh suggests the minimum operator for the intersection (Eq. 1.15, Figure 1.6 left), the maximum operator for the union (Eq. 1.16, Figure 1.6 center) and the complement for the negation (Eq. 1.17, Figure 1.6 right) of fuzzy two sets.

$$(A \cap B)(x) = \min(A(x), B(x)) = A(x) \wedge B(x) \tag{1.15}$$

$$(A \cup B)(x) = \max(A(x), B(x)) = A(x) \vee B(x) \tag{1.16}$$

$$\overline{A}(x) = 1 - A(x) \tag{1.17}$$

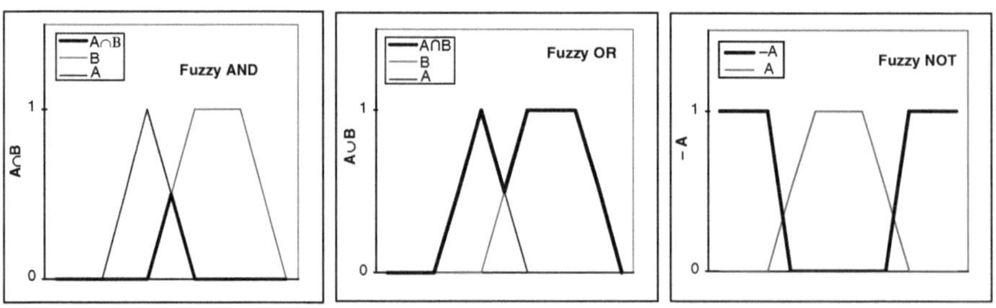

Fig. 1.6. Operations in Fuzzy Sets (from left to right): Fuzzy AND; Fuzzy OR; and Fuzzy NOT

Where the sets A and B are defined in a universe X, and $(A \cap B)(x)$, $(A \cup B)(x)$ denote the membership functions for the intersection and union of sets A and B respectively [13].

This section presented a brief introduction to the key aspects of Fuzzy Sets. Fuzzy sets can be seen as extensions of the classical set theory. Fuzzy sets provide the means for tackling classification problems where *crisp*, more traditional approaches are not feasible given the complexity of the data, or when a conventional mathematical approach does not yield satisfactory results. [3, 12–14] are excellent sources for further reading.

1.2.3 Evolutionary Computation

Evolutionary Computation combines several computer-based problem solving methods inspired by biological mechanisms of natural evolution [15]. Among these techniques we find Genetic Algorithms [16], Evolutionary Programming [17] and Evolution Strategies [18]. Although similar at the highest level, their major differences are in their choices of a) representation for individual structures and b) variation operators. For example, Genetic Algorithms (GAs) traditionally use domain-independent representations, whereas both Evolutionary Strategies (ES) and Evolutionary Programming (EP) use representations tailored to the problem domain. Similarly, both EP and ES use mutation as their main operator while GAs use recombination as their primary operator, and mutation as a secondary operator.

Evolutionary Algorithms are computational analogies that mimic four of the six propositions of modern theory of evolution or *new-Darwinian Theory* [19]: Reproduction, excess, variation and environmental selection. In the computational context, these propositions can be described as follows [20]:

- A computational representation of candidate solutions to the problem at hand;
- A population of candidate solutions;
- Mechanisms for generating new solutions from members of the current population;
- An evaluation method to assess the quality of given solutions;
- A selection method to identify good solutions.

A typical evolutionary algorithm consists of the following steps:

a. An initial population of M individuals at $t = 0$.
b. Evaluate initial population ($t = 0$).
c. Evolve population from generation t to generation $t + 1$ by successive applications of evaluation, selection, recombination and mutation operations.

The remaining of this section focuses on describing the fundamental concepts of Genetic Algorithms – the most widely known paradigm in Evolutionary Computation.

Genetic Algorithms

Developed by John Holland in the 1970s [16], Genetic Algorithms are stochastic search methods that operate over a population of possible solutions. GAs are mainly used for optimization, machine learning and intelligent search, in fields as diverse as medicine, engineering, economics and business. A typical GA consists of the following components:

Representation
An initial population of potential solutions or *chromosomes* is encoded as bit strings, where each *gene* represents a parameter in the universe of possible solutions (Figure 1.7).

Fitness Evaluation
A fitness function is used to determine the quality of candidate solutions or *chromosomes* from the current population.

Reproduction
Genetic operators are applied to the population to create new individuals and introduce diversity to the current population. There are two main types of genetic operators, each with an associated parameter to control the probability of its application:

> Mutation or asexual reproduction. One or more bits in the *chromosome* are flipped: changing a 0 to 1 or vice versa, with a probability given by the *mutation rate* (Figure 1.8). Mutation is considered a secondary operator mainly used to restore lost genetic material. However, some researchers consider the mutation-selection method a powerful search algorithm [21–23].

Chromosome 1	1101100100110110
Chromosome 2	1101111000011110

Fig. 1.7. Chromosomes encoded as bit strings

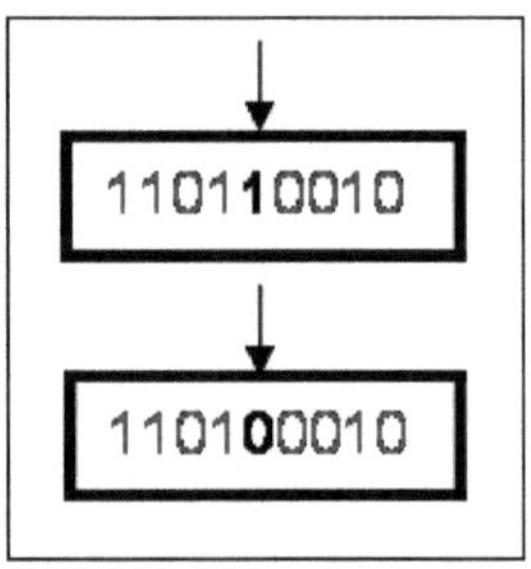

Fig. 1.8. Example of mutation of a chromosome in the 5th bit position

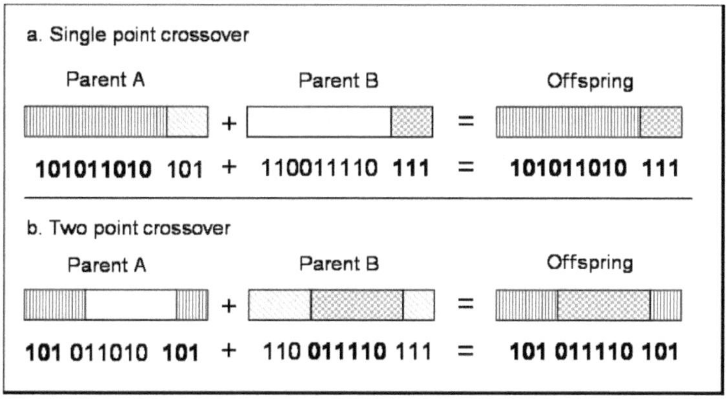

Fig. 1.9. Examples of a) single point and b) two-point crossover

Crossover or sexual reproduction. Considered the main search operator in GAs, recombination or crossover produces offspring by merging portions of two selected parents. Segments of different parents are combined to produce new individuals that benefit from advantageous bit combinations of both parents. As with mutation, crossover is controlled by a *recombination rate*. The most common operators are one-point, multi-point and uniform crossover. In one-point recombination, a single cut-point is randomly selected within two parents and the segments before the cut-points are swapped over. (Figure 1.9a). Multi-point is a generalization of the single cut-point, introducing a higher number of cut-points (Figure 1.9b). In uniform crossover [24] a global parameter is used to indicate the probability of exchanging single bits between parents.

Any efficient optimization algorithm must balance two contradictory forces: *exploration* to investigate new solutions in the search space, and *exploitation* to use the available information to produce better solutions. Selection is the component in GAs that determines the character of the search process: too strong selection means that suboptimal, highly fit individuals (chromosomes) will take over the population, hence reducing the diversity required for further change and progress. On the other hand, too weak selection will result in very slow evolution [20]. There are numerous selection schemes in the literature, the most commonly used are [20]:

- **Proportional Selection.** The reproductive opportunities of an individual are given by its fitness divided by the average fitness of the population.
- **Scaling Methods.** Scaling methods transform the fitness value of an individual into positive numbers to a) keep appropriate levels of competition among individuals and b) satisfy the condition of positive values required by proportional selection.

- **Rank Selection.** Individuals in the population are ranked according to their fitness. The expected number of offspring of each individual depends on its rank rather than on its absolute fitness.
- **Tournament Selection.** n individuals are randomly selected from the population and the fittest is selected for reproduction. All n individuals are then returned to the population and can be selected again. This process is repeated until a new population is filled.

This section introduced the basic concepts of Genetic Algorithms. GAs are powerful tools for optimization and intelligent search. GAs randomly search for optimal, or near optimal, solutions from a search space. Portions of this section are based on the work of Dr. Gabriela Ochoa [20], and were included here with the author's kind permission. [20, 22, 25, 26] are excellent references for further reading.

1.2.4 Synergistic Approaches

The preceding sections introduced the underlying concepts of the three core disciplines of Computational Intelligence. Each approach has advantages and disadvantages. For example, Neural Networks is a robust approach for classification, however, the need for large training datasets, or the risk of getting trapped at *local minima* [7] sometimes precludes the applicability of this technique. Although Fuzzy Logic is very useful for approximate reasoning, the membership function that supports Fuzzy Logic reasoning under uncertain conditions sometimes can produce inaccurate results, since, unlike Probability Theory which indicates the likelihood or probability of something being true, Fuzzy Logic indicates the degree to which something is true. A notable strength of Genetic Algorithms is their robust performance in problems with complex fitness landscapes. That is, problems where the fitness function is discontinuous, noisy or has many local minima [20]. GAs strongly rely on the fitness function as searching mechanism for optimal solutions. However, a "deceptive", ill-defined fitness function could steer the whole search process away from finding the true optimum [25].

Although these approaches are highly successful in solving complex tasks, sometimes their applicability is precluded by their inherent limitations. A step towards more powerful and flexible tools relies on synergistic approaches that embrace the advantages and minimizes the limitations of each methodology alone.

Integration or *coupling* between approaches is of vital importance. Depending on their compatibility and level of interaction, the synergism of these techniques can be classified as loose or tight. Interaction in loosely-coupled synergism is well-defined in time and space. Each tool preserves its own structural and modular identity and works independently with a minimum of communication. In tightly-coupled synergism there is more interaction between modules. Information is not exchanged but shared by the different tools and communication between tools is achieved via common internal structures [27].

Fuzzy Neural Networks (FNN)

Fuzzy Neural Networks (FNN) combine the learning and connectionist structure of Neural Networks with the human-like reasoning of Fuzzy Logic into a hybrid intelligent system that synergizes these two techniques. The main advantage of this approach is its ability to accurately learn from noisy datasets with interpretable outputs [28].

Genetic Evolving Neural Networks

Neuro-GA synergism employs a GA for the optimization of the most important parameters of a Neural Network, namely, the internal structure and initial weights. By optimizing the configuration of nodes in a NN and its weights, training time is reduced while reducing the risk of getting trapped at *local minima* [7].

Fuzzy-GAs

Fuzzy Logic and GAs may synergistically interact in two ways: a) Fuzzy Logic can be used to improve the GA behavior by modeling the GA fitness function or reproduction operators; and b) GAs can be used for optimization of membership functions in Fuzzy classifiers [29].

Neuro-Fuzzy-GAs

"Optimized learning of imprecise data": this summarizes a common synergy of GAs, NN and Fuzzy Logic. This is an advantageous combination where a GA can be used for the optimization of the most important parameters of a Neural Network. The Neural Network is then trained with fuzzy membership distributions defined with Fuzzy Logic [3].

1.2.5 Summary

This section presented a brief introduction to Computational Intelligence. The first part presented a definition of Computational Intelligence, while subsequent sections briefly described its three core technologies. A review of synergistic approaches emphasizes the trend of bringing together different, yet complementary methodologies to produce more robust computational models.

1.3 Applications of Computational Intelligence in Healthcare

Advances in computer and information technology and the amount of data these new technologies generate have created challenging opportunities for the Computational Intelligence (CI) community. This is particularly true in healthcare where computers play an active role in all realms from capturing, storing and processing patient data in all formats at all times. This bears tremendous opportunities for developing effective computational solutions to improve the overall quality of healthcare.

This section presents a review of healthcare applications of the three core Computational Intelligence techniques e.g. Neural Networks [30], Genetic Algorithms, and Fuzzy Logic as well as other emerging techniques. The following sections present a series of examples to illustrate the great potential of these techniques for processing, analysis and mining of complex data acquired from various sources ranging from imaging capture devices to health monitoring systems.

1.3.1 Clinical Diagnosis

Neural networks have been used for assisted screening of Pap (cervical) smears [31], prediction of metastases in breast cancer patients [32], breast cancer diagnosis [33]. Burke et al compared the prediction accuracy of a multilayer perceptron trained with the backpropagation learning algorithm and other statistical models for breast cancer survival [34]. Similarly, neural networks have been used for prognosis and assessment of the extent of hepatectomy of patients with hepatocellular carcinoma [35] and prognosis of coronary artery disease [36].

1.3.2 Signal and Image Analysis and Interpretation

A Backpropagation neural network trained with a robust supervised technique has been used to perform image processing operations such as filtering, and segmentation of brain magnetic resonance images (MRIs) [37]. Aizenberg et al [38] used cellular neural networks to improve resolution in brain tomographies, and improve global frequency correction for the detection of microcalcifications in mammograms. Hall et al compared neural networks and fuzzy clustering techniques for segmentation of MRI of the brain [39]. [40] implemented a self-organizing network multilayer adaptive resonance architecture for the segmentation of CT images of the heart. Däschlein et al implemented a two layer neural network for segmentation of CT images of the abdomen [41].

Olmez and Dokur [42] developed a neural network-based method for the classification of heart sounds, and a hybrid network trained by genetic algorithms for the classification of electrocardiogram (ECG) beats [43].

A Neural Network was successfully applied to enhance low-level segmentation of eye images for diagnosis of Grave's ophthalmopathy [44], segmentation of ultrasound images [45] and endoscopy video-frames of colorectal lesions [46]. Backpropagation (BP) and Radial Basis function (RBF) networks have been used to evaluate the feasibility of using ECG and blood pressure data into a neural network for the classification of cardiac patient states in an ICU setting [47].

A multilayer perceptron was trained to differentiate between Contingent Negative Variation (CNV) evoked responses waveforms of patients with Huntington's disease, Parkinson's disease and schizophrenia [48]. Robert et al used neural networks for classification of electroencephalograms [49]. Sordo et al implemented a knowledge-based neural network (KBANN) for classification of phosphorus (31P) magnetic resonance spectra (MRS) from normal and cancerous breast tissues [50].

Applications of Fuzzy Logic in signal processing range from monitoring and control of electrical and chemical responses of nerve fibers [51], analysis of eye movements [52], clinical monitoring of disease progression [53], and radiation therapy [54]. Fuzzy image enhancing techniques have been used to improve the quality of radiographic images [55]. A fuzzy two-dimensional image restoration tool has been developed for diagnostic and treatment planning of radiation therapy [56]. Similarly, fuzzy logic has been used for segmentation and estimation of intensity inhomogeneities of magnetic resonance images [57]. A neural network with adaptive fuzzy logic has been used for image restoration for quantitative imaging for planar and tomographic imaging [58].

1.3.3 Applications in Healthcare

Several Fuzzy Logic applications have been developed in the field of Anesthesia. Anesthesiology requires monitoring of patient vital signs during the controlled administration of drug infusion to maintain the anesthetic level constant. Examples of applications (extracted from [59]) include depth of anesthesia [60], muscle relaxation [61,62], hypertension during anesthesia [63], arterial pressure control [64], mechanical ventilation during anesthesia [65] and post-operative control of blood pressure [66]. Fuzzy Logic has been applied to computerized clinical guidelines [67], as well as in risk assessment in a healthcare institution [68]. Similarly, knowledge management techniques have been applied to structuring clinical and patient information [69, 70].

1.3.4 Drug Development

Drug development requires understanding of the drug's mechanism of action from its pattern activity against a disease. Several techniques have been implemented in this area. Weinstein et al developed a Neural Network to predict the mechanism of action of an anti cancer drug [71, 72]. Similarly, Langdon et al used genetic programming, decision trees and neural networks to predict behavior of virtual chemicals for the inhibition of a P450 enzyme [73]. Viswanadham et al. developed a knowledge-oriented approach to deploy biochemical information for drug discovery [74].

1.3.5 Disease Treatment

A diseased organism plays a dual active role by being affected by the agent while at the same time unwillingly hosting the noxious agent causing the disease. Hence, disease treatment is mainly a two-fold task: Treatment is targeted at the offending agent, and at the same time directed at restoring the normal physiological state of an individual affected by a disease.

Evolutionary approaches have been applied to chemotherapy scheduling and cancer treatment [75, 76], and in the emergency room [77]. De Luca et al developed a fuzzy rule system for validation and interpretation of genotypic HIV-1 drug resistance based on virological outcomes [78]. Sordo et al developed a state-based model for management of type II diabetes [79].Ying et al developed a fuzzy finite state machine model for treatment regimens, and a genetic-algorithm-based optimizer regimen selection for HIV/AIDS treatment [80].

1.3.6 Summary

This section presented a brief overview of Computational Intelligence techniques in various aspects of healthcare. Some of the techniques focused on diagnosis, from decision support to image and signal processing, treatment of diseases and drug discovery. This review is by no means exhaustive and we encourage the reader to further explore this fascinating and promising field.

1.4 Chapters Included in this Book

This book includes ten chapters. Chapter 1 by Sordo et al. provides an introduction to the three core disciplines of Computational Intelligence, namely Neural Networks, Genetic Algorithms and Fuzzy Logic. It devotes a section to the discussion of a series of Computational Intelligence applications developed over the past several years to aid the healthcare community in various aspects of prevention, diagnosis, treatment, and management of illnesses. The final part of the chapter presents a summary of the latest advances of Computational Intelligence in Healthcare.

Chapter 2 by Kan et al. presents a literature review on Artificial Intelligence applied to optical spectroscopy for detection of cancer based on biochemical and structural changes of normal and cancerous cells. They also present a detailed case study on oral cancer diagnosis using polarized light spectra.

Chapter 3 by Rakus-Andersson focuses on theoretical fuzzy decision-making models as useful tools to estimation of the total effectiveness-utility of a drug when appreciating its positive influence on a collection of symptoms characteristic of a considered diagnosis. The expected effectiveness of a medication is evaluated by a physician as a verbal expression for each distinct symptom. Words describing the effectiveness of the medication are converted into fuzzy sets and then into numbers. These numbers are fed into a utility matrix which is used in a series of computations by different decision algorithms to obtain a sequence of tested medications with a positive influence on symptoms.

Chapter 4 by Ogiela et al. presents semantic reasoning methods for describing the meaning of analyzed objects from spinal cord to bone radiograms. The semantic reasoning procedures are based on the cognitive resonance model. Their research highlights the directions in which modern IT systems as well as medical diagnostic support systems could expand into the field of automatic, computer meaning interpretation of various patterns acquired in image diagnostics.

Chapter 5 by Doukas and Maglogiannis presents the state of the art in intelligent pervasive healthcare applications and enabling technologies. They discuss pervasive healthcare systems in both controlled environments (e.g., hospitals, health care units), and uncontrolled environments where immediate health support is not possible (i.e. patient's home, urban area). They pay particular attention to intelligent platforms for advanced monitoring and interpretation of patient status, aimed at optimizing the whole medical assessment procedure.

Chapter 6 by Rodríguez and Favela focuses on ubiquitous computing in the healthcare. They propose the use of agents to model Healthcare environments and present SALSA, a middleware that enables developers to create autonomous agents that react to contextual elements of a medical environment and communicate with other agents, users and services available in an environment.

Chapter 7 by Hernández-Cisneros et al. describes a system for early detection of breast cancer based on detection and classification of clusters of microcalcifications in mammograms. Their system uses sequential difference of gaussian filters (DoG) and three evolutionary artificial neural networks (EANNs). They show that the use of genetic algorithms (GAs) for finding the optimal architecture and initial weight set for an artificial neural network prior to training it with the Backpropagation algorithm results mainly in improvements in overall accuracy, sensitivity and specificity when compared to other neural networks trained with Backpropagation.

Chapter 8 by Soltysinski presents a combination of multiscale wavelet decomposition and noise reduction for feature extraction of ultrasound images. For noise reduction, the system relies on Bayesian inference for edge detection, and spectral method for contour detection. The proposed segmentation method is tested on 'denoised' cardiac ultrasonographic data and its performance is compared for different noise clipping values. The author also demonstrates the flexibility and adaptability of the proposed method in a number of clinical applications.

Chapter 9 by Homenda describes the role of knowledge based methods in the implementation of user friendly computer programs for disabled people. The author describes in detail a specific computer program to aid blind people interact with music and music notation. The program consists of two main modules: a) information acquisition, and b) knowledge representation and processing. The main task of the information acquisition module is to recognize and store printed music. The knowledge representation and processing module extracts implicit relations between the stored music data by a) identifying symbols and their location, b) extracting relevant features and c) performing a semantic mapping between the identified features and a Braille score output.

Chapter 10 by Anderson and Anderson presents an ethical theory to develop a system that uses machine-learning to abstract relationships between *prima facie* ethical duties from cases of particular types of ethical dilemmas where ethicists are in agreement as to the correct action. Authors argue that their proposed system has discovered a novel ethical principle that governs decisions in a particular type of dilemma that involves three potentially conflicting prima facie duties. Authors describe two prototype systems in the healthcare domain that rely on this principle: one system advises human beings as to the ethically correct action in specific cases of this type of dilemma. The second system uses this principle to guide its own behavior, making it what authors believe may be the first explicit ethical agent.

1.5 Summary

Computers are being seamlessly integrated in all realms of our daily lives and the amount of information they capture is staggering. This poses tremendous challenges to our ability to not only store data, but more importantly, to process such vast information to extract meaningful knowledge. This is particularly true in healthcare where computers have been used to obtain patient information, and assist physicians in making difficult clinical decisions. As portrayed in this chapter, Computational Intelligence rises to the imperative challenge of implementing robust computer applications to foster healthcare safety, quality and efficacy. We certainly appreciate the opportunities for developing novel computational intelligence approaches with the potential to revolutionize healthcare in the coming years. We hope that the latest advances of Computational Intelligence in Healthcare presented in this book will encourage readers to immerse in this field and further explore the exciting opportunities that this field presents to us.

Acknowledgements

We would like to thank Dr. Gabriela Ochoa for her kind permission to include portions of her work on Genetic Algorithms and Evolutionary Computation. We also thank Dr. Ana Macedo for her valuable feedback in writing this manuscript.

References

1. W. Dutch. What is Computational Intelligence and what could it become? In *Challenges for Computational Intelligence*, W. Dutch and J. Mandziuk (Eds.), Springer, 2007.
2. J.C. Bezdek. What is computational intelligence? In *Computational Intelligence Imitating Life*, pp. 1–12, IEEE Press, New York, 1994.
3. A. Konar. *Computational Intelligence. Principles, Techniques and Applications.* Springer, 2005.
4. C. Bishop. *Neural Networks for Pattern Recognition.* Oxford University Press, 1995.
5. F. Rosenblatt. *Principles of neurodynamics: Perceptrons and the theory of brain mechanisms.* Spartan Books, 1962.
6. D. Rumelhart, G. Hinton, R. Williams. Learning Representations by Backpropagating Errors. *Nature*, 323, 533–536. 1986.
7. D. Rumelhart, J. McClelland, et al. *Parallel Distributed Processing. Explorations in the Microstructure of Cognition, Vol. 1: Foundations.* MIT, 1986.
8. J. Hertz, A. Krogh, R.G. Palmer. *Introduction to the Theory of Neural Computation.* Redwood City, CA: Addison Wesley, 1991.
9. I. Aleksander, H. Morton. *An Introduction to Neural Computing.* Chapman & Hall. 1990.
10. P. Wasserman. *Advanced Methods in Neural Computing*, Van Nostrand Reinhold, 1993.
11. T. Masters. *Signal and Image Processing with Neural Networks*, John Wiley & Sons, Inc. 1994.
12. L.A. Zadeh. Fuzzy Sets, *Information and Control*, 8:338–353. 1965.
13. K Cios, W. Pedrycz, R. Swiniarski. *Data Mining Methods for Knowledge Discovery.* Kluwer Academic Publishers. 2000.
14. L.A. Zadeh. The concept of a linguistic variable and its application to approximate reasoning. *Information Sciences*, 8:199–249 (part I); 8:301–357 (part II); 9:43–80 (part III).
15. W.M. Spears, K.A.D. Jong, T. Bäck, D.B. Fogel, H. Garis. An overview of evolutionary computation. In Brazdil, P.B. (Ed.), *Proceedings of the European Conference on Machine* Learning, Vol. 667, of LNAI, pp 442–459 Vienna, Austria, Spinger Verlag, 1993.
16. J.H. Holland. *Adaptation in Natural and Artificial Systems.* University of Michigan Press, Ann Arbor, 1975.
17. L.J. Fogel, A.J. Owens, M.J. Walsh. *Artificial Intelligence through Simulated Evolution.* Wiley Publishing, New York, 1966.
18. I. Rechenberg. *Evolution Strategy: Optimization of Technical Systems by Means of Biological Evolution.* Fromman-Holzboog, Stuttgart, 1973.

19. C. Patterson. *Evolution.* Natural History Museum, London, UK.
20. G. Ochoa. *Error Thresholds and Optimal Mutation Rates in Genetic Algorithms*, PhD Thesis, School of Cognitive and Computing Sciences, University of Sussex, 2000.
21. J.D. Schaffer, L.J. Eshelman. On crossover as an evolutionary viable strategy. In Belew, R.K. & Booker, L.B. (Eds.), *Proceedings of the Fourth International Conference on Genetic Algorithms*, pp. 61–68 San Mateo, California. Morgan Kaufmann Publishers, 1991.
22. D. Fogel. *Evolutionary Computation: Toward a New Philosophy of Machine Learning.* IEEE Press, 1995.
23. T. Bäck, *Evolutionary Algorithms in Theory and Practice.* The Clarendon Press, Oxford University Press, New York, 1996.
24. G. Syswerda. Uniform crossover in genetic algorithms. In Schaffer, J.D. (Ed.), *Proceedings of the Third International Conference on Genetic Algorithms*, pp 2–9 George Mason University. Morgan Kaufmann. 1989.
25. M. Mitchell. *An Introduction to Genetic Algorithms.* MIT Press, 1996.
26. D.E. Goldberg. *Genetic Algorithms in Search, Optimization, and Machine Learning.* Addison-Wesley, Reading, MA. 1989.
27. M. Sordo. *A Neurosymbolic Approach to the Classification of Scarce and Complex Data.* PhD Thesis, School of Cognitive and Computing Sciences, University of Sussex, 1999.
28. B. Kosko, *Neural Networks and Fuzzy Systems: A Dynamical Systems Approach to Machine Intelligence.* Englewood Cliffs, NJ: Prentice Hall, 1992.
29. O. Cordón, F. Herrera, M. Lozano. On the Combination of Fuzzy Logic and Evolutionary Computation: A Short Review and Bibliography. In: *Fuzzy Evolutionary Computation.* Kluwer Academic Pub, pp. 33–56, 1997.
30. M. Sordo. Introduction to Neural Networks in Healthcare. OpenClinical. October 2002. http://www.openclinical.org/docs/int/neuralnetworks011.pdf Accessed October 26, 2007.
31. A.M. Garber. Making the Most of Pap Testing. *JAMA.* 1998;279:240–241.
32. P.L. Choong, C.J.S. deSilva. Breast Cancer Prognosis using EMN Architecture. *Proceedings of the IEE International Conference on Neural Networks.* June 1994.
33. B. Kovalerchuk, E. Triantaphyllou, J.F. Ruiz. The reliability issue of computer-aided breast cancer diagnosis. *Comput Biomed Res,* 33, 296–313. 2000.
34. H. Burke, D. Rosen, P. Goodman. Comparing the Prediction Accuracy of Artificial Neural Networks and Other Statistical Models for Breast Cancer Survival. In Tesauro, G., Touretzky, D., & Leen, T. (Eds.), *Advances in Neural Information Processing Systems*, Vol. 7, pp. 1063–1067. The MIT Press.
35. I. Hamamoto, S. Okada, T. Hashimoto, H. Wakabayashi, T. Maeba, H. Maeta. Prediction of the Early Prognosis of the Hepatectomized Patient with Hepatocellular Carcinoma with a Neural Network. *Comput Bio. Med,* 25(1), 49–59.
36. P. Lapuerta, S.P. Azen, L. LaBree. Use of neural networks in predicting the risk of coronary artery disease. *Comput Biomed Res*, 1995.
37. J.U. Garcia, L. Gonzalez-Santos, R. Favila, R. Rojas, F.A. Barrios. Three-dimensional MRI segmentation based on back-propagation neural network with robust supervised training. *Proc. SPIE* Vol. 3979, pp. 817–824, Kenneth M. Hanson; Eds. 2000.
38. I. Aizenberg, N. Aizenberga, J. Hiltnerb, et al. Cellular neural networks and computational intelligence in medical image processing. *Image and Vision Computing*, 19(4), 177–183. 2001.

39. L. Hall, A. Bensaid, L. Clarke, R. Velthuizen, M. Silbiger, J. Bezdek. A Comparison of Neural Network and Fuzzy Clustering Techniques in Segmenting Magnetic Resonance Images of the Brain. *IEEE Transactions on Neural Networks*, 3(5), 672–682. 1992.
40. J. Rajapakse, R. Acharya. Medical Image Segmentation with MARA. *Proceedings International Joint Conference on Neural Networks*, Vol. 2, pp. 965–972. 1990.
41. R. Däschlein, T. Waschulzik, W. Brauer et al. Segmentation of Computertomographies with Neural Networks Based on Local Features. In Ifeachor, E., & Rosen, K. (Eds.), *International Conference on Neural Networks and Expert Systems in Medicine and Healthcare*, pp. 240–247. 1994.
42. T. Olmez, Z. Dokur. Classification of heart sounds using an artificial neural network. *Pattern Recognition Letters*. Vol. 24, Issue 1–3 pp. 617–629. January 2003.
43. T. Olmez, Z. Dokur. Application of InP Neural Network to ECG Beat Classification. *Neural Computing Applications Journal*. Vol. 11, Num 3–4, pp. 144–155. June 2003.
44. A. Ossen, T. Zamzow, H. Oswald, E. Fleck. Segmentation of Medical Images Using Neural Network Classifiers. In Ifeachor, E., & Rosen, K. (Eds.), *International Conference on Neural Networks and Expert Systems in Medicine and Healthcare*, pp. 427–432. 1994.
45. M.N. Kurnaz, Z. Dokur, T. Ölmez. An incremental neural network for tissue segmentation in ultrasound images. *Computer Methods and Programs in Biomedicine*, v. 85 n. 3, p. 187–195, March, 2007.
46. D.E. Maroulis, D.K. Iakovidis, S.A. Karkanis, D.A. Karras. CoLD: a versatile detection system for colorectal lesions in endoscopy video-frames. *Computer Methods and Programs in Biomedicine*, 2003.
47. M.P. Tjoa, D.N. Dutt, Y.T. Lim, B.W. Yau, R.C. Kugean, S.M. Krishnan, K.L. Chan. Artificial neural networks for the classification of cardiac patient states using ECG and blood pressure data. *The Seventh Australian and New Zealand Conference on Intelligent Information Systems,* 2001.
48. B. Jervis, S. Yu, M. Saatchi, E. Allen. The Sensitivity of Multilayer Perceptrons for Differentiating Between CNV Waveforms of Schizophrenic, Parkinson's Disease and Huntington's Disease Subjects. In Ifeachor, E., & Rosen, K. (Eds.), *International Conference on Neural Networks and Expert Systems in Medicine and Healthcare*, pp. 275–282. 1994.
49. C. Robert, J.F. Gaudy, A. Limoge. Electroencephalogram processing using neural networks. *Clinical Neurophysiology*, 2002.
50. M. Sordo, H. Buxton, D. Watson. A Hybrid Approach to Breast Cancer Diagnosis. In *Practical Applications of Computational Intelligence Techniques*. Jain, L. and DeWilde, P. (Eds.). Kluwer Academic Publishers. 2001.
51. N. Al-Holou, D.S. Joo. Development of a fuzzy logic based system to monitor the electrical responses of nerve fiber. *Biomed Sci Instrum* 1997;33:376–81.
52. J.H. Allum, F. Honegger, M. Troescher. Principles underlying real-time nystagmus analysis of horizontal and vertical eye movements recorded with electro-, infra-red-, or video-oculographic techniques. *J Vestib Res* 1998;8(6):449–63.
53. F. Steimann. The interpretation of time-varying data with DIAMON-1. *Artif Intell Med* 1996;8(4):343–57.

54. E.I. Papageorgiou, C.D. Stylios, P.P. Groumpos. An integrated two-level hierarchical system for decision making in radiation therapy based on fuzzy cognitive maps. *IEEE Transactions on Biomedical Engineering*, Vol. 50(12):1326–1339. 2003.
55. G. Krell, H.R. Tizhoosh, T. Lilienblum, C.J. Moore, B. Michaelis. Enhancement and associative restoration of electronic portal images in radiotherapy. *Int J Med Inf* 1998;49(2):157–71.
56. A. Butt, R. Acharya, C. Sibata, K.H. Shin. Surface matching of multimodality image volumes by a fuzzy elastic registration technique. *Comput Med Imaging Graph* 1998;22(1):13–23.
57. M.N. Ahmed, S.M. Yamany, N. Mohamed, A.A. Farag, T. Moriarty. A modified fuzzy c-means algorithm for bias field estimation and segmentation of MRI data. *IEEE Transactions on Medical Imaging*, Vol. 21(3):193–199, 2002.
58. L.P. Clarke, W. Qian. Fuzzy-logic adaptive neural networks for nuclear medicine image restorations. Engineering in Medicine and Biology Society, 1998. *Proceedings of the 20th Annual International Conference of the IEEE.*
59. M. Mahfouf, M.F. Abbod, D.A. Linkens. A survey of fuzzy logic monitoring and control utilisation in medicine. *Artif Intell Med* 21 (2001) 27–42.
60. M.F. Abbod, D.A. Linkens. Anaesthesia monitoring and control using fuzzy logic fusion. Journal of Biomedical Engineering: Applications, Basis & Communications, *Special Issues on Control Methods in Anaesthesia* 1994;10(4):225–235.
61. D.A. Linkens, M. Mahfouf. Fuzzy logic knowledge based control of muscle relaxation. In: *IFAC Proceedings on Modelling and Control of Systems*, Venice, Italy, 1988. pp. 185–90.
62. D.R. Westenskow. Fundamentals of feedback control: PID, fuzzy logic, and neural networks. *J Clin Anesth* 1997;9(Suppl. 6):33S–5S.
63. S. Oshita, K. Nakakimura, R. Kaieda, T. Murakawa, H. Tamura, I. Hiraoka. Application of the concept of fuzzy logistic controller for treatment of hypertension during anaesthesia. *Masui* 1993;42(2):185–9.
64. A.M. Zbinden, P. Feigenwinter, S. Petersen-Felix, S. Hacisalihzade. Arterial pressure control with isoflurane using fuzzy logic. *Br J Anaesth* 1995;74(1): 66–72.
65. J. Schaublin, M. Derighetti, P. Feigenwinter, S. Petersen-Felix, A.M. Zbinden. Fuzzy logic control of mechanical ventilation during anaesthesia. *Br J Anaesth* 1996;77(5):636–41.
66. H. Ying, L.C. Sheppard. Regulating mean arterial pressure in post-surgical cardiac patients. A fuzzy logic system to control administration of sodium nitroprusside. *IEEE Eng Med Biol-Mag* 1994;13(5):671–7.
67. J. Warren, G. Beliakov, B. van der Zwaag. Fuzzy logic in clinical practice decision support systems. *Proceedings of the 33rd Annual Hawaii International Conference on System Sciences*, 2000.
68. E. Smith, J. Eloff. Cognitive fuzzy modeling for enhanced risk assessment in a healthcare institution. *IEEE Intelligent Systems and their Applications*. Vol. 15(2):69–75, 2000.
69. M. Sordo, T. Hongsermeier, V. Kashyap, R.A. Greenes. An XML-based Schema for Order Sets at Partners Healthcare System. In *Advanced Computational Intelligence Paradigms in Healthcare*. Series: Studies in Computational Intelligence, Vol. 48. Yoshida, H.; Jain, A.; Ichalkaranje, A.; Jain, L.C.; Ichalkaranje, N. (Eds.). Springer-Verlag, Germany, 2007.

70. M. Sordo, M. Palchuk. Grouped Knowledge Elements. In Greenes, RA. (ed.), *Clinical Decision Support: The Road Ahead.* Elsevier, November 2006.
71. J.N. Weinstein, K. Kohn, M. Grever, et al. Neural Computing in Cancer Drug Development: Predicting Mechanism of Action. *Science*, 258, 447–451, 1992.
72. J.N. Weinstein, T.G. Myers, P.M. O'Connor, et.al. An information-intensive approach to the molecular pharmacology of cancer. *Science* **275** 343–349. 1997.
73. W.B. Langdon, S.J. Barrett, B.F. Buxton. Combining Decision Trees and Neural Networks for Drug Discovery. *Proceedings of the* 5th *European Conference, EUROGP2002*, Kinsdale, Ireland, April 2002. LNCS 2278 pp. 78–89.
74. V.N. Vuswanadhan, C. Balan, C. Hulme, J.C. Cheetham, Y. Sun. Knowledge-based approaches in the design and selection of compound libraries for drug discovery. *Curr Opin Drug Discov Devel.* 2002. May, 5(3):400–6.
75. M. Villasana, G. Ochoa. (2004) Heuristic Design of Cancer Chemotherapies. *IEEE Transactions on Evolutionary Computation*, Vol. 8, No. 6, pp. 513–521.
76. G. Ochoa, M. Villasana, and E. K. Burke. An Evolutionary Approach to Cancer Chemotherapy Scheduling, *Genetic Programming and Evolvable Machines Journal* 2007 (to appear).
77. Y. Jinn-Yi, L. Wen-Shan. Using simulation technique and genetic algorithm to improve the quality of care of a hospital emergency department. *Expert Systems with Applications: An International Journal*, Vol. 32(4):1073–1083, 2007.
78. A. De Luca, M. Vendittelli, F. Baldini, S. Di Giambenedetto, et al. Construction, training and clinical validation of an interpretation system for genotypic HIV-1 drug resistance based on fussy rules revised by virological outcomes. *Antivir Ther.* 2004 Aug; 9(4):583–93.
79. M. Sordo, T. Hongsermeier, V. Kashyap, R.A. Greenes. A State-based Model for Management of Type II Diabetes. In *Advanced Computational Intelligence Paradigms in Healthcare.* Series: Studies in Computational Intelligence, Vol. 48. Yoshida, H.; Jain, A.; Ichalkaranje, A.; Jain, L.C.; Ichalkaranje, N. (Eds.). Springer-Verlag, Germany, 2007.
80. H. Ying, F. Lin, R.D. MacArthur, J.A. Cohn, D.C. Barth-Jones, H. Ye, L.R. Crane. A self-learning fuzzy discrete event system for HIV/AIDS treatment regimen selection. *IEEE Trans Syst Man Cybern B Cybern.* 2007 Aug; 37(4): 966–79.

Resources

Books

81. Yoshida, H., et al. (Editors), Advanced Computational Intelligence Paradigms in **Healthcare 1**, Springer, 2007.
82. Vaidya, S., et al. (Editors), Advanced Computational Intelligence Paradigms in **Healthcare 2**, Springer, 2007.
83. Holmes, D. and Jain, L.C. (Editors), Innovations in Machine Learning, Springer, 2006.
84. Silvermann, B., et al. (Editors), Intelligent Paradigms in Healthcare Enterprises, Springer-Verlag, Germany, 2005.
85. Fulcher, J. and Jain, L.C. (Editors), Applied Intelligent Systems, Springer-Verlag, Germany, 2004.

86. Schmitt, M., et al. Computational Intelligence Processing in Medical Diagnosis, Springer, 2002.
87. Jain, L.C. and De Wilde, P. (Editors), Practical Applications of Computational Intelligence Techniques, Kluwer Academic Publishers, USA, 2001.
88. Jain, A., et al. (Editors), Artificial Intelligence Techniques in Breast Cancer Diagnosis and Prognosis, World Scientific Publishing Company, Singapore, 2000.
89. Jain, L.C. and Fanelli, A.M. (Editors), Recent Advances in Artificial Neural Networks: Design and Applications, CRC Press, USA, 2000.
90. Lazzerini, B., et al. Evolutionary Computing and Applications, CRC Press USA, 2000.
91. Lazzerini, B., et al. Fuzzy Sets and their Applications to Clustering and Training, CRC Press USA, 2000.
92. Teodorescu, H.N., et al. (Editors), Soft Computing Techniques in Human Related Science, CRC Press USA, 1999.
93. Jain, L.C. and Martin, N.M. (Editors), Fusion of Neural Networks, Fuzzy Logic and Evolutionary Computing and their Applications, CRC Press USA, 1999.
94. Teodorescu, H.N., et al. (Editors), Fuzzy and Neuro-fuzzy Systems in Medicine, CRC Press USA, 1998.
95. Jain, L.C. (Editor), Soft Computing Techniques in Knowledge-Based Intelligent Engineering Systems, Springer-Verlag, Germany, 1997.

Book Chapters

96. Yoshida, H., Vaidya, S. and Jain, L.C., Introduction to Computational Intelligence in Healthcare, Springer-Verlag, 2007, pp. 1–4, Chapter 1.
97. Jain, L.C. and Konar, A., An Introduction to Computational Intelligence Paradigms, in Practical Applications of Computational Intelligence Techniques, Springer, 2001, pp. 1–38.
98. Teodorescu, H.N., Kandel, A. and Jain, L., Fuzzy Logic and Neuro-Fuzzy Systems in Medicine: A historical Perspective, in Fuzzy and Neuro-Fuzzy Systems in Medicine, CRC Press, 1999, pp. 3–16.

Research Papers

99. Ivancevic, T., Jain, L.C. and Bottema, M. "A New Two-Feature GBAM Classifier for Breast Cancer Diagnosis," Proceedings of the Third International Conference on Knowledge-Based Intelligent Information Engineering Systems, IEEE Press USA, August 1999, pp. 296–299.
100. Ivancevic, T., Jain, L.C. and Bottema, M. "A New Two-Feature FAM-Matrix Classifier for Breast Cancer Diagnosis," Proceedings of the Third International Conference on Knowledge-Based Intelligent Information Engineering Systems, IEEE Press USA, August 1999, pp. 305–308.
101. Halgamuge, S., Herrmann, C.S. and Jain, L.C. "Analysis of EEG Signals with Wavelets and Knowledge Engineering Techniques," Proceedings of The International Conference on Neural Information Processing, Hong Kong, September 1996.

2

AI in Clinical Decision Support: Applications in Optical Spectroscopy for Cancer Detection and Diagnosis

Chih-Wen Kan, Linda T. Nieman, Konstantin Sokolov, and Mia K. Markey

The University of Texas, Department of Biomedical Engineering

Summary. Optical approaches have been studied for the detection and diagnosis of epithelial cancer. Due to the biochemical and structural changes that occur in cancerous cells, malignant, benign, and normal tissues have different spectral properties. Artificial intelligence (AI) methods are being explored to detect and diagnose cancer based on optical imaging and spectra. AI is also used to optimize the design of optical spectroscopy and imaging instrumentation. In this chapter, we review the literature on AI applied to optical spectroscopy for cancer detection and diagnosis and present a detailed case study of research on oral cancer diagnosis using polarized light spectra.

2.1 Optical Spectroscopy in Cancer Detection

Cancer is the second leading cause of death in the United States, exceeded only by heart disease [1]. In 2007, more than 559,650 Americans are expected to die of cancer [1]. Early detection and treatment of cancer is essential to improve the survival rate. Among diagnostic modalities, optical methods stand out since they employ non-ionizing radiation, are non-invasive, and the equipment is moderate in cost.

Optical instrumentation provides information at biochemical, structural, and physiological levels for clinical decision making. Over the past few years, the term "optical biopsy" has been widely used in biomedical optics. "Optical biopsy" is commonly used to describe the idea that a non-invasive optical device could augment biopsy, the removal of tissue for analysis. Alternatively, an optical exam could be used as a screening step to reduce the number of benign biopsies. In other words, optical biopsy would be performed first and only those sites that are positive for disease according to the optical method would be subjected to biopsy.

A review of research on the interaction of light with tissue for disease detection and diagnosis was presented by Richards-Kortum and Sevick-Muraca [2]. As early as 1965, studies revealed the potential to use quantitative fluorescence

C.-W. Kan et al.: *AI in Clinical Decision Support: Applications in Optical Spectroscopy for Cancer Detection and Diagnosis*, Studies in Computational Intelligence (SCI) **107**, 27–49 (2008)
www.springerlink.com

spectroscopy for discriminating normal and malignant tissues [3]. In the past few decades, rapid developments of small light sources, detectors, and fiber optic probes have provided opportunities to quantitatively measure light-tissue interactions. Progress using fluorescence, reflectance, and Raman spectroscopy for cancer detection was reviewed in several recent articles [4–9]. Whereas previous reviews have emphasized the underlying biophysical processes and the design of instrumentation to measure them, this chapter is focused on approaches to analyzing optical spectra in support of clinical decision making.

What is Optical Spectroscopy?

A typical optical fiber based spectroscopic experiment is shown in Figure 2.1. Conceptually it is very simple: an optical fiber delivers light to the tissue region of interest and a second optical fiber collects the remitted photons. The tissue can be illuminated with a single wavelength or a range of wavelengths, such as broad-band visible light. Photons interact with tissue through scattering or absorption. In the visible wavelength range, elastic scattering is often the dominant form of optical-tissue interaction used for cancer detection [10]. Figure 2.2 shows an example of a diagnostic system set-up. The light generated by the excitation source is coupled into a fiber-optic probe for delivery to the tissue. The collected photons are spectrally dispersed by a spectrometer and the spectra, which is a plot of intensity as a function of wavelength, is measured by a camera or other light detector. The information is read out and analyzed using the computer and interface electronics.

Since cancer cells and normal cells have different morphologies, their optical properties are similarly different (Figure 2.3). Changes in architectural and morphological features as a result of cancer progression, including increased

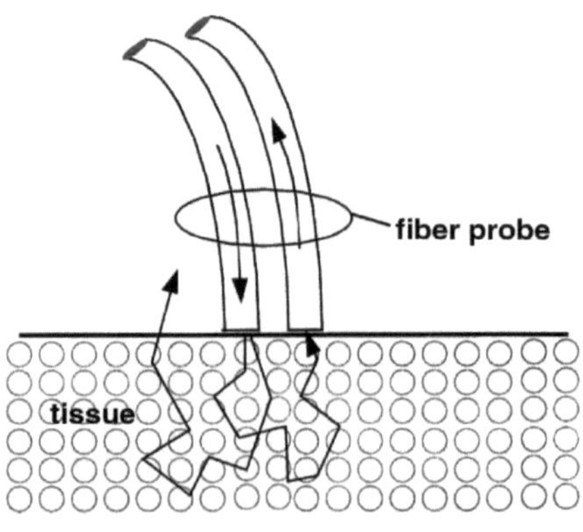

Fig. 2.1. Optical geometry of the fiber-optic probe. The light is delivered into the tissue from an optical fiber probe and interacts with tissue. The remitted light is then collected by another optical fiber for analysis. This figure is reproduced with permission from [21] (©2007 SPIE)

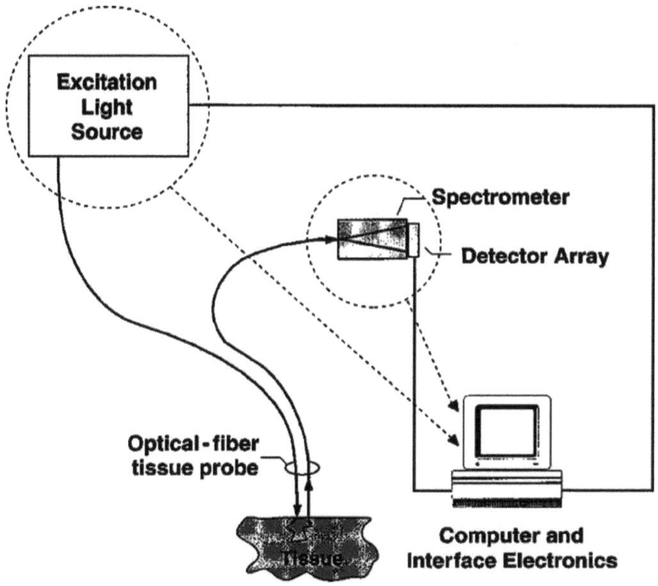

Fig. 2.2. A diagram of a diagnostic system setup. The excitation light source generates photons to impinge on tissue with an optical fiber probe, and the light that leaves the tissue is collected by another fiber and is spectrally dispersed by a spectrometer. The computer and interface electronics control the light source and the spectrometer. This figure is reproduced with permission from [21] (©2007 SPIE)

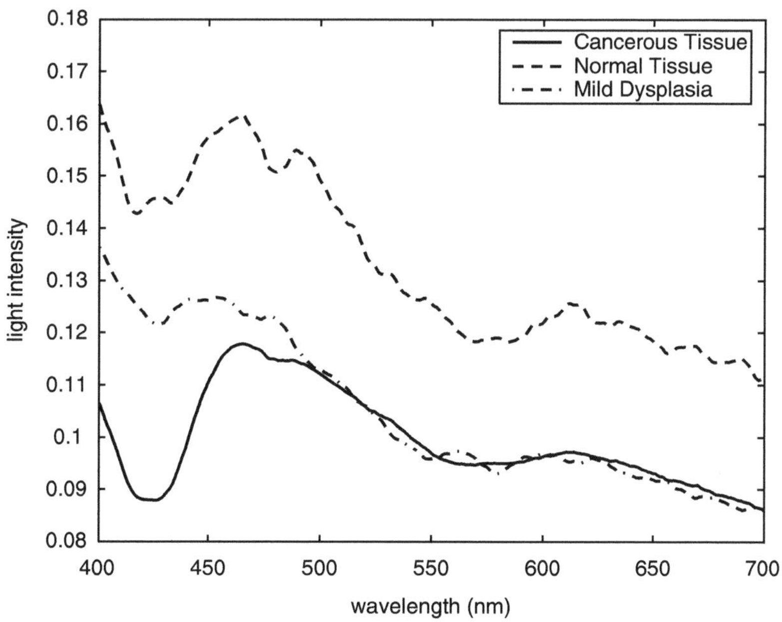

Fig. 2.3. Example diffuse reflectance spectra for normal and malignant sites in oral tissue. The solid curve indicates cancerous oral tissue, while the dash-dotted curve indicates precancerous tissue, and the dashed curve represents normal tissue

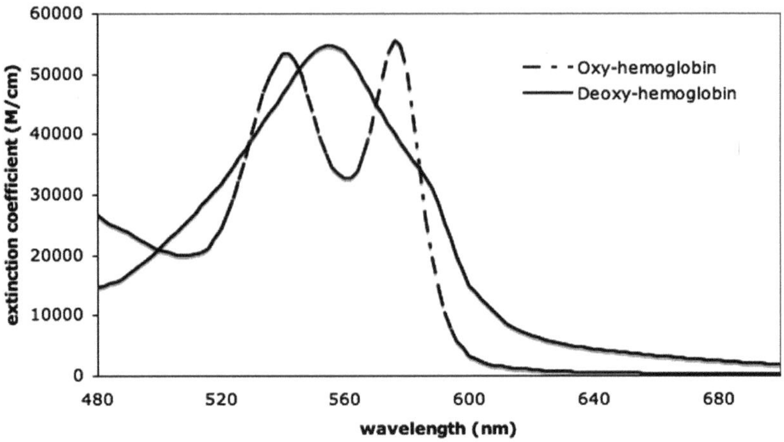

Fig. 2.4. Absorption extinction coefficient of oxy-hemoglobin (dashed curve) and deoxy-hemoglobin (solid curve). The absorption extinction coefficient determines how much light can be absorbed by the object. These two spectra indicate that oxy-hemoglobin absorbs more light at 580 *nm* and deoxy-hemoglobin absorbs more at 560 *nm*

nuclear/cytoplasmic ratio, hyperchromasia, and pleomorphism, affect the nature of the scattering events when light interacts with the tissue. Therefore, these changes complicate the interpretation of spectra as they relate to tissue disease status. For example, cancer cells are well documented to have increased nuclear size, and decreased cell differentiation [11] due to the abnormal duplication of cancerous cells. Larger nuclei result in more backward scattering events, which leads to the collection of more light at the optical fiber [12]. Therefore, the light intensities can be used, to some extent, as features for diagnostic decisions.

The spectral distribution may also be altered by the concentration of hemoglobin. Initially, non-necrotic cancerous tissues contain a higher concentration of hemoglobin due to the increased consumption of more nutrients than normal cells. In Figure 2.4, the extinction coefficients of oxy-hemoglobin and deoxy-hemoglobin are shown. The extinction coefficient is an important optical property as it determines how much light can be absorbed. Clearly, tissues containing different oxy- and deoxy-hemoglobin concentrations will have different spectra.

2.2 AI Methods Used for Spectral Classification

Artificial intelligence (AI) is a key technology for developing clinical decision support systems. AI uses computational techniques to achieve goals that require intelligence. AI methods are used to extract features and to select the features that are most indicative of cancer status in order to classify spectral patterns. In the following sections, we review the general steps taken to develop a clinical decision support system in the context of analyzing optical spectroscopy data. First, preprocessing techniques are applied to the optical spectra to reduce the influences of noise and artifacts and to normalize the spectra of different samples. Second, features are extracted from the spectra to summarize the key information content. Then, feature selection is performed to reduce the number of redundant and irrelevant features. After that, classifiers are trained to distinguish between different histopathology groups. The choice of evaluation metric and testing paradigm is critical to accurately evaluate the performance of a clinical decision support system.

2.2.1 Preprocessing

Preprocessing techniques are needed since real-world data are often noisy, missing, or inconsistent [13]. Biomedical signals are especially notorious in this regard. Hence, it is desirable to have preprocessing techniques to improve the quality of data and the efficiency of data analysis. There are two broad types of preprocessing techniques. *Data cleaning* refers to the removal of noise and imputation of missing data. *Data normalization* transforms the data such that they are standardized. Data normalization may significantly improve the accuracy and efficiency of data analysis [13].

There are several factors that influence optical spectra. Some of these factors are critical for making clinical decisions, such as the structure of the cells and the hemoglobin concentrations, while other factors are not related to disease status. For example, fluctuation of the light source and light detector errors both cause slight changes to the measured optical spectra.

Normalization is a preprocessing step that standardizes the spectral data and enhances spectral features that distinguish between different histopathologies. The simplest approach assumes that the error is uniform in each measurement. In other words, it assumes the same intensity of error at all wavelengths. In this case, the most common normalization method is to divide the spectrum by the baseline intensity of a specific wavelength. The choice of baseline wavelength is often at the extreme ends of a spectrum - either at a short or long wavelength [14], i.e., wavelengths that are outside of the range that usually interact with tissue. Another strategy is to normalize each spectrum by its highest intensity [15]. Normalizing by the peak intensity standardizes the spectra and makes the highest point the same in every spectrum. Unlike normalizing by an extreme wavelength, this method does not make any assumptions of the wavelength ranges that usually interact with tissue. Instead, it chooses the peak intensity to be where the most scattering or absorbing events occur. In a similar manner, one can normalize each spectrum by its lowest intensity, the wavelength at which the least scattering or absorbing events occur. Other researchers have normalized the spectra such that each spectrum has the same area under the plot [15]. Since the area under a spectrum can be viewed as the total energy received by the light collecting probe, this method assumes that the total energy received remains constant and uses this property to reduce the variability between different measurements [15].

Normalization is also key for effective visualization of spectra by clinicians. Noise and artifacts in the spectra may influence the ability of humans to make clinical decisions. Therefore, it is desirable to visually enhance the spectral signatures. Normalization methods used to enhance visualization include smoothing and sharpening of optical spectra and spectral enhancing near a specific wavelength. This is an interesting topic for future work since there are few previous studies addressing normalization for visualization purposes. Moreover, although the normalization goals are different between visualization by humans and analysis by computers, the normalization methods may sometimes be the same.

Other preprocessing methods are used to reduce the noise due to instrumentation, patient, or equipment operator influences. To eliminate the effect that is specific to the patient, a spectrum may be normalized by the spectrum recorded from the contralateral position in the same patient, for example, the breast on the opposite side of the patient [15]. However, a contralateral position measurement is not always available for asymmetric organs or organs that have disease throughout.

Instrumentation effects are composed of various spectral responses from different optical components. To reduce the impact of these interferences, different noise models have been developed [16, 17]. Fawzy *et al.* [16] designed an experiment that measured the true tissue response and the signal reflected from a standard disc for reference. Two linear models were developed to account for the instrument's spectral response.

$$I_{m1}(\lambda) = a_1 I(\lambda) + b_1 I(\lambda) R_{tm}(\lambda) \tag{2.1}$$

where $I(\lambda)$ is the instrument's spectral response and $R_{tm}(\lambda)$ is the true tissue diffuse reflectance to be derived. a_1 and b_1 are the weights of the instrumentation spectral response and that of the true tissue reflected response, respectively. The signal measured from tissue $I_{m1}(\lambda)$ is divided by the reflectance signal measured from a reflectance standard disc to account for instrument spectral response. The reflectance signal measured from the standard disc is

$$I_{m2}(\lambda) = a_2 I(\lambda) + b_2 I(\lambda) R_s \tag{2.2}$$

where $I(\lambda)$ is the instrument's spectral response, and R_s is the reflectivity of the standard disc, which is approximately constant across the whole visible wavelength range, a_2 and b_2 are the weights of the instrumentation spectral response and the spectral response reflected from the standard disc, respectively.

Dividing Eq. 2.1 and Eq. 2.2 and rearranging the equation:

$$R_m(\lambda) = \frac{I_{m1}(\lambda)}{I_{m2}(\lambda)} = a_0 + b_0 R_{tm}(\lambda) \tag{2.3}$$

where $R_m(\lambda)$ is the apparent reflectance spectra measured, $R_{tm}(\lambda)$ is the true tissue diffuse reflectance to be derived, and a_0 and b_0 are additive offset and multiplicative factor, respectively, which depend on the measurement conditions during each *in vivo* measurement. In Eq. 2.3, a_0 and b_0 can be measured by controlled calibration experiments, allowing the true diffuse reflectance, R_{tm}, to be determined. A study conducted by Marín *et al.* pointed out the importance of establishing calibration standards in fluorescence spectroscopy [18]. A consensus calibration standard enables meaningful comparison of data from multiple devices and unambiguous interpretations of experiments.

In the study of Fawzy *et al.* the weights a_0 and b_0 in their noise model can be measured. In some other studies, the weights in the noise models are adjusted such that the effect of instrumentation noise is minimized. To achieve this goal, it is necessary to define a merit function that quantifies the effect of instrumentation noise. Ntziachristos *et al.* (2002) defined a merit function that was a summation of the tumor absorption coefficients and the absorption coefficients of background noise [17]. In other words, the merit function was the difference between the noise estimated by the model and the measured signals. This merit function was minimized by a χ^2 minimization technique. Since the noise components vary by different instruments, operators, and locations of the instrument [18], different noise models are needed for different situations. There exists no single noise model that fits all the cases.

2.2.2 Feature Extraction

To describe ifferent spectral patterns, features are extracted from the spectra. Of course, we can simply use the spectral intensities at each wavelength as the features. But other statistical features, such as the slope of the spectrum, may more efficiently capture information relevant to disease status. There are no features that work "best" in detecting all diseases. Thus, the choice of features is specific to a given diagnostic task.

There are three major categories of feature extraction methods: principal component analysis (PCA), spectral feature extraction, and model-based feature extraction. PCA is a linear transformation technique for reducing the dimensionality of data. Spectral feature extraction describes spectral signatures without prior knowledge of the tissues physical nature, while model based-extraction requires prior knowledge of the physical properties.

Principal Component Analysis (PCA)

PCA is commonly used for feature extraction and reducing the dimensionality of data. PCA is a linear transformation of the data to a new coordinate system such that the data projection on the first principal component has the greatest variance. One can use PCA to reduce the dimensionality of the data by keeping the lower-order principal components and ignoring the higher-order ones. However, PCA transforms the original features into new features without direct physical or biological interpretation. Thus, PCA is not ideal for use in designing a clinical decision support system, in which it is desirable to make decisions based on features that can easily be directly related to the biophysics of the disease process. That being said, several studies have demonstrated the potential of PCA in analyzing optical spectra. Bard *et al.* applied PCA on reflectance spectra on neoplastic lesions of the bronchial tree [14]. In their study, they retained the first 10 principal components that included 99.99% of the total variation of data. Several other studies also retained a pre-determined number of principal components [19–22]. Other studies specified the percentage of the total variances. Mirabal *et al.* retained the principal components that account for 65%, 75%, 85%, and 95% of the total variance as their features [23]. Setting the number of PCs up front has the advantage of fixing the number of inputs to the classifiers being considered. However, the second strategy of selecting the number of PCs that account for a specified percentage of variance controls the amount of information contained in the features.

Spectral Features

In non-model based feature extraction, calculations are made based on the statistical properties of the spectrum. In optical spectroscopy, the spectral intensities themselves are informative since the intensities are related to how many photons are scattered or absorbed. The means of the spectra are commonly used to summarize the amount of light scattered from the tissue [21]. Furthermore, it is possible to divide each spectrum into several spectral bands and calculate the average spectral intensity of each band as a feature [21]. In addition to the first moment of the spectrum, higher order moments, such as the standard deviation, can also be used as features.

Mourant *et al.* (1995) conducted a study on spectroscopic diagnosis of bladder cancer with elastic light scattering [24]. They discovered that the spectral slopes over the wavelength range 330–370 nm have positive values for nonmalignant tissues, and negative values for malignant ones. Bigio *et al.* also used spectral features from a spectral range (330–590 nm) divided into 21 wavelength bands of 20 nm width. Both the average intensities and the slopes of each interval were calculated as spectral features [21].

In feature extraction, one must understand the biophysical properties that underlie optical phenomena. Also, it is well accepted that some wavelengths may be more discriminatory than others. This is because light of different wavelengths behaves differently when interacting with tissues. As the physical interpretation of light-tissue interactions is difficult, feature extraction may help us understand the underlying physics. The advantage of feature extraction is to explicitly encode spectral information in a biophysically meaningful manner.

Model-based Features

Model-based features are extracted by building quantitative models of the tissue and inversely calculating the parameters in the model. These parameters contain important tissue information which may be indicative of the cancer status. For example, the sizes of scatterers in the tissue are typically larger in cancerous tissues; thus, the sizes of scatterers can be used as a feature indicative of cancer status. In these quantitative models, absorption coefficients and scattering coefficients are commonly inversely-determined from optical spectra. However, several other parameters such as tissue blood volume fractions or hemoglobin concentration can also be obtained from these models [22].

Obtaining parameters from quantitative models requires prior knowledge of the tissue and the light used in the system. That is, one must select the model that best approximates the properties of the tissue and the light. For example, the diffusion equation is valid for cases with low to moderate tissue absorption relative to scattering. A rule of thumb is that if

$$\mu_a << 3(1-g)\mu_s \tag{2.4}$$

then diffusion equation should be appropriate, where μ_a is the absorption coefficient $[1/m]$, μ_s is the scattering coefficient $[1/m]$, and g is the anisotropy factor. Therefore, the diffusion equation is suitable for red light and near-infraredlight systems where scattering dominates the light-tissue interaction [25].

Four models are commonly used to numerically and analytically extract the absorption coefficients from diffuse reflectance spectroscopy - radiative transfer theory (RTT), Monte Carlo (MC) modeling, empirical methods, and Mie theory. While the first three methods view light as a flow of photons traveling through a medium, the last method treats light as an electromagnetic wave. These modeling techniques are described below.

Radiative transfer theory (RTT) has been developed largely without reference to electromagnetic theory [26, 27]. It is based on the transfer of energy through a turbid medium. RTT has a stationary form of

$$\hat{s} \cdot \nabla I(\boldsymbol{r}, \hat{s}) + \mu_t(\boldsymbol{r}) I(\boldsymbol{r}, \hat{s}) = \mu_s(\boldsymbol{r}) \int_4 \pi p(\hat{s}, \hat{s}') I(\boldsymbol{r}, \hat{s}') d\omega' + S(\boldsymbol{r}, \hat{s}) \tag{2.5}$$

where $I(\boldsymbol{r}, \hat{s})$ is the radiance $[W/(m^2 \cdot sr)]$ along the $\hat{s}$ direction per unit solid angle and per unit area at location $\boldsymbol{r}$, μ_t is the total extinction coefficient $[1/m]$, μ_s is the scattering coefficient $[1/m]$, p is the scattering phase function $[1/sr]$, and S is the source term that corresponds to the power generated at $\boldsymbol{r}$ in the $\hat{s}$ direction $[W/(m^3 \cdot sr)]$. As there is no general solution available to this equation, an analytical approximation is used to model diffuse scattering. A common analytical approximation of RTT is called the diffusion equation.

Monte Carlo modeling provides a flexible approach to studying light propagation in biological tissues [28]. This method views light as particles and traces three-dimensional random walks of photons in a medium. The two key parameters in Monte Carlo modeling are the scattering angle and the mean free path for a photon-tissue interaction. The mean free path is determined by the probability that a photon is scattered or absorbed after a given step size. This probability is determined by local optical properties: μ_s, the scattering coefficient, and μ_a, the absorption coefficient. Similarly, the scattering angle is determined by the anisotropy factor g. Monte Carlo modeling generates uniformly distributed random numbers and transforms them to follow the distributions of the mean free paths and scattering coefficients. These random attributes are then used to simulate and record the paths of photons. When modeling stratified tissues, multi-layer models are often needed. Each layer is described by its thickness, refractive index n, absorption coefficient μ_a, scattering coefficient μ_s, and anisotropy factor g [29, 30]. Internal reflection or refraction at the medium boundaries can also be simulated.

Another approach to inverse modeling is to use an empirical method. Empirical methods do not make explicit assumptions about the interaction of light and tissue. Instead, the idea is to use a classifier to "learn" the light-tissue interaction from experimental data. For example, Pfefer *et al.* [31] developed an empirical method for the extraction of absorption and scattering coefficients from diffuse reflectance spectra. They trained a neural network with phantoms and then used the network to extract optical parameters from another set of phantoms.

Mie theory is a complete analytical solution of Maxwell's equations for the scattering of electromagnetic radiation by spherical particles [27, 32, 33]. It assumes a homogeneous, isotropic, and optically linear material irradiated by an infinitely extending plane wave. Mie theory assumes that the scatterers are spheres of arbitrary size and have a homogeneous index of refraction. Mie theory is often combined with the other three models for calculating the size of scatterers after obtaining the absorption and scattering coefficients of the tissue [34].

The choice of model depends on the system studied, although it is not uncommon for multiple quantitative models to be employed to elucidate the biophysics of the optical-tissue interaction. The main drawback of all these models, however, is that they either require a priori knowledge of optical parameters or they require simplifying assumptions, such as sphericity of scatterers, which may not be physically realistic. Despite their assumptions, these quantitative models provide valuable insight into the alterations of optical spectra with changing tissue state.

2.2.3 Feature Selection

A large number of features, obtained from quantitative modeling or the measured spectra directly, can be potentially related to health status. Feature selection can aid identification of those optically derived features that are diagnostically relevant and those that are strongly related to each other and thus are redundant. Minimizing the number of features is important to reduce computation complexity, processing time, and to prevent overtraining of classifiers.

Since reflectance spectroscopy measures the combination of the elastic scattering from different organelles, it is not surprising that some wavelengths indicate cancer progression better than others. It is possible that one or several wavelengths contain information on the pathology status. Therefore, it is necessary to select subsets of these features to reduce the redundancy and improve the performance.

There are three main approaches to feature selection: *filters*, *wrappers*, and *embedded methods* [35]. Many feature selection algorithms use filters to select variables by giving ranks to individual features [35]. For example, Marín *et al.* (2005) selected their features using a combination of Principal Component Analysis (PCA) and a two-sample t test. They selected principal component scores (PCS) identified as statistically significant using a two-sample t test for independent samples, with equality of variance between the two groups (positive and negative for dysplasia) based upon an F test [36].

However, it is known that a feature which provides little information by itself can be valuable when combined with others [35]. Therefore, subsets of features can have better predictive power than would be expected by ranking of variables according to their individual predictive power. Thus, wrapper methods have been developed to select feature subsets rather than individual features. Wrapper methods use the prediction performance of a given classifier to assess the relative usefulness of subsets of features. If the number of features is not too large, an exhaustive search can also be considered. An example of a wrapper method is stepwise LDA (Linear Discriminant Analysis). It performs a greedy search of the possible feature combinations [37].

Embedded methods perform feature selection as part of the training process. Thus, they may be more efficient in the training process. For example, decision trees such as CART (Classification and Regression Trees) have a built-in mechanism to perform variable selection [38]. A study conducted by Atkinson *et al.* [39] used CART to analyze fluorescence spectra of suspected cervical intraepithelial neoplasia (CIN) at colposcopy.

2.2.4 Classification

There are two major types of machine learning algorithms: unsupervised learning and supervised learning. In unsupervised learning or clustering, the algorithm identifies clusters in the feature values based on criteria defining the desired properties of groups. Unsupervised learning techniques are useful for assessing the discriminatory power of features. The visualization of the clustering distributions of features provides a qualitative evaluation of their potential for distinguishing between pre-defined categories, such as healthy vs. diseased [20]. In developing clinical decision support systems, supervised learning is more commonly used than unsupervised learning since the task is typically one of prediction, e.g., to predict disease status. Supervised learning refers to an algorithm that uses a training set of items for which target or truth labels are provided to learn a mapping from feature values to target values. In the case of cancer diagnosis, histopathological assessment of a biopsy sample is typically taken as the gold standard for establishing the truth state for classifier training and evaluation. In other words, the task of a supervised learning algorithm or classifier is to use the features provided by the feature extractor and selected in a feature selection step to predict the assignment of the sample to a diagnostic category [43]. Most clinical diagnostic decisions cannot be made based on a single feature; thus, classifiers play an important role in that they determine a function for combining two or more features to make predictions. The most commonly used classifiers for cancer detection/diagnosis from optical spectroscopy are LDA [40] and Artificial Neural Networks (ANN) [41, 42].

The difficulty of a classification task depends on the variability of the feature values within a class relative to the feature variability between classes. For example, suppose the size of a lesion is a feature that we can use to discriminate between benign and malignant lesions. All else being equal, it will be more difficult to distinguish between benign lesions with an average size of 1 mm and malignant lesions with an average size of 2 mm, as compared to the case in which the benign lesion mean size is 1 mm and the malignant lesion mean size is 10 mm. Likewise, for a fixed difference in the class means, the greater the variability within each class, the more challenging the classification task. Therefore, the underlying probability model of the categories determines the difficulty of the classification problem.

Some classifiers are more complex than others in the sense of the range of models that they can describe [43]. For example, a *support vector machine (SVM)* is capable of distinguishing samples by forming a non-linear function of the features, while a linear discriminant analysis (LDA) model is only able to solve linearly separable tasks. However, this does not mean that complex classifiers are always "better" than the simple ones. Complex classifiers suffer from generalization issues, i.e., overtraining. It is very easy to "tune" a complex classifier to the particular training samples, rather than to the real underlying characteristics of the diagnostic categories. A large training set will alleviate generalization issues, but assembling an extensive heterogeneous data set can be challenging. Thus, a simpler classifier may be used to avoid over-training given a limited amount of data. Another motivation for using linear classifiers is that they are more computationally efficient.

The choice of classifier depends on how much prior knowledge we have about the classification task. For example, if we have prior knowledge that the classification problem is linear, it will be most efficient to use a linear classifier rather than a non-linear one. However, in the case where we have little or no prior knowledge about the problem, there is no simple answer as to how to choose the best classifier. The No Free Lunch theorem [44] states that if algorithm A outperforms algorithm B on some cost functions, there must exist exactly as many other functions where B outperforms A. In other words, if one algorithm seems to outperform another in a particular situation, it is because the algorithm is a better fit for that particular problem, not that that algorithm is generally "better" than the other one [43]. Thus, the selection of an algorithm for a practical classification task is an empirical choice because there is typically little prior knowledge of the underlying probability model.

2.2.5 Evaluation

To evaluate the performance of a clinical decision support system, we compare the diagnostic decisions suggested by our system to a gold standard, e.g., biopsy outcome. A performance measure, such as the accuracy, is computed to quantitatively summarize the efficacy of the system.

In two-class classification problems, Receiver Operating Characteristic (ROC) analysis is widely used for analyzing the classifier performance [45]. Sensitivity and specificity indicate the ability of the diagnostic method to distinguish between two groups, e.g., healthy and disease. By varying the threshold, a ROC curve of sensitivity versus (1-specificity) is generated. The area under the ROC curve (AUC) is often used as a metric to quantitatively summarize the performance of a clinical decision support system.

In contrast, for a multi-class classification task, there is not a widely accepted performance metric [46]. Multiple research groups have been working on developing ROC-type analyses for multi-class problems. Several approaches have been proposed, so we briefly review only the most common and refer the reader to other resources for a broader summary [46]. Hand and Till use the average AUCs of the binary one-versus-one comparisons in multi-class problems [47]. Mossman (1999) developed a three-way ROC method [48] that uses the correct classification rates as two separate decision thresholds are varied to form a 3-dimensional plot. The volume under the surface (VUS) of this plot serves as the performance metric. Moreover, Edwards *et al.* creates a ROC hypersurface, which is a two-dimensional plane in a six-dimensional space, and calculates the hypervolume under the hypersurface as a measure of performance [49]. We emphasize that no single metric has been widely adapted.

Generally speaking, three independent sample sets are desired to design and evaluate a classifier [50]. A training set is used for training a classifier. A validation set is used during or after classifier training, in order to adjust the classifier to prevent over-training. A test set is used for evaluating a classifier to report its performance. Ideally, these three sets should be randomly selected from the relevant population. However, there are practical issues to be considered. In particular, since the number of samples available is often limited, it may not be possible to construct truly independent sets, which causes bias. Therefore, sampling techniques such as *cross-validation* [51] and *bootstrap sampling* [52–54] are often necessary in experimental design.

Cross-validation refers to the partitioning of data into non-overlapping subsets of equal size such that the analysis is initially performed on a single subset, while the other subset(s) are retained for subsequent use in confirming and validating the initial analysis [51]. The training/testing process is repeated until each partition has been used in turn as the testing partition. *Leave-one-out cross-validation* is a special case of cross-validation where one sample is assigned to the testing set and the rest are in the training set.

Bootstrap sampling is another technique that can be used to estimate the performance of a classifier. Bootstrap sampling creates a new set by sampling with replacement from the original set [52–54]. Typically, each bootstrap replicate has the same number of observations as the original sample. The process is repeated to create hundreds or thousands of bootstrap replicates. Then, a performance metric is computed from all of the bootstrap replicates and the average performance metric is taken as the estimate of the system performance.

The choice of appropriate evaluation methods is critical. Since clinical studies are often restricted to a small sample size, the analyses can suffer from biased data and little variation between samples [55]. Appropriate evaluation methods enable reliable estimation of system performance, which is essential for designing accurate and reliable clinical decision support systems.

2.3 Case Study: Spectroscopy for Oral Cancer Detection

Oral cancer is a major problem throughout the world. For example, in India, it is the leading cancer in men [56] and in Cuba it is the leading cancer death for women [1]. In developed countries such as the U.S., early detection is low despite regular dental or physical examinations. In this section, we will introduce a case study on developing a clinical decision support system for oral cancer detection and diagnosis using optical spectroscopy.

2.3.1 Clinical Challenges

Currently, oral cancer is usually found by a dentist during a dental check-up or by a general practitioner during a routine physical examination. There are two major challenges to this process. First, suspicious abnormalities must be detected and localized. Even for an experienced clinician, it is difficult to localize an oral lesion. Toluidine blue (TB) dye can be used to help identify the locations that are more probable to be dysplasia or cancer [57]. Unfortunately, although TB dye has a high sensitivity, its specificity is very low [58]. Second, the pathological status of the abnormality must be established, e.g., benign, pre-cancer, or cancer. Clinicians visually assess suspicious abnormalities, but benign inflammatory conditions are difficult to visually distinguish from premalignant lesions. Microscopic histological examination of biopsied tissue by a trained pathologist is the "gold standard" for diagnosis of mucosal abnormalities [57]. A less invasive technique called brush biopsy uses a brush to exfoliate the epithelium of a suspicious lesion. The cells are reviewed by a pathologist using a microscope. The brush biopsy method is painful and can be difficult to scrape the entire epithelium thickness if a keratin layer has formed. Moreover, although brush biopsy has high sensitivity, it is not feasible if the lesion covers a large area. Thus, there is considerable interest in exploring the potential of optical imaging and spectroscopy for detecting, localizing, and non-invasively diagnosing oral lesions.

2.3.2 Design of the Study

Materials

A pilot clinical study was conducted on 27 patients over the age of 18 years that were referred to the Head and Neck clinic at The University of Texas M. D. Anderson Cancer Center (UT MDACC) with oral mucosa lesions suspicious for dysplasia or carcinoma. Spectroscopic measurements were typically performed on 1-2 visually abnormal sites and 1 visually normal site. Biopsies were taken of all measured tissue sites. We measured a total of 57 sites, of which 22 were visually and histopathologically normal (Normal), 13 sites that were visually abnormal but histopathologically normal (Benign), 12 that were visually abnormal sites that proved to be mild dysplasia (MD) on histopathology, and 10 that were visually abnormal sites that proved to be severe high grade dysplasia or carcinoma (SD) after histopathology.

The spectroscopic measurement that was performed was based on Oblique Polarization Reflectance Spectroscopy (OPRS) [59–61]. In each measurement, parallel and perpendicular spectra were collected.

Five spectral signals were used in this study:

1. Parallel signals: $I_{\parallel}$
2. Perpendicular signals: $I_{\perp}$
3. Diffuse reflectance spectrum:

$$I_{diffuse} = I_{\parallel} + I_{\perp} \tag{2.6}$$

4. The ratio of parallel to perpendicular:

$$I_{par/per} = \frac{I_{\parallel}}{I_{\perp}} \tag{2.7}$$

5. The depolarization ratio:

$$I_{depol} = \frac{I_{\parallel} - I_{\perp}}{I_{\parallel} + I_{\perp}} \tag{2.8}$$

We used MATLAB R14 (The MathWorks, Natick, MA) and a neural network toolbox developed by Nabney [62] for data analysis in this case study.

Preprocessing

Two preprocessing steps were are taken in this case study: *Down-sampling* and *Normalization*. Spectra were down-sampled using an averaging window with a spectral width of 5 nm. The purpose of down-sampling is to reduce the computation time and complexity. Moreover, down-sampling reduces the instrumentation noise from the spectrometer. Since the spectrometer resolution was 5 nm, signals within a two data point interval of 5 nm were considered noise. Hence the down-sampling window width was set to be 5 nm. After down-sampling, the spectra were normalized to remove inter-patient variation. Each spectrum was normalized by dividing each intensity value by the intensity at 420 nm.

Feature Extraction and Selection

Three types of features were extracted from each sample. The first and the second types of features were both spectral features, and the third feature type was model-based.

1. spectral intensities of each spectrum: For each spectrum, 64 spectral intensities at 64 different wavelengths were used as features.
2. average spectral intensities: For each spectrum, the average spectral intensity was calculated as a feature.
3. average nuclear size: The average nuclear size of tissue was inversely calculated by fitting the depolarization ratio spectrum to a Mie theory based model [60, 63].

Consequently, for every sample in the database, we had 64 spectral intensities $\times 5$ spectra $+1$ average intensity per each of 5 spectra $+1$ estimate of the average nuclear size $=$ 326 features. As we only had 57 samples, there was a substantial imbalance between the number of samples and the number of features and thus it was critical to reduce the number of features. We did not employ Principal Component Analysis (PCA) since we wanted to preserve the physical meaning of the features. For computational simplicity, we used a filter method to select one spectral intensity from each spectrum. The features were ranked by the area under their ROC curves (AUC). The trapezoid rule was used to compute the AUC under the empirical ROC curve. For each spectrum, the spectral intensity with the highest AUC was selected as the most discriminatory. In this manner, we reduced the number of features to $5+5+1 = 11$. In this case study, a filter method was used for feature selection for computational simplicity. In other work, we are testing a wrapper method that searches for feature combination subsets [61].

Classification and Evaluation

Leave-one-out cross-validation was employed. The classifiers were trained to distinguish between two groups at a time and a series of tests was conducted of different pairwise comparisons, i.e., Normal vs. SD, Normal vs. MD, etc.

A Linear Discrimination Analysis (LDA) and an Artificial Neural Network (ANN) were used to predict the pathology status based on the 11 features. Note that one expects the ANN to learn any model that can be produced by LDA as well as models that have non-linear decision boundaries. However, overtraining is likely to occur with a large number of hidden nodes, especially when the sample size is small. Thus, the ANNs in this analysis used only two hidden nodes so as to reduce the likelihood of overtraining. In this case study, each of the ANNs used in the 6 comparisons was adjusted separately to obtain suitable learning rates, momentum, and iteration cycles. These parameters were adjusted such that the learning was stopped before the mean squared error increased for the held-out cases in the cross-validation.

Classifier performance was evaluated in terms of the area under the Receiver Operating Characteristic curve (AUC). The AUC under the empirical ROC curves was computed using the trapezoid rule. A bootstrapping technique [54] was used to test the hypothesis that the mean difference in the AUC between LDA models and ANN models was zero. P values below the conventional threshold of 0.05 indicate that there is a statistically significant difference between the AUC of the LDA model and that of the ANN model.

2.3.3 Results and Discussion

In this study, we compared LDA and ANN models for classifying optical spectral measurements of oral sites. We observed that the ANN performance was comparable to or higher than that of the LDA for all pairwise classification considered, e.g., Normal vs. Benign, Normal vs. MD, etc (Table 2.1). For example, for the task of distinguishing between Normal and MD sites, the ANN achieved an AUC of 0.83 while the LDA achieved an AUC of 0.65. The potential improvement in classification performance to be gained from using an ANN model rather than a LDA model is most evident when the task was to separate Normal from other disease states. However, the p values generated from the hypothesis test based on bootstrap sampling indicate that only two of the six pairwise classifications have significantly different AUCs ($p < 0.05$). The other four pairs of AUCs are statistically indistinguishable given the available data. While the results of this small pilot study must be interpreted cautiously, our findings are consistent with prior studies that reported that non-linear classifiers were desirable when predicting pathology status from optical spectra of other organ sites [40, 41].

We also noted that both classifiers generally performed best when separating Normal from SD (Table 2.1). This is not unexpected because Normal and SD are pathological extremes. Other groups have also reported good separation of Normal from SD and Normal from dysplasia using other optical

Table 2.1. Classifier performances for pairwise classifications. Data are areas under ROC curve. The first value is for LDA, second value is for ANN, and the third value is the p value obtained from the hypothesis test based on bootstrap sampling. P values below the conventional threshold of 0.05 were regarded as statistically significant

		Class 2			
		Normal	Benign	MD	SD
Class 1	Normal		0.59, 0.70, (p=0.49)	0.65, 0.83, (p=0.04)	0.68, 1.00, (p<0.01)
	Benign			0.61, 0.65, (p=0.75)	0.64, 0.60, (p=0.90)
	MD				0.53, 0.56, (p=0.91)
	SD				

techniques [64–67]. This provides additional evidence that the spectroscopy measurements are capturing meaningful information on the underlying biophysical changes associated with cancer progression.

When using ANNs, one must always be concerned about overtraining. If an ANN is overtrained, its generalization performance can be worse than that of a simpler model, such as LDA. Overtraining often results from trying to learn appropriate values for many network parameters (weights) from a small number of samples. Thus, a common rule of thumb for choosing the maximum number of hidden nodes is to have at least twice as many samples as there are weights in the network. Of course, if the classification problem is complicated, more hidden nodes will be needed and thus more training samples will be required. In this case study, we chose a small number of hidden nodes (2 hidden nodes) to reduce the chance of overtraining since there was a small number of samples available for training. Despite this precaution, very high AUCs were obtained for some classification tasks, which are likely overly optimistic and are not expected to generalize as more data are collected.

In this study, we have shown that optical spectroscopy is capable of discriminating different stages of oral cancer. An ANN model performed better than LDA models at distinguishing oral cancer histopathologies using optical spectroscopy. Moreover, this study verified that optical spectroscopy is better able to distinguish between more histopathologically distinct samples than less histopathologically distinct samples.

In this case study, we have demonstrated that optical spectroscopy has high potential for accurate diagnosis of oral cancer. On the other hand, spectroscopic instruments are not suitable for the detection task since their probing area is small; optical imaging is better suited for that role. More work is needed on combining optical spectroscopy with optical imaging in order to develop systems able to help localize, detect, and diagnose cancer [17].

2.4 Conclusions and Future Works

The intent of this chapter has been to review the literature on AI methods applied to optical spectroscopy for cancer diagnosis. We introduced preprocessing techniques, features extracted from optical spectra to describe key information, feature selection for reducing redundant information, and classifiers trained to distinguish between different histopathology groups. We also reviewed the choice of evaluation metric and testing paradigm for evaluating the performance of a clinical decision support system. Finally, we presented a detailed case study of research on oral cancer diagnosis using polarized light spectra.

It is difficult for a human to visually assess the optical spectra and make a diagnosis despite of the capability of optical spectroscopy for capturing cancer characteristics. The influence of cancer cell morphology on its optical properties is complicated, hence a clinical decision support system is necessary. This chapter shows that AI provides support for clinicians to make diagnostic decisions based on optical spectroscopy. Moreover, AI can also help scientists understand the optical properties of different tissue pathologies. For example, model-based feature extraction enables determining optical parameters of the measured tissue. This example shows how AI methods are used in data mining, which extracts useful information from large databases.

This chapter also indicated the the potential for optical spectroscopy to be extended to optical imaging for detecting epithelial cancer of wide-spread lesions. Optical spectroscopy is not suitable for detection tasks of wide-spread lesions because of its small sampling area; optical imaging is better suited for that. As discussed in preprocessing section, optical spectroscopy can be very useful for selecting optimal imaging wavelengths. However, optical spectroscopy is a practical approach for small lesions, for directing biopsies to limit their number and frequency, and for margin detection during tumor excision. Two-dimensional, or even three-dimensional imaging are both very promising directions for future work.

Acknowledgments

The authors would like to thank Bryan Jiang for his help in the case study, Chris Kite and Arjun Ramachandran for their technical assistance. We also thank Prof. Irving J. Bigio for permission in reproducing certain figures for this chapter.

References

1. Jemal, A.; Cancer Facts & Figures 2007. Atlanta, GA; American Cancer Society; 2007 press, 2007
2. Richards-Kortum, R. & Sevick-Muraca, E.; Quantitative Optical Spectroscopy For Tissue Diagnosis; Annual Review of Physical Chemistry, 1996, 47, 555-606

3. Lycette, R. & Leslie, R.; Fluorescence of malignant tissue.; Lancet, 1965, 40, 436
4. Bigio, I. & Mourant, J.; Ultraviolet and visible spectroscopies for tissue diagnostics: fluorescence spectroscopy and elastic-scattering spectroscopy; Phys. Med. Biol, 1997, 42, 803-814
5. Choo-Smith, L.; Edwards, H.; Endtz, H.; Kros, J.; Heule, F.; Barr, H.; Robinson Jr, J.; Bruining, H. & Puppels, G.; Medical applications of Raman spectroscopy: from proof of principle to clinical implementation; Biopolymers (Biospectroscopy), 2002, 67, 1-9
6. Ramanujam, N.; Fluorescence Spectroscopy of Neoplastic and Non-Neoplastic Tissues; Neoplasia, 2000, 2, 89-117
7. Sokolov, K.; Follen, M. & Richards-Kortum, R.; Optical spectroscopy for detection of neoplasia; Curr. Opin. Chem. Biol, 2002, 6, 651-658
8. Wagnieres, G.; Star, W. & Wilson, B.; In vivo fluorescence spectroscopy and imaging for oncological applications; Photochem. Photobiol, 1998, 68, 603-632
9. Bigio, I. & Bown, S.; Spectroscopic sensing of cancer and cancer therapy: current status of translational research.; Cancer Biol Ther, 2004, 3, 259-67
10. Hu, X. & Lu, J.; Optical Detection of Cancers; Encyclopedia of Biomeaterials and Biomedical Engineering, 2005, 1-10
11. Cotran, R.; Kumar, V. & Robbins, S.; Pathological Basis of Disease Philadelphia: WB Saunders, 1994, 231-240
12. Arifler, D.; Guillaud, M.; Carraro, A.; Malpica, A.; Follen, M. & Richards-Kortum, R.; Light scattering from normal and dysplastic cervical cells at different epithelial depths: finite-difference time-domain modeling with a perfectly matched layer boundary condition Journal of Biomedical Optics, 2003, 8, 484
13. Han, J. & Kamber, M.; Data Mining: Concepts and Techniques. Morgan Kaufmann, 2000
14. Bard, M.; Amelink, A.; Skurichina, M.; den Bakker, M.; Burgers, S.; van Meerbeeck, J.; Duin, R.; Aerts, J.; Hoogsteden, H. & Sterenborg, H.; Improving the specificity of fluorescence bronchoscopy for the analysis of neoplastic lesions of the bronchial tree by combination with optical spectroscopy: preliminary communication Lung Cancer, 2005, 47, 41-47
15. de Veld, D.; Skurichina, M.; Witjes, M.; Duin, R.; Sterenborg, H. & Roodenburg, J.; Clinical study for classification of benign, dysplastic, and malignant oral lesions using autofluorescence spectroscopy Journal of Biomedical Optics, Society of Photo-Optical Instrumentation Engineers, 2004, 9, 940-950
16. Fawzy, Y.; Petek, M.; Tercelj, M. & Zeng, H.; In vivo assessment and evaluation of lung tissue morphologic and physiological changes from non-contact endoscopic reflectance spectroscopy for improving lung cancer detection Journal of Biomedical Optics, 2006, 11, 044003
17. Ntziachristos, V.; Yodh, A.; Schnall, M. & Chance, B.; MRI-Guided Diffuse Optical Spectroscopy of Malignant and Benign Breast Lesions; Neoplasia, 2002, 4, 347-354
18. Marin, N.; MacKinnon, N.; MacAulay, C.; Chang, S.; Atkinson, E.; Cox, D.; Serachitopol, D.; Pikkula, B.; Follen, M. & Richards-Kortum, R.; Calibration standards for multicenter clinical trials of fluorescence spectroscopy for in vivo diagnosis; Journal of Biomedical Optics, 2006, 11, 014010
19. Johnson, K.; Chicken, D.; Pickard, D.; Lee, A.; Briggs, G.; Falzon, M.; Bigio, I.; Keshtgar, M. & Bown, S.; Elastic scattering spectroscopy for intraoperative

determination of sentinel lymph node status in the breast; Journal of Biomedical Optics, 2004, 9, 1122
20. Kamath, S. & Mahato, K.; Optical pathology using oral tissue fluorescence spectra: classification by principal component analysis and k-means nearest neighbor analysis; Journal of Biomedical Optics, 2007, 12, 014028
21. Bigio, I.; Bown, S.; Briggs, G.; Kelley, C.; Lakhani, S.; Pickard, D.; Ripley, P.; Rose, I. & Saunders, C.; Diagnosis of breast cancer using elastic-scattering spectroscopy: preliminary clinical results Journal of Biomedical Optics, 2000, 5, 221
22. Georgakoudi, I.; Jacobson, B.; Van Dam, J.; Backman, V.; Wallace, M.; Muller, M.; Zhang, Q.; Badizadegan, K.; Sun, D. & Thomas, G.; Fluorescence, reflectance, and light-scattering spectroscopy for evaluating dysplasia in patients with Barrett's esophagus Gastroenterology, 2001, 120, 1620-1629
23. Mirabal, Y. N.; Chang, S. K.; Atkinson, E. N.; Malpica, A.; Follen, M. & Richards-Kortum, R.; Reflectance spectroscopy for in vivo detection of cervical precancer; Journal of Biomedical Optics, 2002, 7, 587-594
24. Mourant, J.; Bigio, I.; Boyer, J.; Conn, R.; Johnson, T. & Shimada, T.; Spectroscopic diagnosis of bladder cancer with elastic light scattering. Lasers Surg Med, 1995, 17, 350-7
25. Palmer, G. & Ramanujam, N.; Monte Carlo-based inverse model for calculating tissue optical properties. Part I: Theory and validation on synthetic phantoms Applied Optics, OSA, 2006, 45, 1062-1071
26. Chandrasekhar, S.; Radiative Transfer; Courier Dover Publications, 1960
27. van de Hulst, H.; Light Scattering by Small Particles Light Scattering by Small Particles; New York: John Wiley & Sons, 1957, 1957
28. Rubinstein, R.; Simulation and the Monte Carlo Method; John Wiley & Sons, Inc. New York, NY, USA, 1981
29. Wilson, B. & Adam, G.; A Monte Carlo model for the absorption and flux distributions of light in tissue; Medical Physics, AAPM, 1983, 10, 824
30. Welch, A. & Gemert, M.; Optical-Thermal Response of Laser-Irradiated Tissue Springer, 1995
31. Pfefer, T.; Matchette, L.; Bennett, C.; Gall, J.; Wilke, J.; Durkin, A. & Ediger, M.; Reflectance-based determination of optical properties in highly attenuating tissue Journal of Biomedical Optics, 2003, 8, 206
32. Ungut, A.; Grehan, G. & Gouesbet, G.; Comparisons between geometrical optics and Lorenz-Mie theory; Applied Optics, OSA, 1981, 20, 2911-2918
33. Bohren, C. & Huffman, D.; Absorption and scattering of light by small particles Wiley New York, 1983
34. Perelman, L.; Backman, V.; Wallace, M.; Zonios, G.; Manoharan, R.; Nusrat, A.; Shields, S.; Seiler, M.; Lima, C. & Hamano, T.; Observation of Periodic Fine Structure in Reflectance from Biological Tissue: A New Technique for Measuring Nuclear Size Distribution Physical Review Letters, APS, 1998, 80, 627-630
35. Guyon, I. & Elisseeff, A.; An introduction to variable and feature selection; Journal of Machine Learning Research, MIT Press, 2003, 3, 1157-1182
36. Marín, N.; Milbourne, A.; Rhodes, H.; Ehlen, T.; Miller, D.; Benedet, L.; Richards-Kortum, R. & Follen, M.; Diffuse reflectance patterns in cervical spectroscopy; Gynecologic Oncology, Elsevier, 2005, 99, S116-S120
37. Chan, H.; Sahiner, B.; Lam, K.; Petrick, N.; Helvie, M.; Goodsitt, M. & Adler, D.; Computerized analysis of mammographic microcalcifications in morphological and texture feature spaces; Medical Physics, AAPM, 1998, 25, 2007

38. Breiman, L.; Classification and Regerssion Trees; Chapman & Hall/CRC, 1998
39. Atkinson, E.; Mitchell, M.; Ramanujam, N. & Richards-Kortum, R.; Statistical techniques for diagnosing CIN using fluorescence spectroscopy: SVD and CART; J Cell Biochem Suppl, 1995, 23, 125-30
40. Ge, Z.; Schomacker, K. & Nishioka, N.; Identification of Colonic Dysplasia and Neoplasia by Diffuse Reflectance Spectroscopy and Pattern Recognition Techniques Applied Spectroscopy, Society for Applied Spectroscopy, 1998, 52, 833-839
41. Cirovic, D.; Feed-forward artificial neural networks: applications to spectroscopy TrAC Trends in Analytical Chemistry, Elsevier Science, 1997, 16, 148-155
42. Nayak, G.; Kamath, S.; Pai, K.; Sarkar, A.; Ray, S.; Kurien, J.; D'almeida, L.; Krishnanand, B.; Santhosh, C.; Kartha, V. & Mahato, K.; Principal component analysis and artificial neural network analysis of oral tissue fluorescence spectra: Classification of normal premalignant and malignant pathological conditions Biopolymers, Wiley, 2006, 82, 152-166
43. Duda, R.; Hart, P. & Stork, D.; Pattern Classification Wiley-Interscience, 2000
44. Wolpert, D. & Macready, W.; No free lunch theorems for search; IEEE Transactions on Evolutionary Computation, 1997, 1, 67-82
45. Hanley, J. & McNeil, B.; The meaning and use of the area under a receiver operating characteristic (ROC) curve. Radiology, 1982, 143, 29-36
46. Patel, A. & Markey, M.; Comparison of three-class classification performance metrics: a case study in breast cancer CAD Proc. SPIE, 2005, 5749, 581-589
47. Hand, D. & Till, R.; A Simple Generalisation of the Area Under the ROC Curve for Multiple Class Classification Problems; Machine Learning, Springer, 2001, 45, 171-186
48. Mossman, D.; Three-way ROCs; Medical Decision Making, 1999, 19, 78
49. Edwards, D.; Metz, C. & Nishikawa, R.; Hypervolume under the ROC hypersurface of a near-guessing ideal observer in a three-class classification task; Proceedings of SPIE, 2004, 5372, 128-137
50. Mitchell, T.; Buchanan, B.; DeJong, G.; Dietterich, T.; Rosenbloom, P. & Waibel, A.; Machine Learning; Annual Review of Computer Science, Annual Reviews, 1990, 4, 417-433
51. Kohavi, R.; A study of cross-validation and bootstrap for accuracy estimation and model selection; Proceedings of the Fourteenth International Joint Conference on Artificial Intelligence, Morgan Kaufmann, 1995, 2, 1137-1145
52. Efron, B. & Gong, G.; A Leisurely Look at the Bootstrap, the Jackknife, and Cross-Validation; The American Statistician, JSTOR, 1983, 37, 36-48
53. Efron, B. & Tibshirani, R.; Statistical Data Analysis in the Computer Age; Science, AAAS, 1991, 253, 390
54. Efron, B. & Tibshirani, R.; An introduction to the bootstrap; Chapman & Hall New York, 1993
55. Bland, M.; An introduction to medical statistics; Oxford University Press New York, 2000
56. Ferlay, J.; Bray, F.; Pisani, P. & Parkin, D.; GLOBOCAN 2000: Cancer Incidence, Mortality and Prevalence Worldwide, Version 1.0; IARC CancerBase, 2001
57. Sciubba, J.; Oral cancer and its detection: History-taking and the diagnostic phase of management; The Journal of the American Dental Association, Am Dental Assoc, 2001, 132, 12-18

58. Warnakulasuriya, K. A. & Johnson, N. W.; Sensitivity and specificity of OraScan (R) toluidine blue mouthrinse in the detection of oral cancer and precancer.; Journal Of Oral Pathology & Medicine, 1996, 25, p 97-103
59. Sokolov, K.; Nieman, L.; Myakov, A. & Gillenwater, A.; Polarized reflectance spectroscopy for pre-cancer detection.; Technol Cancer Res Treat, 2004, 3, 1-14
60. Myakov, A.; Nieman, L.; Wicky, L.; Utzinger, U.; Richards-Kortum, R. & Sokolov, K.; Fiber optic probe for polarized reflectance spectroscopy in vivo: Design and performance; Journal of Biomedical Optics, 2002, 7, 388
61. Nieman, L.; Kan, C.; Gillenwater, A.; Markey, M. & Sokolov, K.; Probing the local tissue changes in the oral cavity for the early detection of cancer using oblique polarized reflectance spectroscopy: a pilot clinical trial; Journal of Biomedical Optics (under review), 2007
62. Nabney, I.; NETLAB: Algorithms for Pattern Recognitions; Springer, 2002
63. Sokolov, K.; Drezek, R.; Gossage, K. & Richards-Kortum, R.; Reflectance spectroscopy with polarized light: is it sensitive to cellular and nuclear morphology; Optics Express, OSA, 1999, 5, 302-317
64. Svistun, E.; Alizadeh-Naderi, R.; El-Naggar, A.; Jacob, R.; Gillenwater, A. & Richards-Kortum, R.; Vision enhancement system for detection of oral cavity neoplasia based on autofluorescence; Head & Neck, 2004, 26, 205-215
65. Clark, A. L.; Gillenwater, A.; Alizadeh-Naderi, R.; El-Naggar, A. K. & Richards-Kortum, R.; Detection and diagnosis of oral neoplasia with an optical coherence microscope; Journal of Biomedical Optics, 2004, 9, 1271-1280
66. Wilder-Smith, P.; Krasieva, T.; Jung, W.; Zhang, J.; Chen, Z.; Osann, K. & Tromberg, B.; Noninvasive imaging of oral premalignancy and malignancy; Journal of Biomedical Optics, 2005, 10, 051601
67. Gillenwater, A.; Jacob, R.; Ganeshappa, R.; Kemp, B.; El-Naggar, A. K.; Palmer, J. L.; Clayman, G.; Mitchell, M. F. & Richards-Kortum, R.; Noninvasive Diagnosis of Oral Neoplasia Based on Fluorescence Spectroscopy and Native Tissue Autofluorescence; Arch Otolaryngol Head Neck Surg, 1998, 124, 1251-1258

3

Decision-making Techniques in Ranking of Medicine Effectiveness

Elisabeth Rakus-Andersson

Blekinge Institute of Technology, School of Engineering, Department of Mathematics and Science, S-37179 Karlskrona, Sweden
Elisabeth.Andersson@bth.se

Summary. Theoretical fuzzy decision-making models mostly developed by Zadeh, Bellman, Jain and Yager can be adopted as useful tools to estimation of the total effectiveness-utility of a drug when appreciating its positive influence on a collection of symptoms characteristic of a considered diagnosis. The expected effectiveness of the medicine is evaluated by a physician as a verbal expression for each distinct symptom. By converting the words at first to fuzzy sets and then numbers we can regard the effectiveness structures as entries of a utility matrix that constitutes the common basic component of all methods. We involve the matrix in a number of computations due to different decision algorithms to obtain a sequence of tested medicines in conformity with their abilities to soothe the unfavorable impact of symptoms. An adjustment of the large spectrum of applied fuzzy decision-making models to the extraction of the best medicines provides us with some deviations in obtained results but we are thus capable to select this method whose effects closest converge to the physicians' judgments and expectations.

Keywords: Fuzzy decision-making, fuzzy utility matrix, utilities of medicines, powers of symptom importance, minimization of regret, OWA operators, Choquet integral, Sugeno integral.

3.1 Introduction

Theoretical fuzzy decision-making models mostly developed in [3, 8, 9, 26, 27, 29–31], give rise to successfully accomplished technical applications. However, there are not so many medical applications to decision-making proposals, especially they are lacking in the domain of pharmacy matters.

After visiting of the homepages of some pharmacological concerns, e.g., Astra-Zeneca in Sweden, we realize that the most popular mathematical methods utilized in appreciation of medicine availability in the treatment of patients are statistical tests. In the group of statistical methods adaptable

E. Rakus-Andersson: *Decision-making Techniques in Ranking of Medicine Effectiveness*, Studies in Computational Intelligence (SCI) **107**, 51–73 (2008)
www.springerlink.com

to approximation of drug effectiveness we can recognize descriptive statistics, regression and analysis of variance, a general linear model (GLM) approach, hypothesis tests, continuous statistical distributions including uniform, normal, exponential, chi-squared, student-t, F-ratio, and Weibull distributions, discrete distributions including uniform, binomial, geometric, hypergeometric, Poisson and user-defined distributions, high-quality random number generators, including the Mersenne Twister, classes for working with one-dimensional histograms, Bayes rules, e.g., in [16], Monte-Carlo methods and many others. Statistical tests are very helpful in grading of the curative power of medicines; nevertheless they cannot effectively handle either interactions among medicines or imprecise estimations of the medicine influence on a collection of symptoms that should retreat after the treatment.

Fuzzy set theory, giving the possibility of computing with words [33–36] and solving of systems accommodated to imprecise or vague data, provides us with a mathematical apparatus bringing answers to different posed questions regarding pharmacology. We can list such tools as the adaptation of fuzzy control in medicine models [11], the recognition prime-decision model (RPD) in appreciation of drugs [10] or the process of medicine extraction by the method of midpoints [15]. Other solutions used to estimation of medicine powers and worth mentioning are: classification of medicines by fuzzy matrices [5], rough sets in evaluation of medicines [4] and the use of neuro-fuzzy structures contra rough sets in the possible evaluation of drugs [6].

Anyway, if we formulate the task to solve as determination of a hierarchical ladder in a sample of medicines that affect the same symptoms typical of a considered diagnosis with respect to the choice of the most efficacious medicine then we cannot find any positions in literature except own previously made attempts [17–23]. We thus intend to sum up all results in a survey of fuzzy decision-making models adapted to the selection of the most effective medicine when comparing it to others in the process of the patients' recoveries.

We emphasize that all models discussed below are unique and genuine trials of stating the medicine ranking and therefore we cannot compare the obtained results to other achievements. This comparison will be made for own performances in concluding remarks.

To start with the discussion concerning the choice of drugs we sketch the components of fuzzy decision-making model to introduce the first algorithm designed by Jain [8, 9] in Section 3.2. In section 3.3 we propose algorithms based on max- and min-operators enriched by insertion of weights-powers [3, 27, 30] to extract the best medicine. Finally we perform the aggregation- [12] and OWA-operations [28, 32] to benefit the concepts of Choquet and Sugeno integrals [7, 13, 14, 25] to the same purpose of determining the power of medicines when regarding their influence on clinical symptoms.

3.2 The Jain Decision Algorithm in the Ranking of Medicines

We intend to discuss and compare the functions of different theoretical decision-making models selected as the most appropriate tools adapted to an extraction of the best medicine from a collection of tested drugs with curative effects in a considered diagnosis. Let us first prepare basic notions commonly used in each decision method.

3.2.1 The General Outline of a Drug Decision-Making Model

We introduce the notions of a space of states $X = \{x_1, \ldots, x_m\}$ and a decision space (a space of alternatives) $A = \{a_1, \ldots, a_n\}$. We consider a decision model in which n alternatives $a_1, \ldots, a_n \in A$ act as drugs used to treat patients who suffer from a disease. The medicines should influence m states $x_1, \ldots, x_m \in X$, which are identified with m symptoms typical of the morbid unit considered [17–23].

If a rational decision maker comes to a decision $a_i \in A, i = 1, 2, \ldots, n$, concerning states-results $x_j \in X, j = 1, 2, \ldots, m$, then the decision problem is reduced to the consideration of the ordered triplet (X, A, U), where X is a set of states-results, A – a set of decisions and U – the utility matrix [8, 9, 17–23, 26, 27, 29–31]

$$U = \begin{array}{c} \\ a_1 \\ a_2 \\ \vdots \\ a_n \end{array} \begin{array}{c} \begin{array}{cccc} x_1 & x_2 & \cdots & x_m \end{array} \\ \begin{bmatrix} u_{11} & u_{12} & \cdots & u_{1m} \\ u_{21} & u_{22} & \cdots & u_{2m} \\ \vdots & & \ddots & \vdots \\ u_{n1} & u_{n2} & \cdots & u_{nm} \end{bmatrix} \end{array}, \tag{3.1}$$

in which each element u_{ij}, $i = 1, 2, \ldots, n, j = 1, 2, \ldots, m$, is a representative value belonging to [0, 1] for the fuzzy utility following from the decision a_i with the result x_j.

The theoretical model with the triplet (X, A, U) can find its practical application in the processes of choosing an optimal drug from a sample of tested medicines [17–23].

3.2.2 The Adaptation of Jain's Decision Model to *Drug* – *Symptom* Dependency

Assume now that the state-result is not known exactly and thus proposed to be a fuzzy set $S \subseteq X$ given in the form [8, 9]

$$S = \sum_{j=1}^{m} \mu_S(x_j) \Big/ x_j. \tag{3.2}$$

To solve the decision problem under circumstances introduced above means to find the best decision a_i influenced by all constraints.

The theoretical model with the triplet (X, A, U) and the fuzzy set of states S, thus very shortly sketched, can find its practical application in the processes of choosing an optimal drug. If the diagnosis is recognized by the symptoms accompanying it, then we, by giving a medicine, try to liquidate these symptoms or at least we try to reduce their unfavorable influence upon the patient's health. Not all symptoms retreat after the cure has been carried out. One sometimes can only soothe their negative effects by, for example, the lowering of an excessive level of the indicator, the relief of pain, and the like, but cannot ascertain that the patient is fully free from them. The task of choosing an optimal drug (decision), which soothes the symptoms or has some power to remove them in full, corresponds to the theoretical assumptions presented above.

In order to show the algorithm for finding such a decision let us consider a model with n drugs $a_1, a_2, \ldots, a_n \in A$. Due to the physician's decision, the drugs can be prescribed to the patient (thus may be treated as decisions $a_1, a_2, \ldots, a_n$) with a view to have an effect on m symptoms $x_1, x_2, \ldots, x_m \in X$ representing certain states characteristic of the diagnosis considered. To simplify the symbols let us further assume that each symptom $x_j \in X$, where X is a space of symptoms (states), is understood as the result of the treatment of the symptom after the cure with the drugs $a_1, a_2, \ldots, a_n$ has been carried out.

The relationship between a medicine and a symptom is determined in the term of utility. Let us discuss the formalized technique of stating the representatives of utilities without using intuitive or perceptional estimations.

On the basis of earlier experiments the physician knows how to define in words the curative drug efficiency in the case of considered symptoms. We intend to replace his verbal judgments by numerical expressions to be able to insert them in the mathematical model [1, 2, 33, 34, 36]. In accordance with the physician's advice we suggest a list of terms, which introduces a linguistic variable [33, 35] named "the curative drug effectiveness regarding a symptom" = $\{R_1 =$ "*none*", $R_2 =$ "*almost none*", $R_3 =$ "*very little*", $R_4 =$ "*little*", $R_5 =$ "*rather little*", $R_6 =$ "*medium*", $R_7 =$ "*rather large*", $R_8 =$ "*large*", $R_9 =$ "*very large*", $R_{10} =$ "*almost complete*", $R_{11} =$ "*complete*"$\}$.

Each notion from this list of terms is the name of a fuzzy set. Assume that all sets are defined in the space $Z = [0, 100]$ that is suitable as a reference set to measure a number of patients who have been affected by a medicine in the grade corresponding to each name.

We propose constrains for the fuzzy sets $R_1 - R_{11}$ by applying linear functions [21–23]

$$L(z, \alpha, \beta) = \begin{cases} 0 & \text{for} \quad z \le \alpha \\ \dfrac{z - \alpha}{\beta - \alpha} & \text{for} \quad \alpha < z \le \beta \\ 1 & \text{for} \quad z > \beta \end{cases} \tag{3.3}$$

and

$$\pi(z,\alpha,\gamma,\beta) = \begin{cases} 0 & \text{for} \quad z \le \alpha \\ L(z,\alpha,\gamma) & \text{for} \quad \alpha < z \le \gamma \\ 1 - L(z,\gamma,\beta) & \text{for} \quad \gamma < z \le \beta \\ 0 & \text{for} \quad z > \beta \end{cases} \tag{3.4}$$

where z is an independent variable from $[0,\ 100]$, whereas α, β, γ are parameters.

Let us now define

$$\mu_{R_t}(z) = \begin{cases} 1 - L(z,\alpha_t,\beta_t) & \text{for} \quad t = 1,2,3,4,5 \\ L(z,\alpha_t,\beta_t) & \text{for} \quad t = 7,8,9,10,11 \end{cases} \tag{3.5}$$

and

$$\mu_{R_6}(z) = \pi(z,\alpha_6,\gamma,\beta_6) \tag{3.6}$$

in which α_t, β_t, γ are the borders for supports of the fuzzy sets $R_1 - R_{11}$.

We decide the values of the boundary parameters α_t, β_t, γ in Ex. 1 below.

Example 1

Figure 3.1 collects the graphs of restrictions made for fuzzy sets $R_1 - R_{11}$ that are approved as the terms composing the contents of the effectiveness list.

To each effectiveness, expanded as a continuous fuzzy set, we would like to assign only one value.

Example 2

To find the adequate $z \in [0, 100]$ representing the effectiveness terms $R_1 - R_{11}$ we adopt as z the values α_t for $t = 1,2,3,4,5$, and β_t for $t = 7,8,9,10,11$ in compliance with (3.5), respectively γ due to (3.6). We simply read off

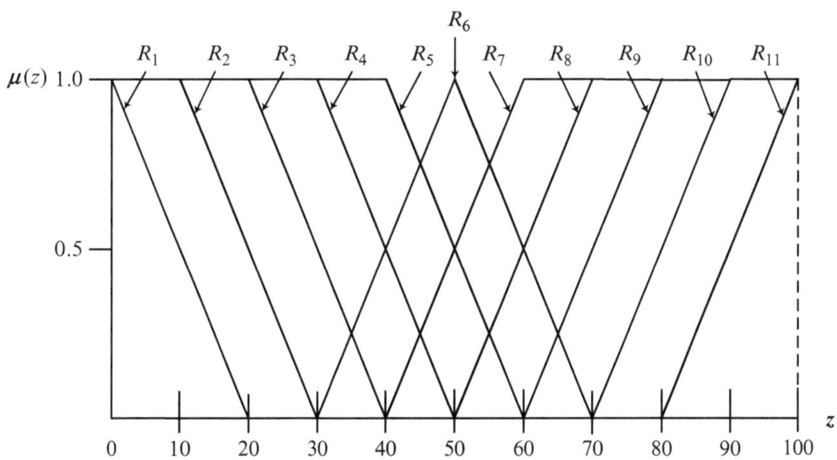

Fig. 3.1. The fuzzy sets $R_1 - R_{11}$

Table 3.1. The numerical representatives of verbal effectiveness

Effectiveness	Representing z-value for effectiveness	$\mu_{effectiveness}(z) = u_{ij}$
none	0	0
almost none	10	0.1
very little	20	0.2
little	30	0.3
rather little	40	0.4
medium	50	0.5
rather large	60	0.6
large	70	0.7
very large	80	0.8
almost complete	90	0.9
complete	100	1

the values of α_t, β_t and γ from Fig. 3.1 in order not to introduce evident calculations. These z-values are elements of the support of a new fuzzy set "$effectiveness$" whose membership function is expressed over the interval [0, 100] by $\mu_{\text{“}effectiveness\text{”}}(z) = L(z, 0, 100)$. For the z-representatives of $R_1 - R_{11}$ we finally compute membership values $\mu_{\text{“}effectiveness\text{”}}(z)$, which replace the terms of effectiveness-utility as quantities u_{ij}. We summarize the obtained results in Table 3.1.

To state a connection between a_i (medicine) and the effectiveness of the retreat of x_j (symptom) the physician uses the word from the list "the curative drug effectiveness regarding a symptom" and this word is "translated" into the quantity u_{ij}, $i = 1, \ldots, n, j = 1, \ldots, m$.

Let us also admit that the physician possesses a general experience as to the "difficulties" in the retreat of the symptoms x_j, $j = 1, 2, \ldots, m$. His medical knowledge, based on observations, can contribute in a classification of symptoms that are harder to treat and symptoms that recede readily during the treatment process. Via the words from the list "the curative drug effectiveness regarding a symptom" one may assign to each symptom a general ability to retreat, fixed, for instance, by observing the cure of many patients with different drugs. For instance, it is commonly known that a fever disappears quicker than some changes in tissues after inflammation. Such a general classification of symptoms found its place in the fuzzy set S [17–19] defined theoretically by (3.2) [8,9], in which the membership degrees $\mu_S(x_j), j = 1, 2, \ldots, m$, correspond now to utilities u_{ij}. These express the mean effectiveness of treatment independently of a prescribed medicine. By the "cure" one can mean the level of the retreating symptom, the decrease of the heightened index, and the like.

In accord with Jain's theory of decision-making, the fuzzy utility [8,9] for each decision-drug $a_i, i = 1, 2, \ldots, n$, with the fuzzy state $S \subseteq X$ characterized by means of the membership degrees $\mu_S(x_j)$ is defined to be a set

$$U_i = \sum_{j=1}^{m} \mu_S(x_j) \Big/ u_{ij} \tag{3.7}$$

for $i = 1, 2, \ldots, n$. The set allows observing of the relationship between the general ability to soothe and this effect in soothing which the drug a_i causes for each symptom x_j. Both the membership degrees $\mu_S(x_j)$ and the elements u_{ij} in the support of the set U_i are the utility values u_{ij} found in the last column of Table 3.1.

3.2.3 The Solution of Jain's Decision Case

The problem of choosing of an optimal decision is solved according to the algorithm developed by Jain [8, 9]. The steps of the action line are listed in the following order.

Algorithm 1

1. We form a non-fuzzy set Y as the union of supports characteristic of U_i, $i = 1, 2, \ldots, n$. This set contains the utilities u_{ij}, which appear in the supports of all sets U_i. Hence, we have access to the range of the common utility expressed as $Y = \bigcup_{i=1}^{n} \mathrm{supp}(U_i)$.
2. We select the maximal element of the set Y, so-called $u_{\max}$.
3. We define the fuzzy sets U_i' as

$$U_i' = \sum_{j=1}^{m} \mu_{U_i'}(u_{ij}) \Big/ u_{ij} \tag{3.8}$$

   for $u_{ij} \in \mathrm{supp}(U_i)$. This means that the supports of U_i' and U_i are the same sets. The membership degrees of U_i' are computed by means of the formula

$$\mu_{U_i'}(u_{ij}) = \frac{u_{ij}}{u_{\max}}, \tag{3.9}$$

   where u_{ij} stands for an element belonging to the support of the set U_i. U_i''s membership degrees evaluate the "deviation" between the support elements of U_i and u_{max} found in the union of all U_i.
4. The next introduced fuzzy set has the form of

$$U_{i0} = \sum_{j=1}^{m} \mu_{U_{i0}}(u_{ij}) \Big/ u_{ij}, \tag{3.10}$$

   provided that the membership degree $\mu_{U_{i0}}(u_{ij})$ is calculated according to the rule

$$\mu_{U_{i0}}(u_{ij}) = \text{mean value}(\mu_{U_i}(u_{ij}), \mu_{U_i'}(u_{ij})). \tag{3.11}$$

   The fuzzy utility U_{i0}, constructed for each medicine a_i, gathers all possible factors that can affect appreciation of the soothing power of a_i.

5. We slowly close the action of Algorithm 1 by the adoption of a new fuzzy set A^* composed of elements $a_1, a_2, \ldots, a_n (a_i \in A, i = 1, 2, \ldots, n)$ and formalized by

$$A^* = \sum_{i=1}^{n} \mu_{A^*}(a_i) \Big/ a_i. \tag{3.12}$$

The membership degree for each a_i is generated by

$$\mu_{A^*}(a_i) = \underset{u_{ij} \in \text{supp}(U_{i0})}{\text{mean value}} (\mu_{U_{i0}}(u_{ij})). \tag{3.13}$$

In practice we compute the arithmetic mean for a sample of membership degrees appearing in each set U_{i0}. This value expresses the decisive character of every a_i in accordance with a rule: the higher value of the membership degree assigned to a_i is found, the better influence of a_i on the patient's health will be expected.
6. To terminate the choice of an optimal decision a^* we accept as a^* this a_i whose membership degree satisfies the equation

$$\mu_{A^*}(a^*) = \max_{1 \leq i \leq n} (\mu_{A^*}(a_i)), \tag{3.14}$$

and we ascertain that the application of the drug a^* should yield the best effects in the retreating process of the symptoms x_j, $j = 1, 2, \ldots, m$.

Example 3

The Jain model is tested on the clinical data coming from the investigation carried out among patients who suffer from D_1 = "*coronary heart disease*" [23]. We consider the most typical symptoms accompanying the illness, i.e., x_1 = "*pain in chest*", x_2 = "*changes in ECG*" and x_3 = "*increased level of LDL-cholesterol*". A physician has recommended a_1 = *nitroglycerin*, a_2 = *beta-adrenergic blockade*, a_3 = *acetylsalicylic acid* (*aspirin*) and a_4 = *statine LDL-reductor* as the medicines expected to improve the patient's state. The physician has also decided that the set S and the matrix U should have the following descriptions

$$S = large/x_1 + medium/x_2 + rather\ large/x_3$$

and

$$U = \begin{array}{c} \\ a_1 \\ a_2 \\ a_3 \\ a_4 \end{array} \begin{array}{c} \begin{array}{lll} \quad x_1 & \quad\quad x_2 & \quad\quad x_3 \end{array} \\ \begin{bmatrix} almost\ complete & very\ large & almost\ none \\ medium & medium & little \\ little & little & very\ little \\ little & little & very\ large \end{bmatrix} \end{array}.$$

We begin the computations with determining of the sets U_i, $i = 1, 2, 3, 4$, as

$$\begin{aligned} U_1 &= {}^{large}\!/_{almost\ complete} + {}^{medium}\!/_{very\ large} + {}^{rather\ large}\!/_{almost\ none} \\ &= {}^{0.7}\!/_{0.9} + {}^{0.5}\!/_{0.8} + {}^{0.6}\!/_{0.1}, \\ U_2 &= {}^{0.7}\!/_{0.5} + {}^{0.5}\!/_{0.5} + {}^{0.6}\!/_{0.3}, \\ U_3 &= {}^{0.7}\!/_{0.3} + {}^{0.5}\!/_{0.3} + {}^{0.6}\!/_{0.2} \end{aligned}$$

and

$$U_4 = {}^{0.7}\!/_{0.3} + {}^{0.5}\!/_{0.3} + {}^{0.6}\!/_{0.8}$$

due to Eq. (3.7).

The non-fuzzy sum of all supports emerges as a set

$$\bigcup_{i=1}^{4} \text{supp}(U_i) = \{0.1, 0.2, 0.3, 0.5, 0.8, 0.9\}$$

in which the largest element is found as $u_{\max} = 0.9$.

Equations (3.8) and (3.9) give rise to creation of new sets U_i', $i = 1, 2, 3, 4$. U_1' – the first set in the sequence – appears as the following fuzzy collection of elements

$$U_1' = {}^{\frac{0.9}{0.9}}\!/_{0.9} + {}^{\frac{0.8}{0.9}}\!/_{0.8} + {}^{\frac{0.1}{0.9}}\!/_{0.1} = {}^{1}\!/_{0.9} + {}^{0.89}\!/_{0.8} + {}^{0.11}\!/_{0.1}.$$

The other sets of U_1''s type, $i = 2, 3, 4$, are expanded as

$$\begin{aligned} U_2' &= {}^{0.56}\!/_{0.5} + {}^{0.56}\!/_{0.5} + {}^{0.33}\!/_{0.3}, \\ U_3' &= {}^{0.33}\!/_{0.3} + {}^{0.33}\!/_{0.3} + {}^{0.22}\!/_{0.2} \end{aligned}$$

and

$$U_4' = {}^{0.33}\!/_{0.3} + {}^{0.33}\!/_{0.3} + {}^{0.89}\!/_{0.8}.$$

We follow the next step of Algorithm 1 in conformity with (3.10) and (3.11) to arrange the sets U_{i0}, $i = 1, 2, 3, 4$ as

$$\begin{aligned} U_{10} &= {}^{\text{mean value}(0.7,1)}\!/_{0.9} + {}^{\text{mean value}(0.5,0.89)}\!/_{0.8} + {}^{\text{mean value}(0.6,0.11)}\!/_{0.1} \\ &= {}^{0.85}\!/_{0.9} + {}^{0.695}\!/_{0.8} + {}^{0.355}\!/_{0.1}, \\ U_{20} &= {}^{0.63}\!/_{0.5} + {}^{0.53}\!/_{0.5} + {}^{0.465}\!/_{0.3}, \\ U_{30} &= {}^{0.515}\!/_{0.3} + {}^{0.415}\!/_{0.3} + {}^{0.41}\!/_{0.2} \end{aligned}$$

and

$$U_{40} = {}^{0.515}\!/_{0.3} + {}^{0.415}\!/_{0.3} + {}^{0.745}\!/_{0.8}.$$

The decision set A^* has been decided as

$$A^* = {}^{0.633}\!/_{a_1} + {}^{0.542}\!/_{a_2} + {}^{0.447}\!/_{a_3} + {}^{0.558}\!/_{a_4}.$$

The magnitudes of the membership degrees give us a hint about priorities of drugs, i.e., a_1 should have the strongest soothing power when regarding the considered symptoms, and it should be accepted as the optimal decision-drug. Moreover, we can state the hierarchy of drugs in the order: $a_1 \succ a_4 \succ a_2 \succ a_3$. The notion $a_i \succ a_l$ indicates that a_i acts better than $a_l, i, l = 1, 2, 3, 4$.

3.3 Unequal States-results in the Choice of Medicines

The purpose of this section is to present other ideas made in the solution of fuzzy decision-making model that still should provide us with the extraction of the most efficacious medicine provided that the particular emphasis is impacted on assigning differing degrees of importance to states-symptoms [21, 27].

3.3.1 The Design of the Bellman-Zadeh Decision Model

We still consider a decision model in which n drugs $a_1, \ldots, a_n \in A$ act as decisions. These affect m symptoms $x_1, \ldots, x_m \in X$ that are typical of a morbid unit under consideration. The utility following each a_i, when treating x_j with it, is a value of u_{ij} constituting the entry of the utility matrix U, $i = 1, \ldots, n, j = 1, \ldots, m$. In conformity with the Bellman-Zadeh and Yager suggestions [3, 26, 27, 29] referring to fuzzy decision-making we form the decision set A^* with the support consisting of drugs $a_1, \ldots, a_n$ as

$$A^* = \sum_{i=1}^{n} \mu_{A^*}(a_i) \Big/ a_i, \tag{3.15}$$

in which the membership degree of each a_i is shaped by an operation

$$\mu_{A^*}(a_i) = \min_{1 \le j \le m} (u_{ij}). \tag{3.16}$$

The best medicine a^* is extracted from the collection A as this a_i for which the membership degree in set A^* is largest (see Eq. (3.14)).

Example 4

We return to the clinical data from Ex. 3 and utilities from the last column of Table 3.1. By adopting singular utilities stated for pairs of associated medicines and symptoms we determine the utility matrix U in the form of

$$U = \begin{array}{c} \\ a_1 \\ a_2 \\ a_3 \\ a_4 \end{array} \begin{array}{c} \begin{array}{ccc} x_1 & x_2 & x_3 \end{array} \\ \begin{bmatrix} 0.9 & 0.8 & 0.1 \\ 0.5 & 0.5 & 0.3 \\ 0.3 & 0.3 & 0.2 \\ 0.3 & 0.3 & 0.8 \end{bmatrix} \end{array}$$

The decision set A^* is stated as

$$A^* = {}^{\min(0.9,0.8,0.1)}/_{a_1} + {}^{\min(0.5,0.5,0.3)}/_{a_2} + {}^{\min(0.3,0.3,0.2)}/_{a_3} + {}^{\min(0.3,0.3,0.8)}/_{a_4}$$
$$= {}^{0.1}/_{a_1} + {}^{0.3}/_{a_2} + {}^{0.2}/_{a_3} + {}^{0.3}/_{a_4}$$

After comparing of the membership degrees of drugs in the decision set A^* we conclude that a_i, $i = 1, \ldots, 4$, are arranged in the sequence $a_2 = a_4 \succ a_3 \succ a_1$.

3.3.2 The Power-Importance of Symptom-States

The last decision seems to be very poor, cautious and contradicts the former decision obtained in Subsection 3.2.3 because of the unfavorable affection of the minimum operator when deciding the degrees of a_i. The use of minimum deprives many data values of their decisive power. We intend to improve the obtained results due to the Bellman-Zadeh decision model by attaching the importance values to the symptoms-states considered.

Let us associate with each symptom x_j, $j = 1, \ldots, m$, a non negative number, which indicates its power or importance in the decision according to the rule: the higher the number is, the more important role of the x_j's retreat will be regarded. We assign $w_1, \ldots, w_m$ as powers-weights to $x_1, \ldots, x_m$ to modify (3.15) as a richer and more extended decision

$$A^*{}_{weighted} = \mu_{A^*_{weighted}}(a_i) \Big/ a_i \tag{3.17}$$

in which the membership degree of each $a_i \in A^*{}_{weighted}$ is computed as [27]

$$\mu_{A^*_{weighted}}(a_i) = \min_{1 \le j \le m} ({u_{ij}}^{w_j}) \tag{3.18}$$

We note that each a_i always takes the value of a membership degree from [0, 1]. If w_j gets bigger then ${u_{ij}}^{w_j}$, $j = 1, \ldots, m$, $i = 1, \ldots, n$, will get smaller, closer to zero. On the contrary, $w_j \to 0$ implies ${u_{ij}}^{w_j} \to 1$. The behaviour of minimum warrants that the minimal value in the sequence of quantities belonging to [0, 1] must be a value coming from the same interval. This time the application of the minimum operator is better motivated as before since we neglect large values of ${u_{ij}}^{w_j}$ corresponding to less important symptoms.

A procedure for obtaining a ratio scale of importance for a group of m elements (symptoms) was developed by Saaty [24].

Assume that we have m objects (symptoms) and we want to construct a scale, rating these objects as to their importance with respect to the decision. We ask a decision-maker to compare the objects in paired comparison. If we compare object j with object k, then we will assign the values b_{jk} and b_{kj} as follows

(1) $b_{kj} = \frac{1}{b_{jk}}$.

(2) If objective j is more important than objective k then b_{jk} gets assigned a number according to the following scheme:

Intensity of importance expressed by the value of b_{jk}	*Definition*
1	Equal importance of x_j and x_k
3	Weak importance of x_j over x_k
5	Strong importance of x_j over x_k
7	Demonstrated importance of x_j over x_k
9	Absolute importance of x_j over x_k
2, 4, 6, 8	Intermediate values

If object k is more important than object j, we assign the value of b_{kj}.

Having obtained the above judgments a $m \times m$ importance matrix $B = (b_{jk})_{j,k=1}^{m}$ is constructed in the drug decision problem sketched above. Matrix B constitutes a crucial part in the procedure of determining of the degrees of importance $w_1, \ldots, w_m$, which affect the decision set $A^*{}_{weighted}$ in the substantial way. The weights are decided as components of this eigen vector that corresponds to the largest in magnitude eigen value of the matrix B.

Example 5

By involving the computation technique suggested in the description of matrix B we try to find the weights for objects x_j, $j = 1, 2, 3$, already introduced in Ex. 3 and Ex. 4.

The physical status of a patient is subjectively better if the pain disappears, which means that at first a physician tries to release the patient from symptom x_1 = "*pain in chest*". The next priority is assigned to x_2 = "*changes in ECG*" and finally, we concentrate our attention on getting rid of x_3 = "*increased level of LDL-cholesterol*". The last symptom does not disappear very quickly and the patient must be cured for some time to be free from it [21–23].

These remarks are helpful when constructing a content of the matrix B as

$$B = \begin{matrix} \\ x_1 \\ x_2 \\ x_3 \end{matrix} \begin{matrix} \begin{matrix} x_1 & x_2 & x_3 \end{matrix} \\ \begin{bmatrix} 1 & 3 & 5 \\ \frac{1}{3} & 1 & 3 \\ \frac{1}{5} & \frac{1}{3} & 1 \end{bmatrix} \end{matrix}$$

The largest eigen value of B has the associated eigen vector $V = (0.93295, 0.30787, 0.18659) \approx (0.93, 0.31, 0.19)$. V is composed of coordinates that are interpreted as the weights w_1, w_2, w_3 sought for x_1, x_2, x_3.

Due to the recommended Eqs. (3.17) and (3.18) the final decision $A^*{}_{weighted}$ is obtained as a fuzzy set

$$
\begin{aligned}
D &= {}^{\min(0.9^{0.93},0.8^{0.31},0.1^{0.19})}\!/_{a_1} + {}^{\min(0.5^{0.93},0.5^{0.31},0.3^{0.19})}\!/_{a_2} \\
&\quad + {}^{\min(0.3^{0.93},0.3^{0.31},0.2^{0.19})}\!/_{a_3} + {}^{\min(0.3^{0.93},0.3^{0.31},0.8^{0.19})}\!/_{a_4} \\
&= {}^{\min(0.906,0.92,0.645)}\!/_{a_1} + {}^{\min(0.525,0.806,0.795)}\!/_{a_2} \\
&\quad + {}^{\min(0.326,0.688,0.736)}\!/_{a_3} + {}^{\min(0.326,0.688,0.958)}\!/_{a_4} \\
&= {}^{0.645}\!/_{a_1} + {}^{0.525}\!/_{a_2} + {}^{0.326}\!/_{a_3} + {}^{0.326}\!/_{a_4}.
\end{aligned}
$$

We conclude that the soothing effect of considered medicines is ranked in the order $a_1 \succ a_2 \succ a_3 = a_4$. This time we have considered effectiveness of drugs by regarding of their action on symptoms and we have paid attention to the priority of symptoms as well. The importance order among the symptoms points out the ones that should disappear first for the reason of their harmful influence on the patient's psychical and physical condition.

3.3.3 Minimization of Regret

The action of the minimum operation in the final decision formulas has provided us with a very cautious prognosis referring to the drug hierarchy. Some high values of utilities, emphasizing a positive effect of medicine on considered symptoms, have no chance of influencing finally computed decision degrees. We can even say that the minimum operation acts as a filter for high values by depriving them of their power.

In the next trial of evaluation of the medicine hierarchy ladder we want to obtain clearer results when applying another fuzzy decision-making technique known as a minimization of regret [30]. We preserve a decision space (a space of medicines) $A = \{a_1, \dots, a_n\}$ and a space of states-symptoms $X = \{x_1, x_2, \dots, x_m\}$. We form a basic payoff matrix (the old U-utility matrix)

$$
C = \begin{array}{c} \\ a_1 \\ \vdots \\ a_i \\ \vdots \\ a_n \end{array}
\begin{array}{c} x_1 \; \dots \; x_j \; \dots \; x_m \\ \left[\begin{array}{ccc} & & \\ & & \\ & c_{ij} & \\ & & \\ & & \end{array} \right] \end{array}, \tag{3.19}
$$

where $c_{ij} = u_{ij}$ is the payoff (utility) to a decision-maker if he connects a_i to x_j, $i = 1, \dots, n, j = 1, \dots, m$.

In a continuation of the proposed approach to the choice of an optimal medicine we first obtain a regret matrix R. Its components r_{ij} indicate the decision-maker's regret in selecting alternative a_i when the state of X is x_j. We then calculate the maximal regret for each alternative.

A procedure of selecting an optimal a_i should follow some steps listed below due to Algorithm 2.

Algorithm 2

1. For each x_j calculate $C_j = \max_{1 \le i \le n} c_{ij}$.
2. For each pair a_i and x_j calculate $r_{ij} = C_j - c_{ij}$.
3. Suppose that matrix B from Subsection 3.3.2 consists of b_{jk}, which still describe the importance scale when comparing states-symptoms x_j and x_k, j, $k = 1, \ldots, m$. The coordinates of this eigen vector that assists the largest in magnitude eigen value of B thus constitute weights $w_1, \ldots, w_m$ assigned to symptoms $x_1, \ldots, x_m$ stated in X. The weights are involved in the computations of estimates $RT_i = w_1 r_{i1} + \cdots + w_m r_{i,m}$ for each a_i. It can be proved that the formulas derived for calculations of RT_i satisfy the conditions of OWA operators [12, 28, 32].
4. Select a^*, such that $RT_{i^*} = \min_{1 \le i \le n} RT_i$.

The values r_{ij} constitute the entries of the matrix R called the regret matrix. We shall refer to C_j as the horizon under x_j.

Example 6

The matrix C remains equal to the matrix U from Ex. 4. We remind of its existence as the table

$$C = \begin{array}{c} \\ a_1 \\ a_2 \\ a_3 \\ a_4 \end{array} \begin{array}{c} \begin{array}{ccc} x_1 & x_2 & x_3 \end{array} \\ \begin{bmatrix} 0.9^* & 0.8^* & 0.1 \\ 0.5 & 0.5 & 0.3 \\ 0.3 & 0.3 & 0.2 \\ 0.3 & 0.3 & 0.8^* \end{bmatrix} \end{array}$$

in which "*" points to the largest element in each column due to Step 1.

The regret matrix R is computed as the next table

$$R = \begin{array}{c} \\ a_1 \\ a_2 \\ a_3 \\ a_4 \end{array} \begin{array}{c} \begin{array}{ccc} x_1 & x_2 & x_3 \end{array} \\ \begin{bmatrix} 0 & 0 & 0.7 \\ 0.4 & 0.3 & 0.5 \\ 0.6 & 0.5 & 0.6 \\ 0.6 & 0.5 & 0 \end{bmatrix} \end{array}.$$

For $w_1 \approx 0.93$, $w_2 \approx 0.31$ and $w_3 \approx 0.19$ (Ex. 5) the values of $RT_i, i = 1, \ldots, 4$, are appreciated as

$$RT_1 = 0.93 \cdot 0 + 0.31 \cdot 0 + 0.19 \cdot 0.7 = 0.133,$$
$$RT_2 = 0.56, \ RT_3 = 0.827, \ RT_4 = 0.713.$$

Finally, due to Step 4 of Algorithm 2 we decide the order of drugs with respect to their curative abilities. We state them in sequence $a_1 \succ a_2 \succ a_4 \succ a_3$, which almost confirms the results obtained by the technique of unequal objectives and the Jain algorithm. Moreover, we notice that the last decision is very clearly interpretable and easy to understand without doubts. This emphasizes an advantage of applying of the OWA weighted operations, which prevent a loss of substantial information. The OWA operations have resulted in the simultaneous engagement of all effectiveness quantities in mean decision-making values involved in the regret model.

3.4 The Drug Hierarchy Made by Mean Operators and Integrals

In the minimization of regret algorithm we have tested the OWA operators as sorts of mean estimates of regret involving each data value. The obtained result seems to be a clear-cut decision that takes into consideration all distinct decisive factors, i.e., the utilities of medicines and powers of symptoms. In this section we intend to expand the techniques of computing of mean values as aggregated utilities of the drug series and even we want to extend the calculations on the concepts of the Choquet and Sugeno integrals [22].

3.4.1 The Utilities of Medicines as Weighted Mean Quantities

Like in Subsections 3.3.2 and 3.3.3, we associate with each state-symptom x_j, $j=1,\ldots,m$, a non negative number that indicates its power or importance in decision making in accordance with the rule: the higher the number is, the greater significance of symptom x_j will be expected, when considering its harmful impact on the patient's condition. If we design $W = \{w_1, w_2, \ldots, w_m\}$ and we assign $w_1, w_2, \ldots, w_m$ as powers-weights to $x_1, x_2, \ldots, x_m, w_j \in W, j = 1, 2, \ldots, m$, where W is a space of weights, then we will modify (3.1) as the weighted matrix [22]

$$U_W = \begin{array}{c} \\ a_1 \\ a_2 \\ \vdots \\ a_n \end{array} \begin{array}{c} \begin{array}{cccc} x_1 & x_2 & \cdots & x_m \end{array} \\ \begin{bmatrix} w_1 \cdot u_{11} & w_2 \cdot u_{12} & \cdots & w_m \cdot u_{1m} \\ w_1 \cdot u_{21} & w_2 \cdot u_{22} & \cdots & w_m \cdot u_{2m} \\ \vdots & & \ddots & \vdots \\ w_1 \cdot u_{n1} & w_2 \cdot u_{n2} & \cdots & w_m \cdot u_{nm} \end{bmatrix} \end{array} \tag{3.20}$$

In compliance with data entries determined in (3.20), the common curative power of a_i is approximated by the quantity $U_W(a_i)$ defined as an OWA operation [28, 32]

$$U_W(a_i) = \sum_{j=1}^{m} w_j \cdot u_{ij}. \tag{3.21}$$

As a final optimal decision a^* we select this a_i that satisfies

$$U_W(a^*) = \max_{1 \leq i \leq n} U_W(a_i), \tag{3.22}$$

i.e., we pick out the decision-drug possessing the highest utility grade with respect to symptoms cured. The distinct utility u_{ij} is comprehended to be the ability of the symptom retreat after medication. In other words, we keep on defining of utility u_{ij} of a_i taken to x_j as effectiveness of drug a_i observed in the case of x_j.

To determine effectiveness-utility of drugs as mathematical expressions taking places in the matrix U_W we recall the investigations accomplished in Subsection 3.2.2 that terminated with results stated in the last column of Table 3.1 as numerical substitutes of verbal expressions.

The weights-powers $w_1, w_2, \ldots, w_m \in W$ corresponding to the symptom importance are still estimated as components of the eigen vector associated with the largest in magnitude eigen value of the matrix B (see Subsection 3.3.2). We normalize the weights w_j by dividing them all by the largest weight $w_{largest}$. We suggest this simple operation to keep all w_j within interval [0, 1] that constitutes a new range of W.

Let us denote the normalized weights by $\hat{w}_j = \frac{w_j}{w_{largest}}$ [22]. Afterwards we reorder $\hat{w}_1, \hat{w}_2, \ldots, \hat{w}_m$ to generate an arrangement of the normalized weights as the ascending sequence $\hat{w}_1^a, \hat{w}_2^a, \ldots, \hat{w}_m^a$ satisfying the condition $0 \leq \hat{w}_1^a \leq \hat{w}_2^a \leq \ldots \leq \hat{w}_m^a = 1$. The symptoms x_j follow the new replacement of associated weights. In order to avoid too many designation signs let us name the ordered and normalized weights $\omega_j = \hat{w}_j^a$ and attached to them symptoms $\chi_j \in X, j = 1, 2, \ldots, m$. The matrix U_W is accommodated to new assumptions as $U_{[0,1]}$ given by

$$U_{[0,1]} = \begin{array}{c} \\ a_1 \\ a_2 \\ \vdots \\ a_n \end{array} \begin{array}{c} \begin{array}{cccc} \chi_1 & \chi_2 & \cdots & \chi_m \end{array} \\ \begin{bmatrix} \omega_1 \cdot \tilde{u}_{11} & \omega_2 \cdot \tilde{u}_{12} & \cdots & \omega_m \cdot \tilde{u}_{1m} \\ \omega_1 \cdot \tilde{u}_{21} & \omega_2 \cdot \tilde{u}_{22} & \cdots & \omega_m \cdot \tilde{u}_{2m} \\ \vdots & & \ddots & \vdots \\ \omega_1 \cdot \tilde{u}_{n1} & \omega_2 \cdot \tilde{u}_{n2} & \cdots & \omega_m \cdot \tilde{u}_{nm} \end{bmatrix} \end{array} \tag{3.23}$$

in which utilities $\tilde{u}_{ij}$ are tied to reorganized symptoms χ_j.

The formula (3.21) has been replaced by

$$U_{[0,1]}(a_i) = \sum_{j=1}^{m} \omega_j \cdot \tilde{u}_{ij} \tag{3.24}$$

in regard to the new order of weights.

We prove new assumptions made in decision-making model in the next exercise.

Table 3.2. The relationship between medicine action and retreat of symptom

$a_i \backslash x_j$	$x_1(w_1 = 0.93)$	$x_2(w_2 = 0.31)$	$x_3(w_3 = 0.19)$
a_1	almost complete, $u_{11} = 0.9$	very large, $u_{12} = 0.8$	almost none, $u_{13} = 0.1$
a_2	medium, $u_{21} = 0.5$	medium, $u_{22} = 0.5$	little, $u_{23} = 0.3$
a_3	little, $u_{31} = 0.3$	little, $u_{32} = 0.3$	very little, $u_{33} = 0.2$
a_4	little, $u_{41} = 0.3$	little, $u_{42} = 0.3$	very large, $u_{43} = 0.8$

Example 7

By referring to Ex. 3 we recall that the following clinical data concerns the diagnosis "*coronary heart disease*". We consider the symptoms x_1 = "*pain in chest*", x_2 = "*changes in ECG*" and x_3 = "*increased level of LDL-cholesterol*". The medicines improving the patient's state are recommended as a_1 = *nitroglycerin*, a_2 = *beta-adrenergic blockade*, a_3 = *acetylsalicylic acid* (*aspirin*) and a_4 = *statine LDL-reductor.*

The physician has already judged the relationship among efficiency of the drugs and retreat of the symptoms. To be able to attach weights (see Ex. 5) to the considered symptoms we express all connections in Table 3.2.

The weights w_1, w_2, w_3 found for x_1, x_2, x_3 in Ex. 5 are now normalized and rearranged in order to obtain $\omega_1 = 0.2$ attached to $\chi_1 = x_3$, $\omega_2 = 0.33$ connected to $\chi_2 = x_2$ and $\omega_3 = 1$ as the power of $\chi_3 = x_1$.

Due to (3.24) we approximate the utilities $U_{[0,1]}(a_i)$ of medicines a_i, $i = 1, 2, 3, 4$ as

$$\begin{aligned}
U_{[0,1]}(a_1) &= 0.2 \cdot 0.1 + 0.33 \cdot 0.8 + 1 \cdot 0.9 = 1.184, \\
U_{[0,1]}(a_2) &= 0.2 \cdot 0.3 + 0.33 \cdot 0.5 + 1 \cdot 0.5 = 0.725, \\
U_{[0,1]}(a_3) &= 0.2 \cdot 0.2 + 0.33 \cdot 0.3 + 1 \cdot 0.3 = 0.439, \\
U_{[0,1]}(a_4) &= 0.2 \cdot 0.8 + 0.33 \cdot 0.3 + 1 \cdot 0.3 = 0.559.
\end{aligned}$$

After placing of the utilities of drugs in the decreasing order (see (3.22)) we establish the hierarchy of medicines as $a_1 \succ a_2 \succ a_4 \succ a_3$, which fits for the results obtained by minimization of regret.

3.4.2 The Choquet Integral as Total Effectiveness

The normalization and the rearrangement of weights have been made in the intention of proving that formula (3.24) can be interpreted as a rule corresponding to the Choquet integral calculation [7,13,14,25].

We know that the symptoms $\chi_1, \ldots, \chi_m \in X$ act as objects in X. To them let us assign the measures $m(\{\chi_j | a_i\}) = \tilde{u}_{ij}$ [22], where the symbols $\chi_j | a_i$ reflect the association between symptom χ_j and medicine $a_i, j = 1, 2, \ldots, m, i = 1, 2, \ldots, n$. The values $m(\{\chi_j | a_i\})$ are listed in the last column of Table 3.1.

The weights ω_j are set as the range values $f(\chi_j)$ of a function $f : X \to [0, 1]$.

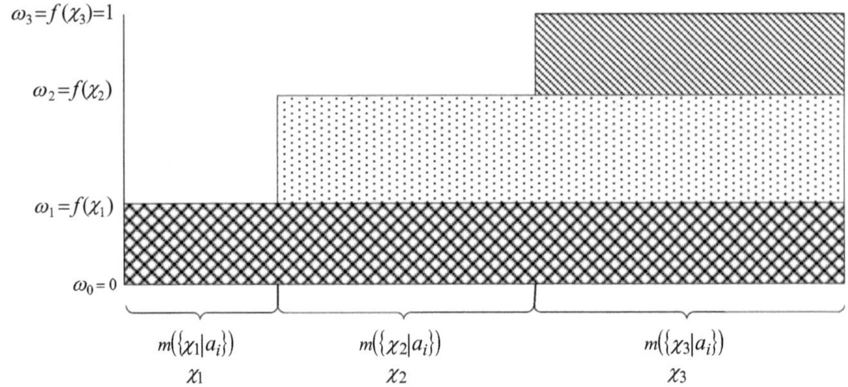

Fig. 3.2. The Choquet integral in evaluation of a_i's total curative effect

By considering the latest suggestions we define the total utility of a_i gathered for all symptoms $\chi_1, \chi_2, \ldots, \chi_m$ as the Choquet integral [22]

$$U_{[0,1]}^{Ch}(a_i) = \int\limits_{X=\{\chi_1,\chi_2,\ldots,\chi_m\}} f(\chi_j)dm(\chi_j\,|a_i\,) \tag{3.25}$$

with respect to the measures $m\,(\{\chi_j\,|a_i\,\})$.

To find a precise calculus formula of integral (3.25) we study Fig. 3.2 made for three symptoms χ_1, χ_2, χ_3. This associates to (3.25) the equation

$$\begin{aligned} U_{[0,1]}^{Ch}(a_i) &= \int\limits_{X=\{\chi_1,\chi_2,\chi_3\}} f(\chi_j)dm(\chi_j\,|a_i\,) \\ &= (\omega_1-\omega_0)\cdot m\,\{\chi_j\,|a_i\,:f(\chi_j)\geq\omega_1\} \\ &\quad+(\omega_2-\omega_1)\cdot m\,\{\chi_j\,|a_i\,:f(\chi_j)\geq\omega_2\} \\ &\quad+(\omega_3-\omega_2)\cdot m\,\{\chi_j\,|a_i\,:f(\chi_j)\geq\omega_3\}\,, \end{aligned} \tag{3.26}$$

which practically explains how to understand the Choquet integral arithmetic. The measures of sets consisting of elements $\chi_j\,|a_i$, defined by properties $f(\chi_j)\geq\omega_1$, $f(\chi_j)\geq\omega_2$ and $f(\chi_j)\geq\omega_3$, are estimated as sums of utilities corresponding to respective $\chi_j\,|a_i$ fulfilling conditions above.

The general formula of the Choquet integral is revealed in the form

$$\begin{aligned} U_{[0,1]}^{Ch}(a_i) &= \int\limits_{X=\{\chi_1,\chi_2,\ldots,\chi_m\}} f(\chi_j)dm(\chi_j\,|a_i\,) \\ &= \sum_{j=1}^{m}(\omega_j-\omega_{j-1})\cdot m\,\{\chi_k\,|a_i\,:f(\chi_k)\geq\omega_j\} \end{aligned} \tag{3.27}$$

for $\omega_0=0, j,k=1,2,\ldots,m, i=1,2,\ldots,n$.

Let us recall that m is a utility measure with values in {0, 0.1, 0.2, 0.3, 0.4, 0.5, 0.6, 0.7, 0.8, 0.9, 1} (the set of u_{ij}-values standing for effectiveness) defined for symptoms after treating them by medicines. If the utility is *none* then its measure will be equal to zero. For the total utility *complete* we reserve the measuring quantity of one. The physician can decide the common utility of a medicine for two symptoms being less than the sum of utilities for distinct symptoms, e.g., the effectiveness of a_2 for *"changes in ECG"* and *"increased level of LDL-cholesterol"* together is judged as 0.4 while the separate measures of effectiveness emerge 0.5 and 0.3 (see Table 3.2). The last remark reveals the non-additive property of the effectiveness measure m. Without any formal proofs made for confirmation of effectiveness as a fuzzy measure, we intend to use it in Choquet integrals constructed for the sample of medicines to approximate their remedial effects.

In the next example we compute the entire effectiveness of medicines from Ex. 3 by adopting the Choquet integral calculus.

Example 8

Let us involve formula (3.27) together with Fig. 3.2 to estimate

$$\begin{aligned}
U^{Ch}_{[0,1]}(a_1) &= \int\limits_{X=\{\chi_1,\chi_2,\chi_3\}} f(\chi_j)dm(\chi_j\,|a_1) \\
&= (0.2-0)\cdot m\{\chi_j\,|a_1 : f(\chi_j)\geq 0.2\} \\
&\quad +(0.33-0.2)\cdot m\{\chi_j\,|a_1 : f(\chi_j)\geq 0.33\} \\
&\quad +(1-0.33)\cdot m\{\chi_j\,|a_1 : f(\chi_j)\geq 1\} \\
&= 0.2\cdot m\{\chi_1\,|a_1, \chi_2\,|a_1, \chi_3\,|a_1\} \\
&\quad +0.13\cdot m\{\chi_2\,|a_1, \chi_3\,|a_1\} + 0.67\cdot m\{\chi_3\,|a_1\} \\
&= 0.2\cdot(0.1+0.8+0.9)+0.13\cdot(0.8+0.9)+0.67\cdot 0.9 = 1.184, \\
U^{Ch}_{[0,1]}(a_2) &= 0.2\cdot(0.3+0.5+0.5)+0.13\cdot(0.5+0.5)+0.67\cdot 0.5 = 0.725, \\
U^{Ch}_{[0,1]}(a_3) &= 0.2\cdot(0.2+0.3+0.3)+0.13\cdot(0.3+0.3)+0.67\cdot 0.3 = 0.439
\end{aligned}$$

and

$$U^{Ch}_{[0,1]}(a_4) = 0.2\cdot(0.8+0.3+0.3)+0.13\cdot(0.3+0.3)+0.67\cdot 0.3 = 0.559.$$

The results are identical with calculations obtained in Ex. 7, which confirms the proper interpretation of the Choquet integral in the drug ranking $a_1 \succ a_2 \succ a_4 \succ a_3$.

3.4.3 The Sugeno Integral in Hierarchical Drug Order

To be able to introduce the Sugeno-like integral in the calculations leading to the choice of an optimal medicine, we normalize the measures

$m\{\chi_k |a_i : f(\chi_k) \geq \omega_j\}$ from (3.27), $j, k = 1, 2, \ldots, m$, when dividing them all by the largest value in the sequence. This operation provides us with the quantities $\hat{m}\{\chi_k |a_i : f(\chi_k) \geq \omega_j\}$ belonging to [0, 1].

As the next estimate of a_i's entire utility we propose a formula [7, 13, 14, 22, 25]

$$\begin{aligned} U^S_{[0,1]}(a_i) &= \int\limits_{X=\{\chi_1,\chi_2,\ldots,\chi_m\}} f(\chi_j) dm(\chi_j |a_i) \\ &= \max_{1\leq j\leq m} (\min(\omega_j, \hat{m}\{\chi_k |a_i : f(\chi_k) \geq \omega_j\})) \end{aligned} \tag{3.28}$$

for $j, k = 1, 2, \ldots, m$, $i = 1, 2, \ldots, n$.

Example 9

The measures $m\{\chi_k |a_1 : f(\chi_k) \geq 0.2\} = 1.8$, $m\{\chi_k |a_1 : f(\chi_k) \geq 0.33\} = 1.7$ and $m\{\chi_k |a_1 : f(\chi_k) \geq 1\} = 0.9$ found for a_1 in Ex. 8 are now divided by the largest value of m equal to 1.8 to generate their normalized versions $\hat{m}\{\chi_k |a_1 : f(\chi_k) \geq 0.2\} = 1$, $\hat{m}\{\chi_k |a_1 : f(\chi_k) \geq 0.33\} = 0.944$ and $\hat{m}\{\chi_k |a_1 : f(\chi_k) \geq 1\} = 0.5$. In the scenario of (3.28) we estimate the utility of a_1 as

$$\begin{aligned} U^S_{[0,\,1]}(a_1) &= \int\limits_{X=\{\chi_1,\chi_2,\chi_3\}} f(\chi_j) dm(\chi_j |a_1) \\ &= \max(\min(0.2, 1), \min(0.33, 0.944), \min(1, 0.5)) = 0.5 \end{aligned}$$

For a_2 we get the utility value

$$U^S_{[0,\,1]}(a_2) = \max(\min(0.2, 1), \min(0.33, 0.769), \min(1, 0.384)) = 0.384,$$

while a_3 and a_4, respectively, possess the affection grades on symptoms from X approximated as

$$U^S_{[0,\,1]}(a_3) = \max(\min(0.2, 1), \min(0.33, 0.75), \min(1, 0.375)) = 0.33$$

and

$$U^S_{[0,\,1]}(a_4) = \max(\min(0.2, 1), \min(0.33, 0.428), \min(1, 0.214)) = 0.33.$$

Even the application of the Sugeno integral provides us with almost the same hierarchy ladder of medicines upgraded in the order $a_1 \succ a_2 \succ a_4 = a_3$. We should mention that the utility values in the last computations are comparable to the "ideal" utility equal to one that can be reached in the state of absolute absence of all symptoms.

3.5 Conclusions

We have presented the adaptations of some fuzzy decision making models to the conditions attributed to the process of selecting of the most efficacious medicine. The decision patterns should be particularly helpful in doubtful cases when we observe unequal remedial abilities of different medicines acting on the same symptoms.

As a primary method of fuzzy decision-making we have adjusted the Jain model to the process of extraction of the best medicine from the collection of proposed remedies. The basis of investigations has been not only restricted to judgment of the distinct medicine influence on a clinical symptom but even extended to estimation of general ability of the symptom retreat.

In the next methods we have also employed the indices of the symptoms' importance to emphasize the essence of additional factors in the final decision. We have estimated the regret following utilities of pairs (medicine, symptom) to be furnished with the medicine order totally confirmed by a physician.

By interpreting the utilities of drugs as measures we have inserted concepts of the Choquet and Sugeno integrals to successfully revise the ranking of drugs.

Except from Bellman-Zadeh model that provides us with the decision based on the strict minimum operator we have produced the results absolutely acceptable from the medical point of view, which confirms the reliability of adaptation of tested decision cases to medical assumptions. After accomplishing of the close analysis of results we should admit that the utilization of mean values or OWA operators in numerical computations yields the most significant effects. All algorithms are based on simple calculations that allow testing of large databases without cumulating of approximation errors.

In the end, we assure that all medical adaptations constitute own original contributions in fuzzy decision-making, which have already been published one by one in many international sources [17–23].

References

1. Adlassnig, K. P.: A Fuzzy Logical Model of Computer-assisted Medical Diagnosis. Methods of Information in Medicine 19, nr 3 (1980) 141–148
2. Adlassnig, K. P.: Fuzzy Modeling and Reasoning in a Medical Diagnostic Expert System. EVD in Medizin und Biologie 17, 1/2 (1986) 12–20
3. Bellman, R. E., Zadeh, L. A.: Decision Making in a Fuzzy Environment. Management Sci. Vol. 17, nr 4 (1970) 141–164
4. Chad-Ton Su, Chien-Hsin Yang, Kuang-Hung Hsu, Wen-Ko Chiu: Data Mining for the Diagnosis of Type II Diabetes from Three-dimensional Body Surface Anthropometrical Scanning Data. Computers & Mathematics with Applications, vol. 51, issues 6–7 (2006) 1075–1092
5. Chen Shi-quan: Fuzzy Classification of Acute Toxicity of Poisons. Fuzzy Sets and Systems, vol. 27, issue 3 (1988) 255–260

6. Gorzałczany, M. B., Piasta, Z.: Neuro-fuzzy Approach Versus Rough-set Inspired Methodology for Intelligent Decision Support. Inf. Sci., vol. 120, issues 1–4 (1999) 45–68
7. Grabisch, M., Murofushi, T., Sugeno, M., Kacprzyk, J.: Fuzzy Measures and Integrals. Theory and Applications. Physica Verlag, Berlin Heidelberg (2000)
8. Jain, R.: Decision Making in the Presence of Fuzzy Variables. IEEE Trans. Syst. Man and Cybern. SMC-6 (1976) 698–703
9. Jain, R.: A Procedure for Multi-aspect Decision Making Using Fuzzy Sets. Int. J. Syst. Sci. 8 (1977) 1–7
10. Ji, Y., Massanari, R. M., Ager, J., Yen, J., Miller, R., Ying, H.: A Fuzzy Logic Based on Computational Recognition-primed Decision Model. Inf. Sci., vol. 177 (2007) 4338–4353
11. Kumar, K. J.: Fuzzy Logic and Modern Analytical Tool Coupling in Comprehensive Evaluation of Traditional and Complementary Medicine. Pharmacognosy Magazine, vol. 2 (2006) 202–203
12. Mesiar, R., Calvo, T., Yager, R. R.: Quantitative Weights and Aggregation. IEEE Transactions on Fuzzy Systems 12 (2004) 62–69
13. Mirofushi, T., Sugeno, M.: An Interpretation of Fuzzy Measures and the Choquet Integral as an Integral with Respect to a Fuzzy Measure. Fuzzy Sets and Systems 29 (1989) 201–227
14. Mirofushi, T., Sugeno, M.: Fuzzy Measures and Fuzzy Integrals. In: Grabisch, M., Murofushi, T., Sugeno, M., Kacprzyk, J. (eds.): Fuzzy Measures and Integrals. Theory and Applications. Physica Verlag, Berlin Heidelberg (2000) 3–34
15. Nieto, J. J., Torres, A.: Midpoints for Fuzzy Sets and Their Application in Medicine. Artificial Intelligence in Medicine, vol. 27 (2003) 81–101
16. O'Hagan, A., Stevens, J. W.: Bayesian Methods for Design and Analysis of Cost-effectiveness Trials in the Evaluation of Health Care Technologies. Statistical Methods in Medical Research, vol. 11 (2002) 469–490
17. Rakus-Andersson, E.: A Fuzzy Decision Making Model Applied to the Choice of the Therapy in the Case of Symptoms not Disappearing after the Treatment. In: deBaets, B., Fodor, J., Kóczy, L. T. (eds.): Proc. of EUROFUSE-SIC'99, University of Veterinary Science – Department of Biomathematics and Informatics, Technical University of Budapest – Department of Telecommunications and Telematics, Budapest (1999) 298–303
18. Rakus-Andersson, E., Gerstenkorn, T.: A Comparison of Different Fuzzy Decision Making Models Supporting the Optimal Therapy. In: Szczepaniak, P., Lisboa, P.J., Tsumoto, S. (eds.): Studies in Fuzziness and Soft Computing Series, Springer-verlag, Berlin Heidelberg New York (1999) 561–572
19. Rakus-Andersson, E.: A Fuzzy Group-Decision Making Model Applied to the Choice of the Optimal Medicine in the Case of Symptoms not Disappearing after the Treatment. In: Dubois, D. (ed.): The International Journal of Computing Anticipatory Systems, University of Liège, Chaos, Liège (1999) 141–152
20. Rakus-Andersson, E.: A Choice of Optimal Medicines by Fuzzy Decision Making Including Unequal Objectives. Issues in the Representation and Processing of Uncertain and Imprecise Information, EXIT – The publishing House of The Polish Academy of Sciences (2005) 307–321
21. Rakus-Andersson, E.: Minimization of Regret versus Unequal Multi-objective Fuzzy Decision Process in a Choice of Optimal Medicines. Proceedings of the

XIth International Conference IPMU 2006 – Information Processing and Management of Uncertainty in Knowledge-based Systems, vol. 2, Edition EDK, Paris-France (2006) 1181–1189
22. Rakus-Andersson, E., Jogreus, C.: The Choquet and Sugeno Integrals as Measures of Total Effectiveness of Medicines. In: Theoretical Advances and Applications of Fuzzy Logic and Soft Computing (Proceedings of IFSA 2007, Cancun, Mexico), eds: Castillo, O., Melin, P., Ross, O. M., Cruz, R. S., Pedrycz, W., Kacprzyk, J., Springer-verlag, Berlin Heidelberg (2007) 253–262
23. Rakus-Andersson, E.: The Fuzzy and Rough Techniques in Medical Diagnosis and Medication. Springer-verlag, Berlin Heidelberg, 2007
24. Saaty, T. L.: Exploring the Interface between Hierarchies, Multiplied Objectives and Fuzzy Sets. Fuzzy Sets and Systems 1 (1978) 57–68
25. Sugeno, M.: Fuzzy Measures and Fuzzy Integrals – a Survey. In: Gupta, M. M., Saridis, G. N., Gaines, B. R. (eds.): Fuzzy Automata and Decision Processes, New York North-Holland (1977) 89–102
26. Yager, R. R.: Multiple Objective Decision-Making Using Fuzzy Sets. Int. J. Man-Machine Studies 9 (1977) 375–382
27. Yager, R. R.: Fuzzy Decision Making Including Unequal Objectives. Fuzzy Sets and Systems 1 (1978) 87–95
28. Yager, R. R., Kacprzyk, J.: The Ordered Weighted Averaging Operators: Theory and Applications. Kluwer, Norwell, MA (1997)
29. Yager, R. R.: Modeling Uncertainty Using Partial Information. Inf. Sci. vol. 121 (1999) 271–294
30. Yager, R. R.: Decision Making Using Minimization of Regret. Int. J. of Approximate Reasoning 36 (2004) 109–128
31. Yager, R. R.: Uncertainty Modeling and Decision Support. Reliability Engineering and System Safety, vol. 85 (2004) 341–354
32. Yager, R. R.: Generalized OWA Aggregation Operators. Fuzzy Optimization and Decision Making 3 (2004) 93–107
33. Zadeh, L. A.: The Concept of a Linguistic Variable and its Application to Approximate Reasoning. Inf. Sci. 8 (1975) 199–249
34. Zadeh, L. A.: Calculus of Fuzzy Restrictions. Fuzzy Sets and Their Applications to Cognitive and Decision Processes. Academic Press, London (1975)
35. Zadeh, L. A.: Test-score Semantics as a Basis for a Computational Approach to the Representation of Meaning. Literary and Linguistic Computing 1 (1986) 24–35
36. Zadeh, L. A.: From Computing with Numbers to Computing with Words – From Manipulation of Measurements to Manipulation of Perceptions. IEEE Transactions on Circuits and Systems 45 (1999) 105–119

4

Cognitive Categorizing in UBIAS Intelligent Medical Information Systems

Lidia Ogiela[1], Ryszard Tadeusiewicz[2], and Marek R. Ogiela[2]

[1] AGH University of Science and Technology, Faculty of Management
Al. Mickiewicza 30, PL-30-059 Kraków, Poland
{logiela}@agh.edu.pl
[2] AGH University of Science and Technology, Institute of Automatics
{rtad, mogiela}@agh.edu.pl

Summary. This chapter will demonstrate that artificial intelligence methods based on linguistic mechanisms for semantic meaning reasoning can be used to develop new classes of intelligent information systems, and can be applied quite successfully to conduct in-depth meaning analyzes in the presented DSS (Diagnostic Support Systems) information systems as well as in a subclass of intelligent, cognitive systems used to analyze images: UBIAS (Understanding Based Image Analysis Systems). The study will present an IT mechanism for describing the meaning of analyzed objects using selected examples of analyzes of medical images, including those of the spinal cord and bone radiograms. The presented semantic reasoning procedures are based on the cognitive resonance model and have been applied for the job of interpreting the meaning of a selected type of diagnostic images of the central nervous system as well as images of the bone system. The solutions and applications presented here are of a research nature and show the directions in which modern IT systems as well as medical diagnostic support systems expand into the field of automatic, computer meaning interpretation of various patterns acquired in image diagnostics.

4.1 Introduction

Intelligent, cognitive information systems used to analyze varied, often extremely complex medical images have been developing extremely fast for many years as scientists and researchers try to answer the question how much the efficiency of this type of systems will allow humans to be replaced in making the final decision and whether this type of process is at all practicable. The whole class of computer systems designed for analyzing various types of images as well as the whole class of diagnostic support systems have overstepped their originally set functional limits which restricted the operation of such systems to visualizing and classifying patterns. At first it was thought that those systems would be used only for diagnostic jobs, so their operations

L. Ogiela et al.: *Cognitive Categorizing in UBIAS Intelligent Medical Information Systems*, Studies in Computational Intelligence (SCI) **107**, 75–94 (2008)
www.springerlink.com

would boil down to making simple statements without the practical possibility of verifying those. This type of IT systems were not sufficient for meaning interpretation jobs and for analyzing complex medical data, which would require imitating the thought processes of diagnosticians and taking steps towards understanding the semantics of the analyzed images. Consequently, within the broad class of IT systems, a subclass of systems was developed which were oriented towards jobs of analyzing various medical patterns, with the capability of conducting semantic reasoning based on the meaning information contained in the analyzed image. This is the UBIAS (Understanding Based Image Analysis Systems) class, the functional structure of which the authors have defined [11, 14].

DSS systems and UBIAS systems are currently very popular due to their wide diagnostic possibilities. In this paper we shall show an example of a system that was prepared not only to diagnose, but one that is also oriented towards the issues of cognitive analysis and the understanding pathological lesions taking place in the area of central nervous system. Particular attention is paid to disease lesions in the spinal cord.

Every medical image constituting a type of primary component for diagnostic IT systems is subject to analysis. The objective is to determine whether there is any important disease lesions observed in the patient's analyzed organ or whether there are no such changes (i.e. the patient is healthy). If there are any such lesions, their type is analyzed and the system directs its functions towards determining what disease the patient has. DSS systems operate on the basis of three main rules:

- Image transformation in order to obtain the best possible content quality and substance which the image carries,
- Image analysis in order to get the image properties in the form of a feature vector,
- Image recognition in order to classify all features of the analyzed image.

DSS systems proposed in earlier research were used, among others, for pancreas as well as for kidney and heart disease diagnosis. Their functioning is based on medical image recognition methods [10, 19] (Figure 4.1).

Due to the fact that DSS systems develop very rapidly, an attempt was made to construct a new class of such systems using in their operation the

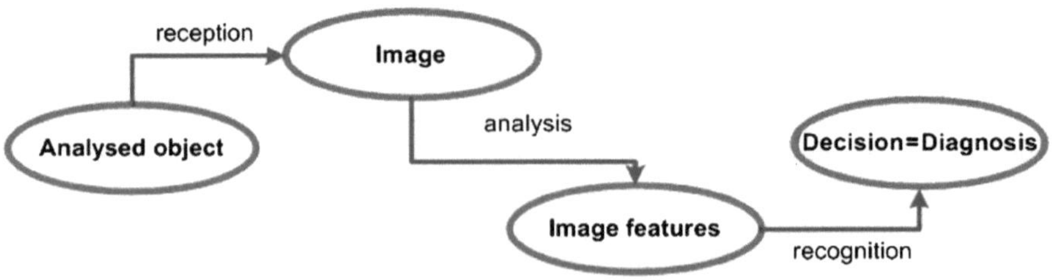

Fig. 4.1. Medical image recognition diagram

mechanisms of cognitive analysis (UBIAS systems). The said are to be directed at attempts to automatically understand the semantics of analyzed images, and therefore at their content meaning interpretation.

UBIAS cognitive information systems were thus developed on the basis of intelligent IT systems whose purpose was not just the simple analysis of data by storing, processing and interpreting it, but mainly an analysis based on understanding and reasoning of an about the semantic contents of the processed data. This is a significant extension of the capabilities of previous information systems.

Every information system which analyzes a selected image or information based on certain characteristic features of it contains in its database the knowledge indispensable for performing the correct analysis or reasoning, which forms the basis for generating the system's expectations of the analysis conducted. Combining the actual features of the analyzed image with the expectations of the semantic contents of the image generated based on the knowledge (about the pattern studied), brings about a phenomenon called the cognitive resonance. This phenomenon has been described more broadly in the publication [19, 24], but the notion behind it will also be presented in the next subsection.

UBIAS cognitive information systems are based on methods which lay down structural reasoning techniques to fit patterns [15,20,25]. Consequently, the structure of the image being analyzed is compared during the analysis process to the structure of the image representing such a pattern. The comparison is conducted using sequences of derivation rules which allow this pattern to be generated unanimously. These rules, sometimes called productions, are defined in a specially introduced grammar, which in turn defines a certain formal language or a so-called image language. The image (information) recognized in this way is assigned to the class which contains the pattern representing it. The analysis and reasoning process is conducted using the phenomenon of cognitive analysis, whose main element and also one of its foundations is the cognitive resonance phenomenon.

4.2 Using the Cognitive Analysis Method in the Medical Image Interpretation Process

Cognitive analysis is the main element of the correct operation of cognitive information systems designed for analyzing and drawing conclusions in the field of medical diagnostic systems.

Cognitive analysis used in IT systems is very often based on the syntactic approach [2, 7]. For the purpose of meaning image interpretation it first uses a pre-processing operation usually composed of:

- Image coding by means of terminal elements of the introduced language,
- Analyzed object shape approximation, as well as
- Filtration and pre-processing of the input image.

As a result of the execution of such stages it is possible to obtain a new image representation in the form of hierarchic semantic tree structures and subsequent production steps of this representation from the initial grammar symbol [6, 9]. An intelligent cognitive system distinguishing at the stage of pre-processing image data must, in the majority of cases, perform image segmentation, identify primitive components and determine spatial as well as semantic relations between them. An appropriate classification (also machine perception) is based on the recognition of whether a given representation of the actual image belongs to a class of images generated by languages defined by one of possible number of grammars. Such grammars can be considered to belong to sequential, tree and graph grammars while recognition with their application is made in the course of a syntactic analysis performed by the system [19].

In the most recent research on intelligent information systems it was observed that the recognition of an analyzed image alone is insufficient since more and more frequently there is a postulate to direct the intelligent information systems' possibilities so that they are able to perform the operation of automatically understanding image semantics. In order to enable such reasoning, the techniques of artificial intelligence are used. Apart from a simple recognition of an image they enable one that also extracts important semantic information allowing for a meaning interpretation, i.e. machine understanding.

This process relates only to cognitive information systems and it is a lot more complex than with pure recognition. This is due to the fact that in this case the flow of information goes clearly in two directions. In this model the stream of empirical data, as contained in the sub-system and aimed to register and analyze the image, interferes with the stream of generated expectations [10, 19] (Figure 4.2).

Between the stream expectation, generated for every hypothetical image and the data steam that is obtained by means of analysis of the currently considered image, there must be a special interference. As a result of this some coincidences (of expectations and features found on the image) gain on importance while others (both compliant and non compliant) lose their importance. This interference leads to a cognitive resonance, which confirms

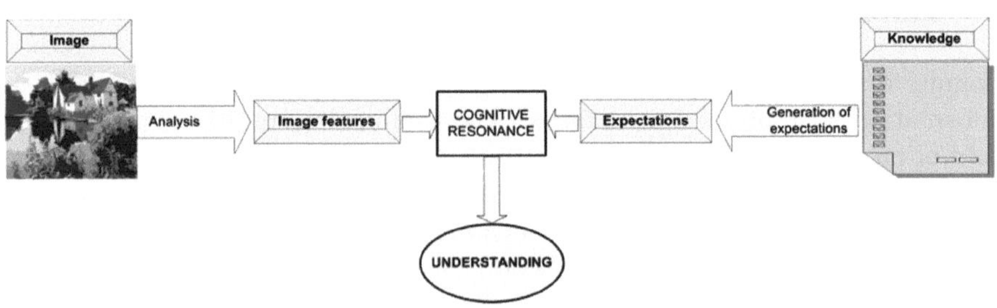

Fig. 4.2. Cognitive resonance in visual data analysis

one of certain possible hypotheses (in the case of an image whose content can be understood) or makes it possible to determine that there is a discordance, which cannot be removed, between the currently perceived image and all other gnostic hypotheses with an understandable interpretation. The second case stands for a failure of automatic image understanding.

Cognitive information systems function based on the cognitive resonance phenomenon which belongs only to these systems and differentiates them from other intelligent IT systems [8,9,24]. The application and use of such systems can be multiple due to wide possibilities offered to them by contemporary science. Nevertheless the greatest possibilities for the use of cognitive IT systems are currently offered by the medicine. This is due to the fact that there are more and more diseases in on-going pathological processes in individual organs and a growing number of detection cases as well as diagnosing these diseases. Medical images belong to some of the most varied data and they contain extremely deep and important (among others, for the patient's fate) meaning interpretation. Cognitive information systems could certainly also serve many other fields of science and everyday life, should an attempt be made to develop intelligent information systems in the field of economics, marketing, management, logistics, military affairs by adding the process of understanding the analyzed information or data.

Here it is worth noting another new class of systems developing very fast at present, which is used to analyze economic data. This class includes UBMSS (Understanding Based Managing Support Systems) which also use reasoning and cognitive resonance, but to analyze a specific type of data, namely that necessary to take strategic corporate decisions. The operation of UBMSS systems is presented in Figure 4.3, while the detailed description of the system presented is available in publications of [12,23].

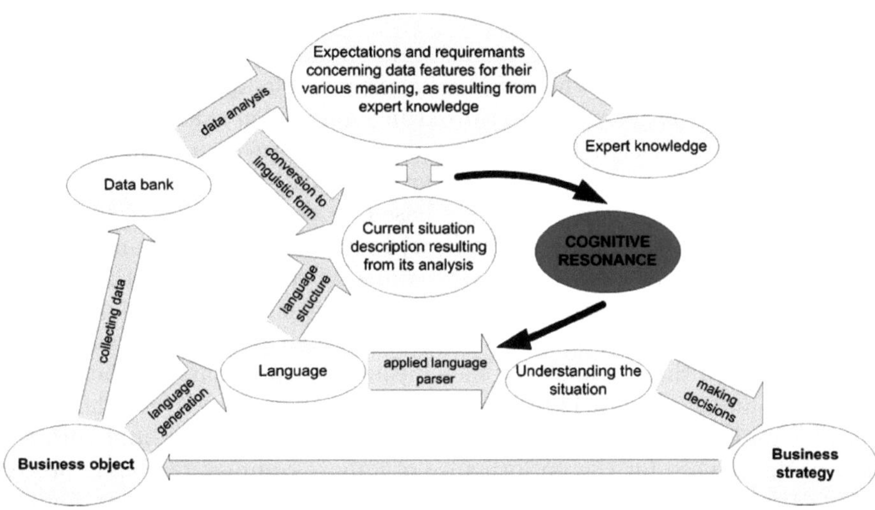

Fig. 4.3. Understanding Based Managing Support Systems

The idea of introducing UBMSS is based on the expansion of the already existing DSS (Decision Support Systems) in which the company must select the right economic strategy. A company, wanting to select the right economic strategy, collects a data pool of sufficient information to analyze the studied phenomenon. Simultaneously, it performs a number of operations aimed at selecting the right (from the IT point of view) language to describe the company's current situation. During data analysis the knowledge of experts generating certain expectations and requirements with regard to the studied phenomenon is included in the entire process. The characteristic features of the data described, which are yielded by the system, are confronted with the features produced by a panel of experts. This, as a consequence, leads to cognitive resonance which, as a result, leads to interference between the expectations generated by the system and the features produced for a given phenomenon. This interference, of course, aims to define important links between the features and the expectations, however, the entire process of analysis may yield irrelevant links. Cognitive resonance in the system leads to a stage of understanding the phenomenon, its causes, development and characteristic features. As a result, it becomes one of the most important stages in strategic decision-making for a given company. Cognitive analysis based on the process of cognition and understanding enables inference with regard to the future connected with the selection of the right economic strategy. Of course, such conclusions may be general and just indicate the weaknesses of the strategy implemented before as well as the benefits following another improved company strategy.

4.3 Artificial Intelligence Techniques in UBIAS Medical Systems

The information systems using cognitive data analysis, which are discussed in this chapter, vary due to the broad range of possible applications of individual techniques. Image-type data stored in information systems is nowadays broadly analyzed by signal processing aimed at improving the quality of data (e.g. images), their meaning analysis and classification.

The idea of introducing UBIAS is based on the expansion of the already existing DSS (Decision Support Systems) in which the pattern analysis tasks are transformed and expanded to the semantic description of the analyzed medical images leading to the understanding of such images. The human mind has incomparably greater perception capacities than a computer even with the best software so that it can reach such meanings appropriate for the observed objects or analyzed data infinitely better than a machine. Nevertheless also machine understanding techniques are slowly being improved and with time they could be used for the performance of a more complex reasoning process, one relating to the significance of data collected rather than just for their simple analysis. In order to enable IT systems such semantic reasoning based on data, advanced IT techniques are used. These techniques, apart from simple information analysis and possible classification (recognition) of data destined for analysis, make it possible also to extract important semantic information from them, ones that point to meaning interpretation. At the current stage of development, data semantic analysis is always set in some pre-determined context. It is impossible for a computer to discover simultaneously the analysis objective and its result. This means that systems currently built can undertake an attempt at understanding data with some a priori pre-definition of what the understanding is supposed to serve. This must be differentiated from a situation in which a human being, coming across a new situation analyzes it in many respects; the outcome of the analysis could be completely unexpected conclusions standing for a complete mental consideration of a given situation, i.e. its complete understanding. Referring to a frequently quoted example of semantic analysis of some specified medical images one can expect that the computer, after an analysis of X-ray image will 'understand' that the patient suffers from some kind of disease. This would not be achievable applying only the technique of automatic image recognition. On the other hand, a human being looking at the same image can, of course, do the same by diagnosing (the diagnosis being the same as the computer would have made or a different one). However, only a man can understand something totally unexpected, for example that an image is bad in quality because the X-ray machine was out of focus and that the examination must be repeated. The first type of understanding is well set in the context of medical examination. It is therefore available both for a medical doctor and for an appropriately programmed computer. The latter requires going outside the framework of an a priori defined scenario and for the time being it is available only for humans.

The main objective of the considerations presented in this paper is to focus the Reader's attention only at the first, easier way of interpreting data understanding process (for example, of images). Still even this process is a lot more complex than just data analysis and their possible recognition. Information flow in the second case is clearly two-sourced and two-directional (just like in the cognitive understanding process model, as taking place during eye perception). In the model considered here, the empirical data stream is collected and stored in a sub-system whose objective is to register and analyze the data the which the analyzed IT stores and processes in accordance with its destination; this interferes with a stream of automatically generated expectations concerning some selected features and data properties. The source of this expectation stream is the knowledge resources located in the system. It is a basis for the generation of semantic hypothesis while the knowledge source are people (experts), from whom the knowledge was obtained and adjusted appropriately for being used in automatic reasoning process.

The terms and conceptual basis of the above-defined approach is a new knowledge field, the so-called cognitive analysis. Currently it is better known in the context of psychological scientists' analyzes examining human cognitive processes. It is also known in the context of hypotheses about the nature of reason and rationality, as examined by philosophers dealing with the epistemology, gnoseology and semiotics foundations as well as criteriology by D. J. Mercier and other advanced intellectual trends. To a smaller degree, however, was it so far used in science itself [1, 10].

4.4 UBIAS System Model for Cognitive CNS Image Analysis

In this section we shall propose, as an example of intelligent IT system, a medical model of IT system supporting diagnosing. The selected system conducts intelligent analysis of image data relating to pathological lesions in the central nervous system, related both to selected disease units of the spinal cord [3, 4, 11]. This model will be based on the construction and the operating rule of UBIAS systems. Due to the fact that the issue of occurrence of disease units in the spinal cord is extremely extensive, some selected pathological phenomena, representative of central nervous system disease types will be presented.

The main element of a correctly functioning IT system supporting the medical image diagnostics is, in accordance with the concept presented in this paper, analysis preparation of a cognitive method of disease units and pathological lesions as occurring in the spinal cord. The cognitive analysis contained in the DSS-CNS system is aimed to propose an automatic correct interpretation method of these extremely complicated medical images, ones resulting from imaging parts of the nervous system. Such images are difficult to interpret due to the fact that various patients have various morphologies of the imaged organs. This is true both of the correct state and if there are any disease lesions. The nervous system, similarly as most elements of the human body, is not always correctly built and fully developed from the birth. The anatomy and pathomorphology differentiate between a number of developmental defects of the central nervous system. It often occurs that this system for the first couple of years functions correctly and only after some time there are some troubles with its functioning, demonstrated by the child's behaviour and feeling: seen either as a single symptom or as a widespread disease. All kinds of troubles occurring in the central nervous system, identified with disease units of the spinal cord are clinically diagnosed and subject to diagnostic procedure based mainly on image diagnostics. Due to small differentiation in the absorption of X-rays by the distinguished medical structures of the brain (for example, by the while and grey substance) as well as due to the fact that the whole central nervous system is hidden behind bones (of the scull and backbone) which strongly attenuate X-rays, the main role in image examinations of the central nervous system is customary assigned to NMR topography (Nuclear Magnetic Resonance) labelled also zeugmatography or most frequently the MRI method (Magnetic Resonance Imaging) – imaging based on the nuclear magnetic resonance phenomenon.

Magnetic resonance makes it possible to obtain maps of density distribution (the so-called topography) primarily of hydrogen atom nuclei (protons) and of these protons' relaxation time. Owing to the application of a projection corresponding to the tomography technique (computational reconstruction of the examined parameter distribution based on many multi-directional probing) the NMR image can be obtained on any cross-section of the body. Hydrogen is a constituent of water making up 60–70% of living organisms; it is also a constituent of all organic compounds. It is worth remembering that fats have an extremely high amount of hydrogen. Information obtained about its distribution inside the organism is the basis for image construction: the images differentiate tissues with regards to the degree of their hydration or fat content. Proton density and their relaxation times can be mirrored by brightness (i.e. greyness degree) of points on the given map. The method of magnetic resonance offers a lot more contrasting soft tissue images then X-ray images. In the case of many diseases it can also show more precisely the difference between a healthy tissue and one that was changed by disease.

All the analyzed images of spinal cord were, before their proper recognition, subject to segmentation and filtration procedures. Their aim was to extract from among other image elements important elements of the spinal cord [4, 10, 18]. Structures shown in this way were then subject to cognitive analysis stages using the grammar described below. In order to analyze disease lesions of the spinal cord, the following attributed grammar has been proposed – figure 4.4.

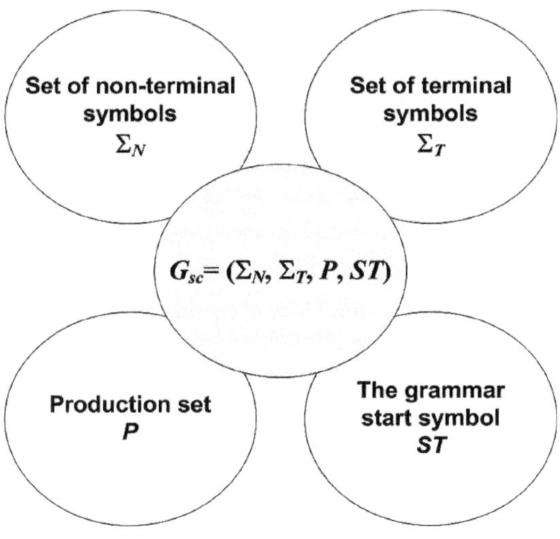

Fig. 4.4. Attributed grammar G_{SC} for spinal cord lesions analysis

The following definitions have been adopted for individual sets defined in G_{SC} sequence grammar:

$$\Sigma_N = \{SPINE\_LESION, SPINAL\_STENOSIS, SPINAL\_DILATATION, SPINAL\_TUMOR, N, D, S\},$$
$$\Sigma_T = \{n, d, s\}$$

Apart from these, the following meaning was given to terminal elements present in the description: $n \in [-11°, 11°]$, $d \in (11°, 180°)$, $s \in (-180°, -11°)$,

$$ST = SPINE\_LESION$$

The production set P has been presented in fig. 4.5 where grammar rules and semantic actions have been defined for individual pathological changes.

The proposed grammar makes it possible to detect various kinds of spinal cord or meningeal stenoses characteristic for neoplastic lesions and inflammatory processes of the spinal cord. Figure 4.6a presents an image of the spinal cord with a visible deformation; figure 4.6b shows the spinal cord image after binarising while figure 4.6c depicts the diagram of the spinal cord. The red area represents the area of occurrence of the anomalies within the structure of the spinal cord. The set of yellow chords, cross-cutting the spinal cord in subsequent points perpendicularly to its axis, as shown on figure 4.6c which demonstrates how the width diagram was made.

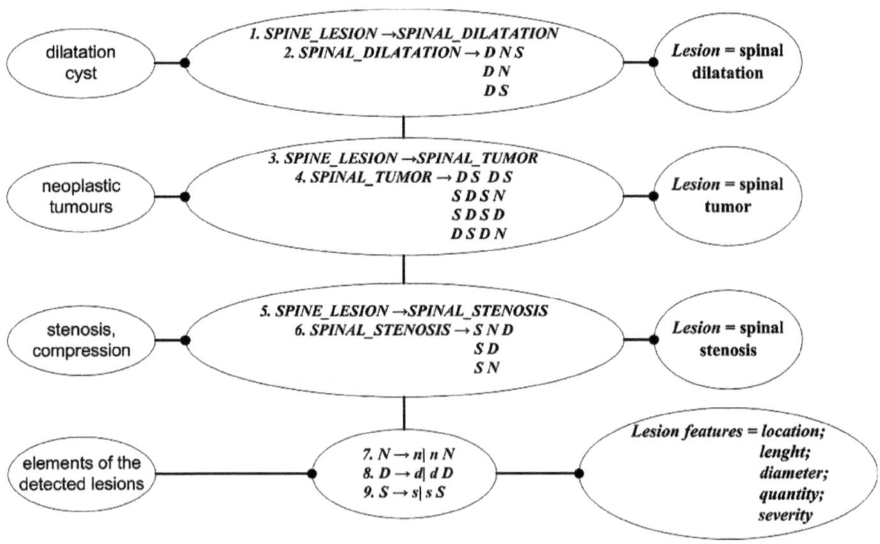

Fig. 4.5. The production set defining changes in the G_{SC} grammar

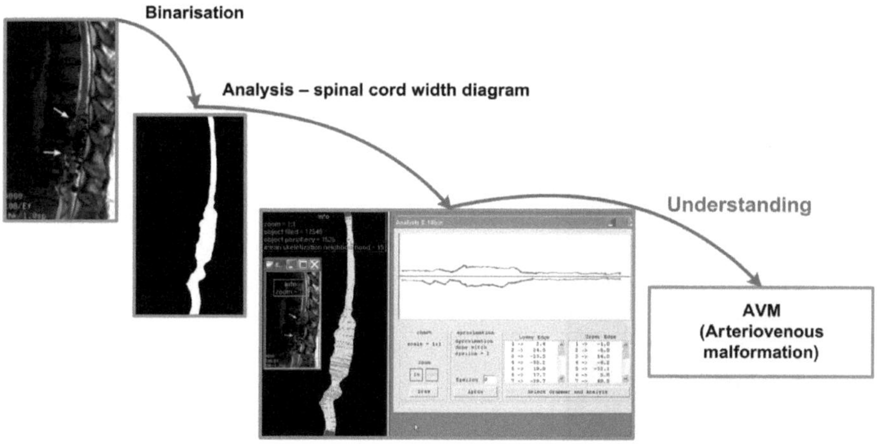

Fig. 4.6. Spinal cord: deformed, after binarising, spinal cord width diagram

Spinal cord width diagram (Figure 4.6) presents, in the most concise form, the results of spinal cord morphology analysis. It is the most precious source of information when one is looking for pathological lesions and it contains all-important data about the examined fragment of central nervous system. At the same time it ignores all spinal cord image details unimportant from the diagnostic point of view, as presented on figure 4.6.

To give an example, the spinal cord MR image, as presented above in figure 4.6 will be subject to (on Figure 4.7a) a diagnostic description of pathological lesions detected in the spinal cord. Image 4.7a presents an example of results obtained by the author in the course of examinations for a given disease case. The results presented here have been achieved by the application of attribute grammar and they are an example of the cognitive approach to the medical data considered here. The type of lesion detected here has been assigned based on its location and on morphometric parameters determined by the grammar semantic procedures.

Figure 4.7b shows an example diagnosis and a description of the lesion obtained by cognitive analysis and semantic reasoning which detects and describes the paraganglioma. This description, just as the description shown in Figure 4.7a, was generated using cognitive analysis applied in a UBIAS system.

The examples above (and many others, obtained as a result of research [13–17]) present the results of semantic meaning interpretation of the analyzed and detected pathological lesions occurring in the spinal cord.

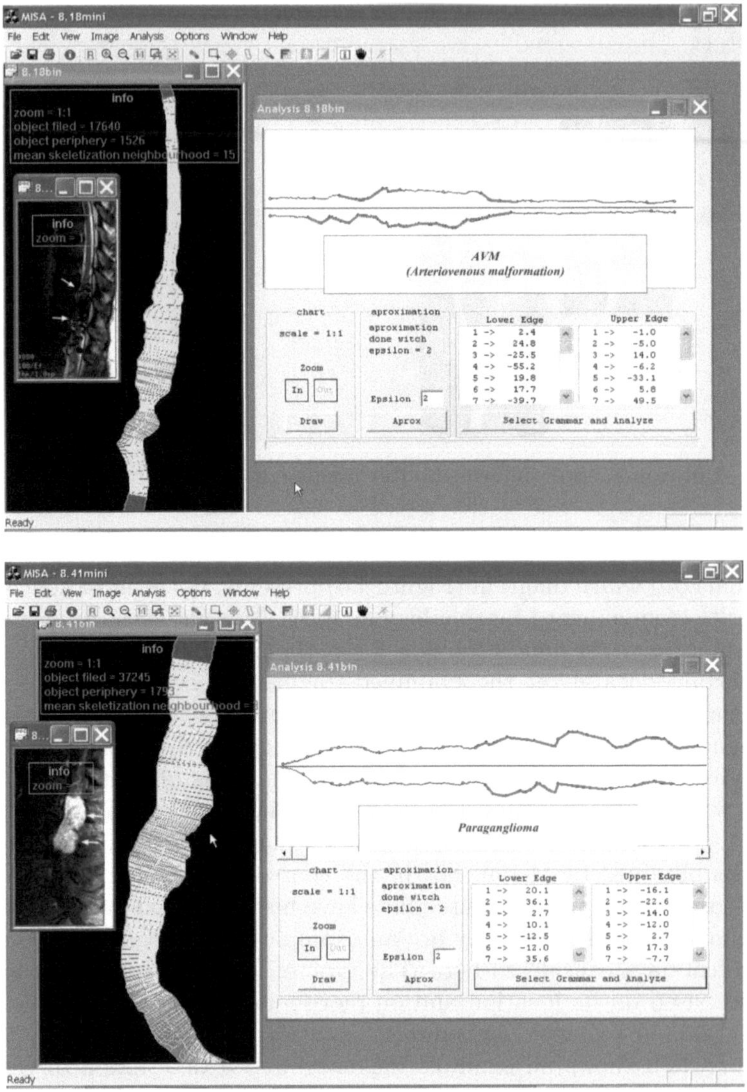

Fig. 4.7. Diagnostic descriptions of spinal cord lesions **A**) Spinal cord lesions with AVM syndrome detected as a result of cognitive analysis, **B**) Spinal cord with paraganglioma detected by the system

4.5 Cognitive Analysis Effectiveness in UBIAS Systems

In order to perform meaning analysis on spinal cord images with the use of a linguistic mechanism as described in this paper, the MISA (Medical Image Syntax Analyzer) computer system has been developed. This enables the analysis and classification of spinal cord images analyzed in this paper.

Table 4.1. The efficiency of cognitive analysis methods directed towards discovering and understanding selected disease phenomena in the central nervous system

Lesion	Number of images	Recognised images	Efficiency [%]
Spinal cord dilation	2	2	100
Cysts	18	17	94
Neoplastic tumours	27	25	93
Stenoses and compression	14	12	86
Degeneration	23	20	87
Total	84	76	**90,5**

The application efficiency of cognitive analysis procedures, using this system, has been presented in a table and it is directed towards comparing the results obtained from the use of this system with those that one can consider as a correct diagnosis (table 4.1).

These results are obtained as a result of the application of semantic analysis algorithms conducted in reasoning modules of the proposed system and based on semantic actions assigned to structural rules. The proposed approach exhibits significant scientific novelty features and is applied in diagnostic analysis using DSS medical information systems and UBIAS systems.

The research conducted by the authors, based on the analysis of images with pathological lesions in a part of the central nervous system, the spinal cord, have demonstrated that cognitive data analysis can be a factor that significantly enriches the possibilities of contemporary information systems. In particular, the described research has demonstrated that an appropriately built image grammar enables the conduct of precise analysis and the description of medical images from which important semantic information can be gained on the nature of processes and pathological lesions as found in the patient's spinal cord. It is worth emphasizing that the results described in this paper have been obtained following the cognitive process, simulating an experts' method of thinking: if one observes a deformation of the organ shown by the medical image used, then one tries to understand the pathological process that was the reason for the appearance of deformations found. One does not perform a mechanic classification for the purpose of pointing out more similar samples on the pathological image. Moreover, the research conducted has demonstrated that for cognitive analysis attempts (on the central nervous system) it is possible to apply it on sequential grammar-based linguistics.

4.6 An Example Application of Cognitive Analysis to Problems of Interpreting Long Bone Fractures

Another example of application of structural formalism for semantic categorization of medical images is lesion analysis in case of leg bones abnormalities or injuries interpretation. Such analysis is possible both for arm and leg bones, but further will be presented example of interpretation of various types (shapes) of leg bones fracture, and stages of theirs recovery. For detection of the most common leg bone fractures the following attributed grammar has been proposed (figure 4.8):

where:

VN = {RESULT, FRACTURE, FISSURE, TRANSVERSE, SPIRAL, ABHESION, DELAYED_UNION, DISPLACED_M1, DISPLACED_M2, DISPLACED1, DISPLACED2, LONGITUDINAL, A, B, C, D, E, F, G, H}

VT = {'a', 'b', 'c', 'd', 'e', 'f', 'g', 'h'} where symbols defined as follows: $a \in [-10°, 10°]$, $b \in (10°, 70°]$, $c \in (70°, 110°]$, $d \in (110°, 170°]$, $e \in (170°, -170°)$, $f \in (-110°, -170°]$, $g \in (-70°, -110°]$, $h \in (-10°, -70°]$.

STS = RESULT. A production set SP is presented in Table 4.2.

The proposed grammar is designed not just for simple image analysis, but also becomes the starting point for conducting a semantic reasoning about the analyzed fractures. The examples of bone fractures described by the authors have been subjected to a descriptive analysis leading to making a medical diagnosis, but an attempt has also been made to reason out the substantive and semantic content of the analyzed image presenting a long bone fracture. An example result of bone fracture detection and analysis is presented in fig. 4.9.

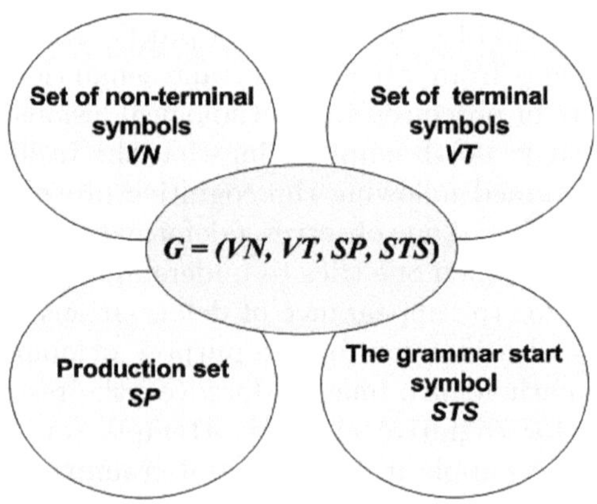

Fig. 4.8. Attributed grammar for leg bones fracture analysis

Table 4.2. Set of grammar rules defining types of fractures

Lesion	Grammar rules
Fissure fracture	RESULT → FRACTURE → A FISSURE A FISSURE → H B | H A B
Transverse fracture	RESULT → FRACTURE → A H E | A TRANSVERSE E | A G F E | A TRANSVERSE H E TRANSVERSE → H G | H F
Spiral fracture	RESULT → FRACTURE → A SPIRAL A SPIRAL → ABHESION F | ABHESION G F | ABHESION F E | ABHESION F G | H F | G F | F G | F H | F ABHESION → B A H | B H
Displaced fracture	RESULT → FRACTURE → DISPLACED_M1 F | DISPLACED1 F | DISPLACED_M2 D | DISPLACED2 D DISPLACED_M1 → B A | B G | B H DISPLACED_M2 → H G | H F | H E DISPLACED1 → B A H G | B A H | B A G | B A G H DISPLACED2 → H G F E | H G E
Delayed union fracture	RESULT → FRACTURE → A DELAYED_UNION A DELAYED_UNION → ABHESION ABHESION | ABHESION A ABHESION | ABHESION G ABHESION | ABHESION C ABHESION | ABHESION G A ABHESION | ABHESION G C ABHESION | ABHESION G A C ABHESION | ABHESION A C ABHESION | ABHESION B C ABHESION ABHESION → B A H | B H
Longitudinal fracture	RESULT →FRACTURE → A LONGITUDINAL E LONGITUDINAL → TRANSVERSE TRANSVERSE | TRANSVERSE E TRANSVERSE | TRANSVERSE E H | H E TRANSVERSE | H E H
Adhesion	RESULT → FRACTURE → A ABHESIONE ABHESION → B A H | B H
Elements of the detected lesions	A → 'A' A | 'A' B → 'b' B | 'b' C → 'c' C | 'c' D → 'd' D | 'd' E → 'e' E | 'e' F → 'f' F | 'f' G → 'g' G | 'g' H → 'h' H | 'h'

Figure 4.9a presents a limb fracture after a certain time of union, together with the periosteum growing around it. The UBIAS system has recognised this lesion as a bone fracture at the phase of hard bone matter growth. The fracture is visible in the image, but the analyzed area is partially filled with periosteum. Figure 4.9b presents the bone fracture with the spiral fracture automatically detected by the UBIAS system.

The UBIAS systems presented here, designed for analyzing images of lower and upper limb fractures, serve to analyze various types of fractures, including spiral, longitudinal, displaced ones, factures at the phase of bone reconstruction and at the phase of hard bone matter growth. The jobs of analyzing the lesions and pathologies in the field of long bone fractures make use of cognitive

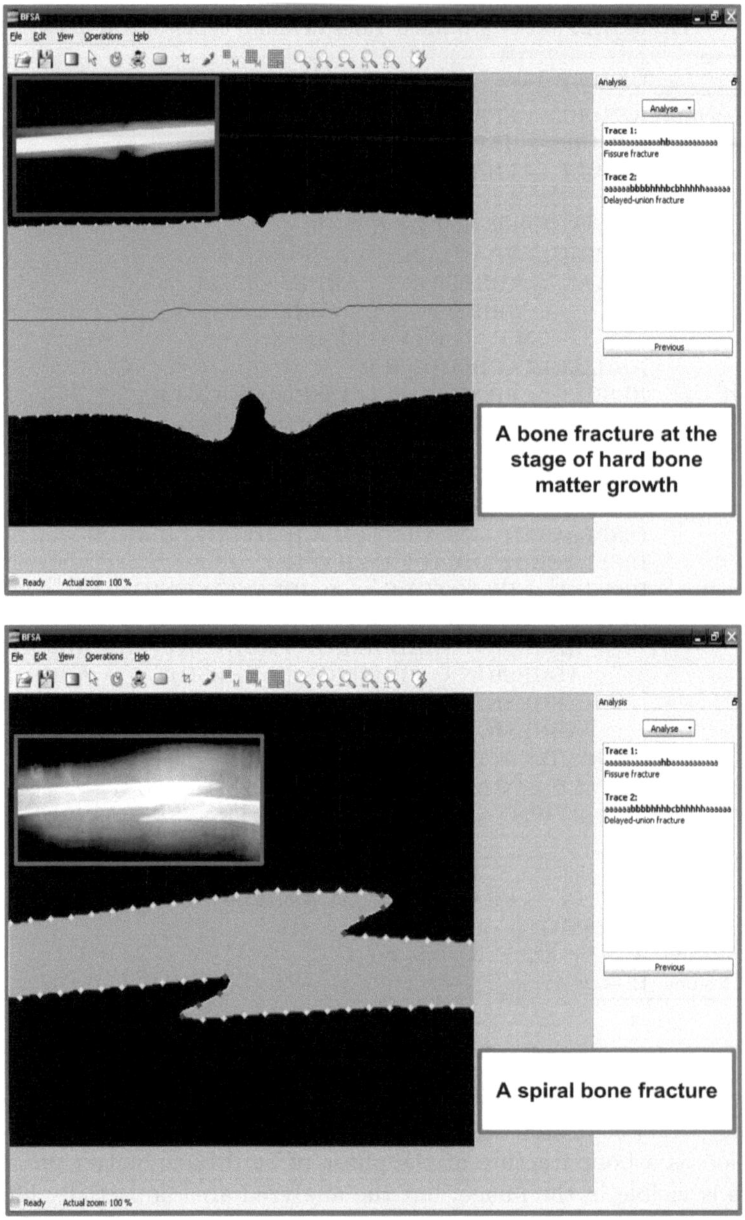

Fig. 4.9. Bone fracture analysis **A)** A description of a bone fracture; the marked fragment shows the bone fracture at the phase of hard bone matter growth detected by the system, **B)** Description of spiral fracture

analysis on the basis of which the system for cognitive analysis and interpretation of image-type data conducts reasoning and analysis using semantic information contained in the image under consideration.

4.7 Conclusions

The authors have illustrated the methodology of cognitive analysis presented in the publication as a tool supporting the development of new generation IT systems mainly with examples of problems of image analysis, particularly of medical images. Cognitive analysis applied in the context, presented here, of interpreting the meaning of selected types of medical images allows a new class of intelligent information systems to be developed, including the UBIAS class of systems described in this publication.

The cognitive analysis methods proposed here for pathological phenomena shown in medical images are a double achievement. Firstly, if we treat them literally and consider them only in the context of their utilitarian purpose, they are a successful attempt at developing medical information systems and systems helping to diagnose selected disease entities. Within this scope, the publication offers new results which can be considered and assessed with regards to their practical utility. However, a much more important objective of the authors was to show the capabilities offered by cognitive analysis treated as a tool for obtaining valuable knowledge components (and not just data) from modern information systems. By developing a system for the automatic understanding of medical images, it has been empirically proven that modern artificial intelligence methods make it possible to cross the barrier between the form of data collected in the information system and its substantive content necessary to understand its meaning. Obviously, the cognitive analysis of a different type of data (e.g. those needed by a UBMSS-class system presented in Chapter 4.2 for managing a corporation) will require a different type of preprocessing of this data, other procedures for its analysis and other languages in which this data will be described and which will later make it possible to extract itssubstantive sense. So using the results from this publication in a broader context requires solving many difficult specific problems.

Cognitive analysis methods proposed by the authors of this publication to develop cognitive information systems may represent an additional, precise tool very useful for many other purposes. It is worth noting the support for the early diagnosis of irregularities of the central nervous system in the medicine of developmental defects of children. The application of these systems in PACS (Picture Archiving and Communication Systems) is also worth considering.

The very high computational efficiency of the algorithms developed as part of this project for the semantic interpretation of images (which algorithms are of a multinomial complexity) makes the proposed cognitive analysis methods exceptionally useful in practice. It could be said that as a side effect of the scientific research, this publication offers medical practice a practical tool for extracting, recognising and understanding the diagnostic features of the analyzed medical image.

The semantic information on the disease factor extracted during the syntactic reasoning is mainly used to formulate the correct diagnosis, but it may also have further uses. In particular, it could be used to:

- follow the progress of the therapeutic process, including the definition of its direction and type;
- forecast the disease progress and the future condition of the patient;
- construct a description which indexes image data in a specialised medical database;
- streamline the processes of context-sensitive searching for semantic image information by a process of automatic formulation of queries to the system of multimedia database indexing.

The UBIAS systems presented here, which represent cognitive systems for the intelligent analysis and semantic reasoning on the basis of analyzed data, are applied not only in the broad and in-depth analysis of medical images, but are also quite successfully used for interpreting economic problems. These jobs are performed by another sub-class of DSS systems called UBMSS.

Acknowledgement

This work has been supported by the Ministry of Science an d Higher Education, Republic of Poland, under project number N516 025 32/2881 decision No. 2881/T02/2007/32.

References

1. Albus J. S., Meystel A. M.: Engineering of Mind – An Introduction to the Science of Intelligent Systems. A Wiley-Interscience Publication John Wiley & Sons Inc (2001)
2. Branquinho J. (eds.): The Foundations of Cognitive Science, Clarendon Press, Oxford (2001)
3. Brejl M., Sonka M.: Medical image segmentation: Automated design of border detection criteria from examples, Journal of Electronic Imaging, Vol. 8, No 1, (1999) pp. 54–64
4. Burgener F. A., Meyers S. P., Tan R. K., Zaunbauer W.: Differential Diagnosis in Magnetic Resonance Imaging Georg Thieme Verlag (2002)
5. Chomsky N.: Language and Problems of Knowledge: The Managua Lectures, MIT Press, Cambridge, MA (1988)
6. Davis L. S. (eds.): Foundations of Image Understanding, Kluwer Academic Publishers (2001)
7. Duda R. O., Hart P. E., Stork D. G.: Pattern Classification, Second Edition, A Wiley-Interscience Publication John Wiley & Sons, Inc. (2001)
8. Klopotek M. A., Wierzchon S. T., Trojanowski K. (eds.): Intelligent Information Processing and Web Mining, Proceedings of the International IIS: IIP WM'04 Conference Held in Zakopane, Springer, Poland, May 17–20 (2004)
9. Meystel A. M., Albus J. S.: Intelligent Systems – Architecture, Design, and Control, A Wiley-Interscience Publication John Wiley & Sons, Inc., Canada (2002)

10. Ogiela L.: Usefulness assessment of cognitive analysis methods in selected IT systems, Ph. D. Thesis. AGH Kraków (2005)
11. Ogiela L.: Cognitive Understanding Based Image Analysis Systems (UBIAS) of the Diagnostic Type, IEEE International Workshop on Imaging Systems and Techniques – IST, Krakow, Poland, May 4–5, CD-ROM (2007)
12. Ogiela L.: UBMSS (Understanding Based Managing Support Systems) as an Example of the Application of Cognitive Analysis in Data Analysis, CISIM 2007, IEEE Proceedings 6th International Conference CISIM'07 – Computer Information Systems and Industrial Management Applications, Elk, Poland, 28–30 June 2007, (2007) pp. 77–80
13. Ogiela L., Tadeusiewicz R., Ogiela M.: Cognitive Analysis In Diagnostic DSS-Type IT Systems, in: L. Rutkowski et al. (eds.), ICAISC 2006, LNAI 4029, Springer-Verlag Berlin Heidelberg, (2006) pp. 962–971
14. Ogiela L., Tadeusiewicz R., Ogiela M. R.: Cognitive Approach to Visual Data Interpretation in Medical Information and Recognition Systems, IWICPAS, LNCS 4153, Springer-Verlag Berlin Heidelberg (2006), pp. 244–250
15. Ogiela M. R., Tadeusiewicz R., Ogiela L.: Intelligent Semantic Information Retrieval In Medical Pattern Cognitive Analysis. Computational Science and Its Applications – ICCSA (2005), 3483, 852–857
16. Ogiela M. R., Tadeusiewicz R., Ogiela L.: Image languages in intelligent radiological palm diagnostics, Pattern Recognition 39 (2006), Elsevier Ltd., pp. 2157–2165
17. Ogiela M. R., Tadeusiewicz R., Ogiela L.: Graph image language techniques supporting radiological, hand image interpretations, Computer Vision and Image Understanding 103 (2006), Elsevier Inc., pp. 112–120
18. Tadeusiewicz R., Ogiela L., Ogiela M. R.: Cognitive Analysis Techniques in Business Planning and Decision Support Systems, in: L. Rutkowski et al. (eds.), ICAISC 2006, LNAI 4029, Springer-Verlag Berlin Heidelberg, (2006) pp. 1027–1039
19. Tadeusiewicz R., Ogiela M. R.: Medical Image Understanding Technology, Artificial Intelligence and Soft-Computing for Image Understanding. Springer-Verlag Berling Heildelberg (2004)
20. Tadeusiewicz R., Ogiela M. R.: New Proposition for Intelligent Systems Design: Artificial Understanding of the Images as the Next Step of Advanced Data Analysis after Automatic Classification and Pattern Recognition, in: Kwasnicka H., Paprzycki M. (eds.): Intelligent Systems Design and Applications, IEEE Computer Society Press, Los Alamitos, Washington, Brussels, Tokyo, 2005, pp. 297–300, Proceedings 5th International Conference on Intelligent Systems Design and Application – ISDA 2005, September 8–10, Wroclaw (2005)
21. Tadeusiewicz R., Ogiela M. R.: Automatic Image Understanding – A New Paradigm for Intelligent Medical Image Analysis (opening article), BIO-ALGORITHMS AND MED-SYSTEMS, Vol. 2, No. 3, (2006) pp. 5–11
22. Tadeusiewicz R., Ogiela M. R.: Why Automatic Understanding?, LNCS Vol. 4432, 2007, Springer-Verlag Berlin Heidelberg (2007) pp. 477–491
23. Tadeusiewicz R., Ogiela M. R., Ogiela L.: A New Approach to the Computer Support of Strategic Decision Making in Enterprises by Means of a New Class of Understanding Based Management Support Systems, CISIM 2007 – IEEE 6th International Conference on Computer Information Systems and Industrial Management Applications Elk, Poland, June 28–30, 2007, in K. Saeed, A. Abraham, R. Mosdorf (eds.) IEEE Computer Society, (2007) pp. 9–13

24. Tadeusiewicz R., Ogiela M. R.: Automatic Understanding of Images, in Adipranata R., S. Rostianingsih, Ballangan, Itan R. (eds.): Proceedings of International Conference on Soft Computing, Intelligent System and Information Technology (ICSIIT 2007), Bali – Indonesia 26–27 July 2007, Special Book for Keynote Talks, Informatics Engineering Department, Petra Christian University, Surabaya, (2007) pp. 13–38
25. Tanaka E.: Theoretical aspects of syntactic pattern recognition, Pattern Recognition, Vol. 28, (1995) pp. 1053–1061
26. Zhong N., Raś Z. W., Tsumoto S., Suzuki E. (eds.): Foundations of Intelligent Systems, 14th International Symposium, ISMIS 2003, Maebashi City, Japan (2003)

5

Intelligent Pervasive Healthcare Systems

Charalampos Doukas and Ilias Maglogiannis

Dep. of Information & Communication Systems Engineering,
University of the Aegean Samos, Greece
{doukas, imaglo}@aegean.gr

Summary. The chapter presents the state of the art in intelligent pervasive healthcare applications and the corresponding enabling technologies. It discusses pervasive healthcare systems in either controlled environments (e.g., health care units or hospitals), or in sites where immediate health support is not possible (i.e. the patient's home or an urban area). Special focus is raised on intelligent platforms (e.g., agents, context-aware and location-based services, and classification systems) that enable advanced monitoring and interpretation of patient status and environment optimizing the whole medical assessment procedure.

5.1 Introduction

In this era of ubiquitous and mobile computing the vision in biomedical informatics is towards achieving two specific goals: the availability of software applications and medical information anywhere and anytime and the invisibility of computing [41]. Both aforementioned goals lead to the introduction of pervasive computing concepts and features in e-health applications. Applications and interfaces that will be able to automatically process data provided by medical devices and sensors, exchange knowledge and make intelligent decisions in a given context are strongly desirable. Natural user interactions with such applications are based on autonomy, avoiding the need for the user to control every action, and adaptivity, so that they are contextualized and personalized, delivering the right information and decision at the right moment [42]. All the above pervasive computing features add value in modern pervasive e-healthcare systems.

These technologies can support a wide range of applications and services including mobile telemedicine, patient monitoring, location-based medical services, emergency response and management, pervasive access to medical data, and personalized monitoring. Wireless technology enables ambulance personnel to send real-time data about a patient's condition to a hospital while en route. In some cases, paramedics can electronically retrieve the patient's

C. Doukas and I. Maglogiannis: *Intelligent Pervasive Healthcare Systems*, Studies in Computational Intelligence (SCI) **107**, 95–115 (2008)
www.springerlink.com

medical records, including known allergies or preexisting conditions, from the hospital database. In medical facilities equipped with wireless local area networks (LANs), doctors and staff can review and update a patient's medical record from any location using a handheld device. Entering diagnostic information and taking notes electronically eliminates the need for time-consuming manual dictation and errors associated with handwritten instructions. In addition, physicians can generate and wirelessly transmit prescriptions to a pharmacy, which also saves time and increases accuracy.

With remote monitoring, patients undergoing postoperative care who are no longer in acute danger but are still subject to a relapse or other complications can be safely transferred earlier to other units within a hospital. Many can move to less costly assisted care facilities or even return home more quickly. Healthcare providers can use location-based tracking services to supervise elderly patients or those with mental illnesses who are ambulatory but restricted to a certain area. For example, an assisted care facility could use network sensors and radiofrequency ID badges to alert staff members when patients leave a designated safety zone. Network or satellite positioning technology also can be used to quickly and accurately locate wireless subscribers in an emergency and communicate information about their location. Proximity information services can direct mobile users to a nearby healthcare facility; voice-activated systems could provide such instructions to blind persons.

Both patients and healthcare providers would benefit from pervasive access to lifetime clinical records. During a check-up, for example, patients could use a handheld device to upload their personal medical history and insurance data into their healthcare provider's database, reducing the effort required to enter such detailed information manually. Alternatively, such information could be downloaded from a Web-based health information system with proper authentication. Patients could likewise use mobile devices to update their personal and family medical information and physician contacts, receive alerts to take prescribed medications, check for drug interactions, or dynamically change restrictions on who can access their health data. Wireless service providers or healthcare providers could use such capabilities to make any information they store sharable only with the user's consent.

Numerous portable devices are available that can detect certain medical conditions—pulse rate, blood pressure, breath alcohol level, and so on—from a user's touch. Many such capabilities could be integrated into a handheld wireless device that also contains the user's medical history. It may even be possible to detect certain contextual information, such as the user's level of anxiety, based on keystroke patterns. After analyzing data input, the device could transmit an alert message to a healthcare provider, the nearest hospital, or an emergency system if appropriate.

The development of pervasive health-care systems is a very promising area for commercial organizations active in the health monitoring domain. The considered pervasive infrastructure creates numerous business opportunities for players like emergency medical assistance companies, the telecommunication operators, insurance companies, etc. The pervasive paradigm creates added value for all these actors in the business chain. Currently, the cost effective provision of quality healthcare is a very important issue throughout the world since healthcare faces a significant funding crisis due to the increasing population of older people and the reappearance of diseases that should be controllable. The pervasive healthcare systems are capable of attacking all these challenges in an efficient, ubiquitous and cost-effective way. Pervasive hardware and software is gradually becoming cost-affordable, can be installed and operated in numerous sites (frequently visited by patients), can be interfaced to a wide variety of medical information systems (e.g., patient databases, medical archives), thus involving numerous actors. Hence, the pervasive e-health systems present a truly scalable architecture covering a wide spectrum of business roles and models [31].

This chapter aims at presenting the use of such intelligent pervasive systems in the medical sector. It is structured as follows: Section 5.2 discuses the technologies that enable the use of pervasive healthcare computing (i.e., patient data acquisition methods and tools, networking technologies, positioning methods and context-awareness frameworks). Section 5.3 overviews the intelligent aspect that can be applied in electronic healthcare systems. Section 5.4 presents pervasive healthcare applications in controlled environments, such as health care units or hospitals, while Section 5.5 provides examples of applications in sites where immediate health support is not possible (i.e. the patient's home or a remote area). Finally, Section 5.6 presents the challenges of the near future and concludes this chapter.

5.2 Pervasive HealthCare Enabling Technologies

Applications that conform to the pervasive computing paradigm are continuously running and always available. Pervasive applications are characterized by adaptation of their functionality subject to their current environment. Such environment may refer to the physical location, orientation or a user profile. In a mobile and wireless environment, changes of location and orientation are frequent. Apart from collecting patient-related data, sensing the user's identity, environment characteristics and location in e-health applications is quite important for adapting the provided to the physician or patient, services in an intelligent manner. This Section discusses methods and technologies for data acquisition, networking, and location provision.

5.2.1 Patient Biosignals and Acquisition Methods

A broad definition of a signal is a 'measurable indication or representation of an actual phenomenon', which in the field of biosignals, refers to observable facts or stimuli of biological systems or life forms. In order to extract and document the meaning or the cause of a signal, a physician may utilize simple examination procedures, such as measuring the temperature of a human body or have to resort to highly specialized and sometimes intrusive equipment, such as an endoscope. Following signal acquisition, physicians go on to a second step, that of interpreting its meaning, usually after some kind of signal enhancement or 'pre-processing', that separates the captured information from noise and prepares it for specialized processing, classification and decision support algorithms.

Biosignals require a digitization step in order to be converted into a digital form. This process begins with acquiring the raw signal in its analog form, which is then fed into an analog-to-digital (A/D) converter. Since computers cannot handle or store continuous data, the first step of the conversion procedure is to produce a discrete-time series from the analog form of the raw signal. This step is known as 'sampling' and is meant to create a sequence of values sampled from the original analog signals at predefined intervals, which can faithfully reconstruct the initial signal waveform. The second step of the digitization process is quantization, which works on the temporally sampled values of the initial signal and produces a signal, which is both temporally and quantitatively discrete; this means that the initial values are converted and encoded according to properties such as bit allocation and value range. Essentially, quantization maps the sampled signal into a range of values that is both compact and efficient for algorithms to work with. The most popular biosignals utilized in pervasive health applications ([1,3,4,10,11,18,19,24,25,31]) are summarized in the Table below.

In addition to the aforementioned biosignals, patient physiological data (e,g., body movement information based on accelerometer values), and context-aware data (e.g., location, environment and age group information) have also been used by pervasive health applications ([1–4,6,13–15,23,25,27,32]). The utilization of the latter information is discussed in the following sections.

Table 5.1. Broadly used biosignals with corresponding metric ranges, number of sensors required and information rate [51]

Biomedical Measurements (Broadly Used Biosignals)	Voltage range (V)	Number of sensors	Information rate (b/s)
ECG	0.5–4 m	5–9	15000
Heart sound	Extremely small	2–4	120000
Heart rate	0.5–4 m	2	600
EEG	2–200 μ	20	4200
EMG	0.1–5 m	2+	600000
Respiratory rate	Small	1	800
Temperature of body	0–100 m	1+	80

In the context of pervasive healthcare applications, the acquisition of biomedical signals is performed through special devices (i.e. sensors) attached on the patients body (see Fig. 5.1) or special wearable devices (see Fig. 5.2). The transmission of the collected signals to the monitoring unit is performed through appropriate wireless technologies discussed in Section 5.2.2. Regarding the contextual information, most applications are based on data collected from video cameras, microphones, movement and vibration sensors.

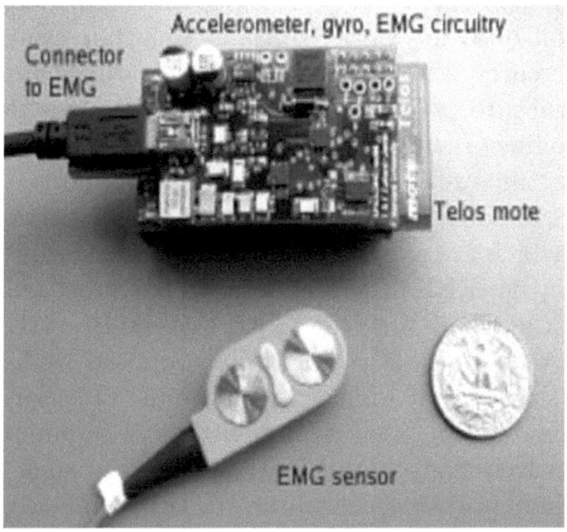

Fig. 5.1. Accelerometer, gyroscope, and electromyogram (EMG) sensor for stroke patient monitoring [9]

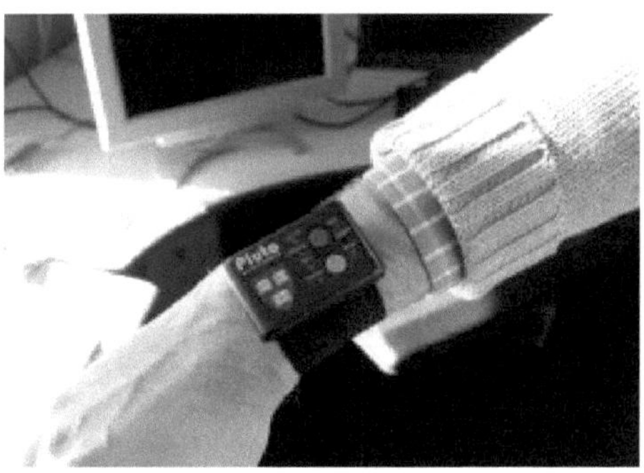

(a)

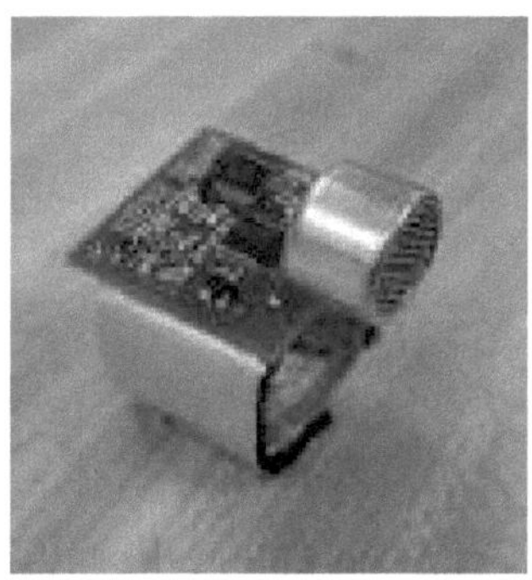

(b)

Fig. 5.2. Wearable medical sensor devices: **(a)** A 3-axis accelerometer on a wrist device enabling the acquisition of patient movement data [9], **(b)** A ring sensor for monitoring of blood oxygen saturation [22]

5.2.2 Communication Technologies

Regarding communication, there are two main enabling technologies according to their topology: on-body (wearable) and off-body networks. Recent technological advances have made possible a new generation of small, powerful, mobile computing devices. A wearable computer must be small and light enough to fit inside clothing. Occasionally, it is attached to a belt or other accessory, or is worn directly like a watch or glasses. An important factor in wearable computing systems is how the various independent devices interconnect and share data. An off-body network connects to other systems that the user does not wear or carry and it is based on a Wireless Local Area Network (WLAN) infrastructure, while an on-body or Wireless Personal Area Network (WPAN) connects the devices themselves; the computers, peripherals, sensors, and other subsystems and runs at ad hoc mode. Table 5.2 presents the characteristics of wireless connectivity and mobile networking technologies correspondingly, which are related to off-body and on-body networks. WPANs are defined within the IEEE 802.15 standard. The most relevant protocols for pervasive e-health systems are Bluetooth and ZigBee (IEEE 802.15.4 standard). Bluetooth technology was originally proposed by Ericsson in 1994, as an alternative to cables that linked mobile phone accessories. It is a wireless technology that enables any electrical device to communicate in the 2.5-GHz ISM (license free) frequency band. It allows devices such as mobile phones, headsets, PDAs and portable computers to communicate and send data to each other without the need for wires or cables to link the devices together.

Table 5.2. Wireless connection technologies for pervasive health systems

Technology	Data rate	Range	Frequency
IEEE 802.11a	54 Mbps	150 m	5 GHz
IEEE 802.11b	11 Mbps	150 m	2.4 GHz ISM
Bluetooth (IEEE 802.15.1)	721 Kbps	10 m–150 m	2.4 GHz ISM
HiperLAN2	54 Mbps	150 m	5 GHz
HomeRF (Shared Wireless Access Protocol, SWAP)	1.6 Mbps (10 Mbps for Ver.2)	50 m	2.4 GHz ISM
DECT	32 kbps	100 m	1880–1900 MHz
PWT	32 kbps	100 m	1920–1930 MHz
IEEE 802.15.3 (high data rate wireless personal area network)	11–55 Mbps	1 m–50 m	2.4 GHz ISM
IEEE 802.16 (Local and Metropolitan Area Networks)	120 Mbps	City limits	2–66 GHz
IEEE 802.15.4 (low data rate wireless personal area network), Zigbee	250 kbps, 20 kbps, 40 kbps	100 m–300 m	2.4 GHz ISM, 868 MHz, 915 MHz ISM
IrDA	4 Mbps (IrDA-1.1)	2 m	IR (0.90 micro-meter)

It has been specifically designed as a low-cost, low-size, and low-power radio technology, which is particularly suited to the short range of a Personal Area Network (PAN). The main features of Bluetooth are: a) Real-time data transfer usually possible between 10–15 m, b) Support of point-to-point wireless connections without cables, as well as point-to-multipoint connections to enable ad hoc local wireless networks, c) data speed of 400 kb/s symmetrically or 700–150 kb/s of data asymmetrically. On the other hand, ZigBee (IEEE 802.15.4 standard) has been developed as a low data rate solution with multi-month to multiyear battery life and very low complexity. It is intended to operate in an unlicensed international frequency band. The maximum data rates for each band are 250, 40, and 20 kbps, respectively. The 2.4 GHz band operates worldwide while the sub-1-GHz band operates in North America, Europe, and Australia.

Pervasive healthcare systems set high demanding requirements regarding energy, size, cost, mobility, connectivity and coverage. Varying size and cost constraints directly result in corresponding varying limits on the energy available, as well as on computing, storage and communication resources. Low power requirements are necessary also from safety considerations since such systems run near or inside the body.

Mobility is another major issue for pervasive e-health applications because of the nature of users and applications and the easiness of the connectivity to other available wireless networks. Both off-body and personal area networks must not have line-of-sight (LoS) requirements. The various communication modalities can be used in different ways to construct an actual communication network. Two common forms are infrastructure-based networks and ad hoc networks. Mobile ad hoc networks represent complex systems that consist of wireless mobile nodes, which can freely and dynamically self-organize into arbitrary and temporary, "ad hoc" network topologies, allowing devices to seamlessly inter-network in areas with no pre-existing communication infrastructure or centralized administration. The effective range of the sensors attached to a sensor node defines the coverage area of a sensor node. With sparse coverage, only parts of the area of interest are covered by the sensor nodes. With dense coverage, the area of interest is completely (or almost completely) covered by sensors. The degree of coverage also influences information processing algorithms. High coverage is a key to robust systems and may be exploited to extend the network lifetime by switching redundant nodes to power-saving sleep mode.

5.2.3 Location Based Technologies

Positioning of individuals provides healthcare applications with the ability to offer services like supervision of elderly patients or those with mental illnesses who are ambulatory but restricted to a certain area. In addition, assisted care facilities can use network sensors and radiofrequency ID badges to alert staff members when patients leave a designated safety zone. Network or satellite positioning technology also can be used to quickly and accurately locate wireless subscribers in an emergency and communicate information about their location. Proximity information services can direct mobile users to a nearby healthcare facility. Location-based health information services can help find people with matching blood types, organ donors, and so on. A more extensive list of location-based health services can be found in [44].

Positioning techniques can be implemented in two ways: Self-positioning and remote positioning. In the first approach, equipment that the user uses (e.g., a mobile terminal, or a tagging device) uses signals, transmitted by the gateways/antennas (which can be either terrestrial or satellite) to calculate its own position. More specifically, the positioning receiver makes the appropriate signal measurements from geographically distributed transmitters and uses these measurements. Technologies that can be used are satellite based (e.g., the Global Positioning System (GPS) and assisted-GPS), or terrestrial infrastructure-based (e.g., using the cell id of a subscribed mobile terminal).

The second technique is called remote positioning. In this case the individual can be located by measuring the signals traveling to and from a set of receivers. More specifically, the receivers, which can be installed at one or more locations, measure a signal originating from, or reflecting off, the object to be positioned. These signal measurements are used to determine the length and/or direction of the individual radio paths, and then the mobile terminal position is computed from geometric relationships; basically, a single measurement produces a straight-line locus from the remote receiver to the mobile phone. Another Angle Of Arrival (AOA) measurement will yield a second straight line, the intersection of the two lines giving the position fix for this system. Time delay can also be utilized: Since electromagnetic waves travel at a constant speed (speed of light) in free space, the distance between two points can be easily estimated by measuring the time delay of a radio wave transmitted between them. This method is well suited for satellite systems and is used universally by them. Popular applications that are based on the latter technique for tracking provision are the Ekahau Positioning Engine [45], MS RADAR [46] and Nibble [47]. More information regarding positioning techniques and systems can be found in [43].

5.3 Introducing Intelligence in Electronic Healthcare Systems

This section presents technologies that enable the introduction of intelligence in electronic healthcare systems. Context-awareness, intelligent software agents, and advanced classification methods for medical data are discussed to cover this aspect.

5.3.1 Context Awareness

Context awareness is the capability of the networking applications to be aware of the existence and characteristics of the user's activities and environments. In rapidly changing scenarios, such as the ones considered in the fields of mobile, pervasive, or ubiquitous computing, systems have to adapt their behavior based on the current conditions and the dynamicity of the environment they are immersed in ([48]). A system is context-aware if it can extract, interpret and use context information and adapt its functionality to the current context of use. The challenge for such systems lies in the complexity of capturing, representing and processing contextual data. To capture context information generally some additional sensors and/or programs are required [28].

The way context-aware applications make use of context can be categorized into the three following classes: presenting information and services, executing a service, and tagging captured data.

Presenting information and services refers to applications that either present context information to the user, or use context to propose appropriate selections of actions to the user.

Automatically executing a service describes applications that trigger a command, or reconfigure the system on behalf of the user according to context changes.

Attaching context information for later retrieval refers to applications that tag captured data with relevant context information.

5.3.2 Intelligent Agents

Intelligent agents can be viewed as autonomous software (or hardware) constructs that are proactively involved in achieving a predetermined task and at the same time reacting to its environment. According to [49], agents are capable of:

- performing tasks (on behalf of users or other agents).
- interacting with users to receive instructions and give responses.
- operating autonomously without direct intervention by users, including monitoring the environment and acting upon the environment to bring about changes.
- showing intelligence – to interpret monitored events and make appropriate decisions.

Agents can be proactive, in terms of being able to exhibit goal-directed behavior, reactive; being able to respond to changes of the environment, including detecting and communicating to other agents, autonomous; making decisions and controlling their actions independent of others. Intelligent agents can be also considered as social entities where they can communicate with other agents using an agent-communication language in the process of carrying out their tasks.

In the context of pervasive healthcare, intelligent agents can contribute by analyzing patient and contextual information, distributing tasks to responsible individuals, inform users regarding special actions and circumstances.

5.3.3 Patient Data Classification Methods

Data classification is important problem in a variety of engineering and scientific disciplines such biology, psychology, medicine, marketing, computer vision, and artificial intelligence [50]. Its main object is to classify objects into a number of categories or classes. Depending on the application, these objects can be images or signal waveforms or any type of measurements that need to be classified. Given a specific data feature, its classification may consist of one of the following two tasks: a) supervised classification in which the input pattern is identified as a member of a predefined class; b) unsupervised classification in which the pattern is assigned to a hitherto unknown class.

In statistical data classification, input data are represented by a set of n features, or attributes, viewed as a n-dimensional feature vector. The classification system is operated in two modes: training and classification. Data preprocessing can be also performed in order to segment the pattern of interest from the background, remove noise, normalize the pattern, and any other operation which will contribute in defining a compact representation of the pattern. In the training mode, the feature extraction/selection module finds the appropriate features for representing the input patterns and the classifier is trained to partition the feature space. The feedback path allows a designer to optimize the preprocessing and feature extraction/selection strategies. In the classification mode, the trained classifier assigns the input pattern to one of the pattern classes under consideration based on the measured features.

There is a vast array of established classification techniques, ranging from classical statistical methods, such as linear and logistic regression, to neural network and tree-based techniques (e.g., feed-forward networks, which includes multilayer perception, Radial-Basis Function networks, Self-Organizing Map, or Kohonen-Networks), to the more recent Support Vector Machines. Other types of hybrid intelligent systems are neuro-fuzzy adaptive systems which can comprise of an adaptive fuzzy controller and a network-based predictor. More information regarding data classification techniques can be found in [50].

In the context of intelligent pervasive health systems, input classification data can be both biomedical signals, physiological and contextual data. Generated classification results can contain information concerning the status of a patient, suggested diagnosis, behavioral patterns, etc. In the following sections, pervasive healthcare systems that use such intelligent technologies are presented.

5.4 Intelligent Pervasive Healthcare Systems in Controlled Environments

Pervasive healthcare systems in controlled environments (i.e. in hospital or treatment centers) are mostly used for the advanced management of health information (e.g., patient health records, pharmaceutical information, etc.) and provision of location and context-aware services.

5.4.1 Intelligent Health Information Management

The transformation of healthcare intuitions to sophisticated computerized environments has resulted in the generation and transaction of volumes of healthcare information and knowledge for routine healthcare activities. Notwithstanding issues pertaining to the storage of volumes of healthcare information, there is an imminent need to address issues regarding effective information/knowledge utilization and management [5]. Pervasive healthcare information systems include services like:

- Secure user access to medical records at any time;
- Support for user queries about the medical centers, medical units, or doctors available in a certain area;
- Online booking for appointments with specialist doctors, whose offices, in turn, automatically receive the appropriate medical records for reference and updating.

Both patients and healthcare providers can benefit from pervasive access to healthcare information like lifetime clinical records. During a check-up, for example, patients could use a handheld device to upload their personal medical history and insurance data into their healthcare provider's database, reducing the effort required to enter such detailed information manually. Alternatively, such information could be downloaded from a Web-based health information system with proper authentication.

On the other hand, data like a single patient's healthcare history, workflows (i.e. procedures carried out on that patient), and logs (i.e. recording of meaningful procedural events) are often distributed among several heterogeneous and autonomous information systems. Different healthcare actors—including general practitioners, hospitals, and hospital departments—administer these information systems, form disconnected islands of information. Communication and coordination between organizations and among medical team members permits information sharing and distributed decision making. Thus, intelligent health information systems are essential in order to support such communication and information management. Agent-based techniques [7] often support this communication; modelling application components as somewhat autonomous agents easily reflects healthcare institutions' decentralized networks. Mobile and ubiquitous agent interfaces ([5, 31]) provide continuous and more direct access to the aforementioned information. A common

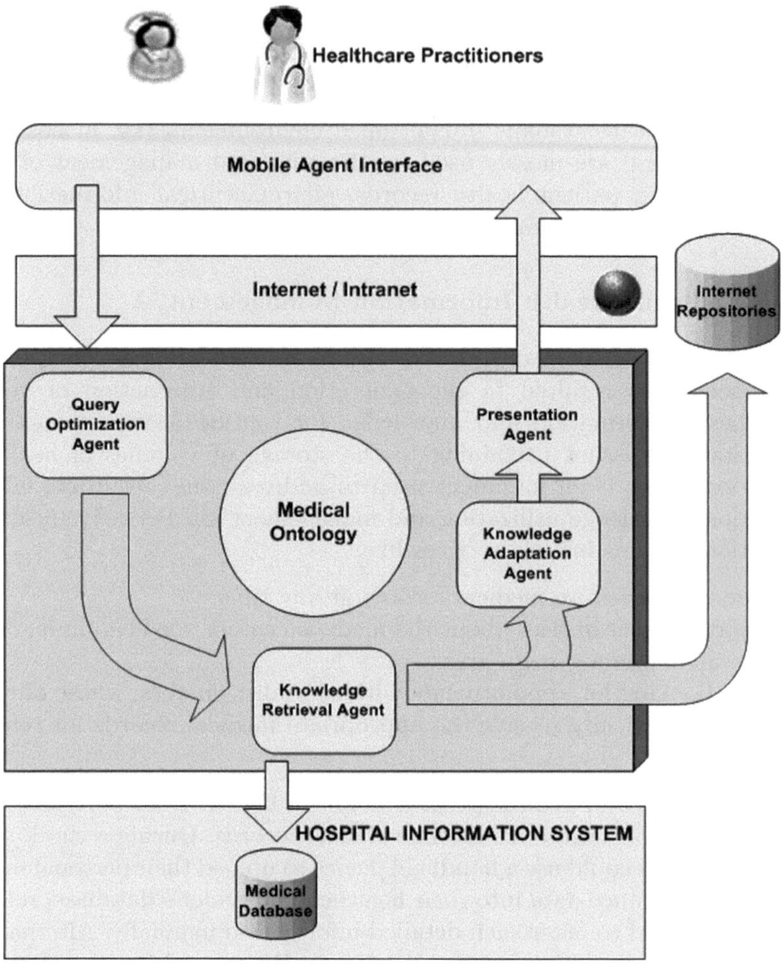

Fig. 5.3. An Intelligent Health Information Management System

architecture of an intelligent health management system is illustrated in Fig. 5.3. Software agents installed either on mobile devices (e.g., PDAs) or on interactive devices within the treatment center (e.g., LCD monitors, or smart walls [11]). Information retrieval and presentation can be either performed by user request or reactively (e.g., based on user's location or patient's state). Queries regarding patient data or medical information (e.g., medication procedures, diseases symptoms, etc.) are parsed through specific agents (i.e. query optimization agents) and forwarded to knowledge retrieval agents for research. The information retrieval can be performed either from the local hospital information system or remote medical knowledge repositories. Information retrieval, knowledge adaptation and presentation to the user are performed by related agents using medical ontologies for proper knowledge data representation [8].

Using such advanced knowledge representation and medical data retrieval methods, access to multiple healthcare information is feasible, even from mobile devices. Proper access restriction to sensitive information can be applied and direct access to important information in cases of emergency can be established [40].

5.4.2 Location and Context-aware Services

Location and context-aware services can optimize the treatment process by proper allocation of physicians according to the patients' status and location. Figure 5.4 illustrates the architecture of an intra-hospital intelligent pervasive system based on the aforementioned services. Location provision based on RFID and Bluetooth technology enables the intelligent distribution of medical personnel among patients which in turn, helps the nurses to gain time, which can be dedicated to the care of special patients, to learn or to prepare

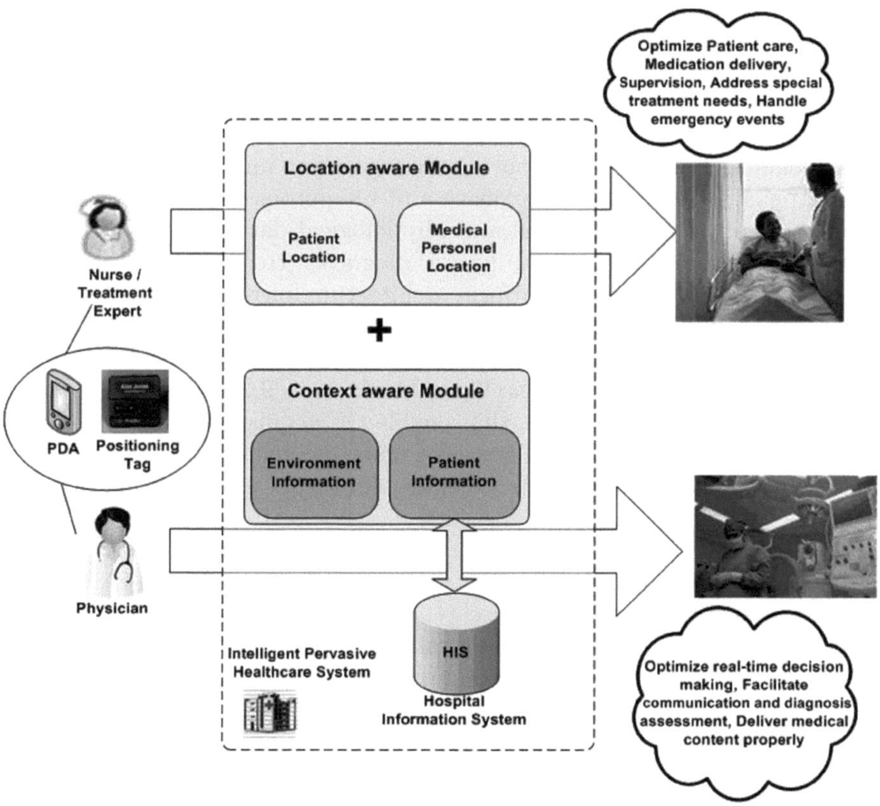

Fig. 5.4. Architecture of an intra-hospital intelligent pervasive system enabling location and context-aware services

new activities [1]. The time spent on supervision and control tasks is reduced substantially, as well as the time spent attending false alarms, while the time for direct patient care has been increased. Real-time decision making can be improved using mobile devices that facilitate communication between medical experts using location services and intelligent agents for smart retrieval of patient health records [2, 3]. Intra-hospital exchange of medical multimedia content between medical experts can be also facilitated through context-awareness. The QoS DREAM framework [4] is based on emergency event notification and location of patients/physicians in order to perform proper multimedia content (e.g., video and voice calls, patient image and video data, etc.) streaming. Using location and patient identification services, special entertainment can be delivered to the patients in addition to medication assistance (see "Context-aware Hospital Bed" and "Context-aware Pill Container" in [37]).

5.5 Intelligent Remote and Home-care Systems

Telemedicine systems enable the remote monitoring and treatment of patients and can be deployed either within the patient's environment (e.g., home), on areas where fully equipped medical facilities are unreachable (e.g., isolated areas, islands, etc.) and even on mobile treatment units (e.g., ambulances). The latter systems use also pervasive and ubiquitous devices for continuous monitoring of patient biological and physiological data. Intelligent technologies can be incorporated for the proper diagnosis, treatment and interaction with the patients. A typical platform architecture for remote treatment of patients, using intelligent pervasive technologies, is illustrated in Fig. 5.5. The major components are analyzed hereafter:

On-Body Monitoring Devices: Wearable devices ([9,22]) or sensors attached to the patient's body ([19, 25]), that enable the acquisition of biological data (e.g., ECG, temperature, blood pressure, blood oxygen saturation, respiration, etc.) ([10,16,18,23,26,36]) or physiological data (e.g., movement, location and weight) ([16, 23, 24, 26, 27, 30]).

Patient Area Devices: Devices like video cameras, microphones, proximity and temperature sensors, vibration sensors and respiration devices can be used for tracking a patient's state ([11, 13, 15, 18, 20, 21, 24]), location and behavior ([12, 13, 17, 24]). Smart interactivity devices (e.g., the Smart Table and Smart Frame in Fig. 5.6) can be used for advanced interaction with the patients, special tasks performance (e.g., medication program followup) and emergency communication [30].

Status Monitoring Module: Software modules or applications responsible for intelligent classification of the sensor data and emergency events detection. Adaptive neuro-fuzzy inference systems have been used in order to combine biological (i.e. ECG) and physiological data (i.e. physical activity) as an advanced method of measurement and prevention of cardiovascular diseases [16].

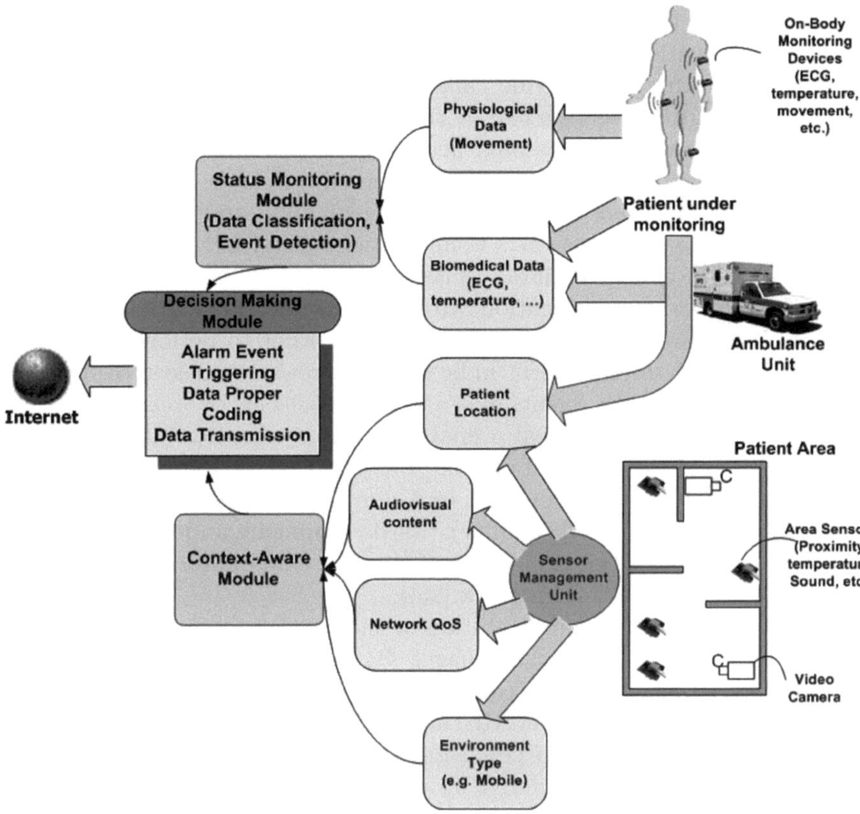

Fig. 5.5. A typical platform architecture for remote patient monitoring using intelligent pervasive systems

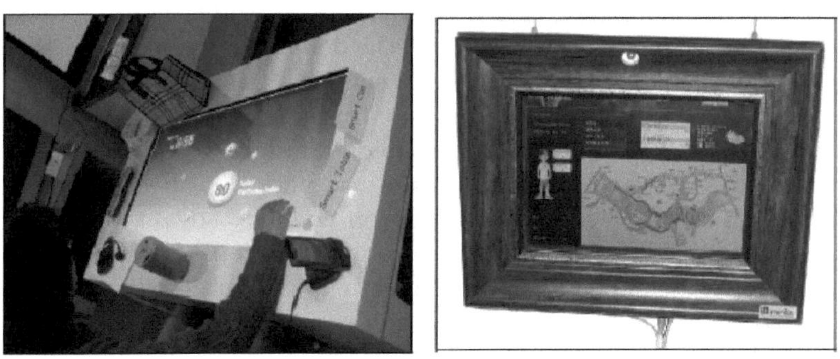

Fig. 5.6. Smart Table and Smart Frame prototypes for advanced pervasive interaction with the patient in a home environment [11]

Intelligent healthcare agents in combination to respiratory waveform ontology and fuzzy recognition agents, have been used in order to classify the respiratory waveform [21]. Home spirometers can be also used for periodically screening sirpometric data and detecting changes and trends that may indicate lung dysfunction [18]. Accelerometer data can be used to classify patient's daily activity and provide contextual information. ECG analysis and more precisely, QRS detection can be thus improved by dynamically selecting the leads with best SNR classified according to the activity type [23]. Additionally, intelligent processing of movement data can be successfully used for detection of emergency events (e.g., patient falls) and for general classification of movement types [27]. Using patient electronic health records in combination with biological data, decision making and alarm event triggering is possible. Proper communication with related care providers is also facilitated [10]. Software agents can also be used in order to perform distributed analysis of vital data and alarm indication to previously-selected physicians and family members [11]. Agents may also assist patients or treatment experts to perform basic tasks like meal preparation and medication [11, 12].

Context-Aware Module: Intelligent software that collects and interprets data from the patient's environment (e.g., environment type, location, audiovisual context, and network quality). Its development and deployment can be performed through the utilization of special middleware components and software agents (AGAPE framework [35]).

The presentation and interpretation of the contextual information can be done through domain-specific languages [34] or through ontological modeling ([36, 39]). Using the latter context information, detection of behavioral patterns of daily activity using Mixture models can assist diagnosis in conjunction to a person's health condition [13]. Special patterns can be built based on movement data acquired by motion sensors placed on site. Visual information consisting of body orientation calculated from posture extraction can trace periods of inactivity indicating an emergency status [15]. The latter information can also be used for tracking the actions of elders with dementia and assisting them in their daily activities [32]. Additionally, location and activity classification can be utilized for the detection of abnormalities in special groups, like the elderly [24]. Activity classification is also feasible from the measurement of floor vibration signals and usage of advanced signal processing techniques [20]. Collection of physiological signals and mapping of the latter to emotional states can synthesize the patient's affective information for the health-care provider [17]. Based on context, advanced collaborative environments can allow the optimized communication between sensitive patient groups (e.g., children) with treatment experts and family members [14]. Location tracking can provide information regarding the current ambient air quality of the patient's area and thus prevent possible morbidity of asthma during the patient's outdoor activities [26]. Similarly, patient tracking when traveling abroad can provide information regarding nearby treatment centers in case of an emergency [38].

Decision Making Module: It is the interface to a networked e-health system since it makes decision regarding the alarm event triggering, the patient data proper coding and the proper transmission of the latter to the monitoring units [33]. Based on information collected from the status monitoring and the context aware modules, selective transmission of the data is performed (e.g., only in cases of emergency), utilizing thus network and other (e.g., power) resources [28]. Furthermore, based on contextual information like network quality and patient state, proper data coding can be performed (e.g., compression or encryption) using advanced coding techniques (e.g., scalable video compression using H.264 coding [29]).

5.6 Conclusions and Future Challenges

The technological advances of the last few years in mobile communications, location- and context-aware computing has facilitated the introduction of pervasive healthcare applications. Healthcare can benefit from pervasive computing benefits in at least four ways:

- Enabling distributed access and processing of medical data;
- Lowering costs by getting appropriate care to the people who need it much faster than previously possible;
- Making expert care accessible to more people, thereby increasing the scale at which first-rate healthcare is applied; and
- Making healthcare more personalized, prompting individuals to take more responsibility for maintaining their health.

Location and Context-aware services in conjunction with intelligent patient status interpretation can offer advanced medical services to both patients and treatment practitioners. As discussed within this chapter, detection of emergency events can be performed in more sophisticated and direct ways, patient treatment can be optimized and transferred out of the hospital into the patient's site, collaboration between medical experts can optimize decision making, retrieval of patient information can be done in intelligent and ubiquitous ways, utilization of network and other resources can be achieved optimizing the whole telemedicine procedure.

However there are still issues and challenges that have to be addressed: First, most existing implementations do not interoperate sufficiently, resulting in segmented solutions. Moving to a fully pervasive system would be a complex transition requiring several steps and incremental budgetary increases to create the necessary infrastructure. This process should not interfere with the basic functioning of the current systems. Thus, usage of intelligent systems and methods, like context-awareness and agent environments must be enhanced with options and methods for overcoming such interoperability and collaboration issues. Privacy and security are also potential problems. Healthcare data should be available anytime anywhere, but only to authorized persons. Location privacy is also an important issue that is not sufficiently addressed in the development of pervasive healthcare systems. The usability of pervasive healthcare solutions is another challenge, at least in the near future. Those who are less technically savvy are generally willing to use intelligent mobile devices if these devices enrich their lives, give them more independence, and offer intuitive interfaces. Training healthcare professionals as well as patients to use such devices will become less problematic as handhelds and other wireless products become commonplace in society.

Regardless the remaining challenges, intelligent pervasive healthcare systems are anticipated to be expanded in the near future by using the most recent technological advances in a more active and direct way for offering more comprehensive and higher quality health services to citizens.

References

1. Juan M. Corchado, Javier Bajo, Yanira de Paz, Dante I. Tapia: Intelligent Environment for monitoring Alzheimer patients, agent technology for healthcare, to be published in Decision Support Systems, article available online at www.sciencedirect.com
2. Moushumi Sharmin, Shameem Ahmed, Ahamed S.I., Haque M.M., Khan A.J.: Healthcare aide: Towards a virtual assistant for doctors using pervasive middleware, In Proc. of Fourth Annual IEEE International Conference on Pervasive Computing and Communications Workshops (2006) 6–12.
3. Paganelli F., Spinicci E., Mamelli A., Bernazzani R., Barone P.: ERMHAN: A multi-channel context-aware platform to support mobile caregivers in continuous care networks, In Proc. of IEEE International Conference in Pervasive Technologies (2007) 355–360.
4. Scott Mitchell, Mark D. Spiteri, John Bates and George Coulouris: Context-Aware Multimedia Computing in the Intelligent Hospital, In Proc. SIGOPS EW2000, the Ninth ACM SIGOPS European Workshop (2000).
5. Zafar Iqbal Hashmi, Syed Sibte Raza Abidi, Yu-N Cheah: An Intelligent Agent-based Knowledge Broker for Enterprise-wide Healthcare Knowledge Procurement, 15th IEEE Symposium on Computer-Based Medical Systems (CBMS'02) 173.
6. A. Choudhri, L. Kagal, A. Joshi, T. Finin and Y. Yesha. PatientService : Electronic Patient Record Redaction and Delivery in Pervasive Environments. In Fifth International Workshop on Enterprise Networking and Computing in Healthcare Industry (2003).
7. Kifor, T., Varga, L., Vazquez-Salceda, J., Alvarez, S., Miles, S. and Moreau, L: Provenance in Agent-Mediated Healthcare Systems, *IEEE Intelligent Systems*, vol. 21, 6 (2006) 38–46.
8. Antonio Moreno, Aida Valls, David Isern, David Sanchez: Applying Agent Technology to Healthcare: The GruSMA Experience, *IEEE Intelligent Systems*, vol. 21, 6 (2006) 63–67.
9. David Malan, Thaddeus Fulford-Jones, Matt Welsh, and Steve Moulton: Code-Blue: An Ad Hoc Sensor Network Infrastructure for Emergency Medical Care, International Workshop on Wearable and Implantable Body Sensor Networks (2004).
10. Gouaux F., Simon-Chautemps L., Adami S., Arzi M., Assanelli D., Fayn J., Forlini M.C., Malossi C., Martinez A., Placide J., Ziliani G.L., Rubel P.: Smart

devices for the early detection and interpretation of cardiological syndromes, In 4th International IEEE EMBS Special Topic Conference on Information Technology Applications in Biomedicine (2003) 291–294.
11. Youngho Jeen, Jiyoung-Kim, Jaeil Park, Peom Park: Design and implementation of the Smart Healthcare Frame Based on Pervasive Computing Technology, In The 9th International Conference on Advanced Communication Technology (2007) 349–352.
12. Camarinha-Matos L.M., Vieira W.: Intelligent mobile agents in elderly care, Robotics and Autonomous Systems, 27 (1999) 59–75.
13. Tracy S. Barger, Donald E. Brown and Majd Alwan: Health-Status Monitoring Through Analysis of Behavioral Patterns, In IEEE Transactions on Systems, Man and Cybernetics, 35, 1 (2005) 22–27.
14. Starida K., Ganiatsas G., Fotiadis D.I., Likas A.: CHILDCARE: a collaborative environment for the monitoring of children healthcare at home, In 4th International IEEE EMBS Special Topic Conference on Information Technology Applications in Biomedicine (2003) 169–172.
15. Jansen Bart, Deklerck Rudi: Context aware inactivity recognition for visual fall detection, In Pervasive Health Conference and Workshops (2006) 1–4.
16. Jatoba L., Grossmann U., Ottenbacher J., Stork W., Muller-Glaser K.: Development of a Self-Constructing Neuro-Fuzzy Inference System for Online Classification of Physical Movements, In 9th International Conference on e-Health Networking, Application and Services (2007) 332–335.
17. C. Lisetti, F. Nasoz, C. LeRouge, O. Ozyera and K. Alvarez: Developing multimodal intelligent affective interfaces for tele-home health care International Journal of Human-Computer Studies 59 (2003) 245–255.
18. Jannett T.C., Prashanth S., Mishra S., Ved V., Mangalvedhekar A., Deshpande J.: An intelligent telemedicine system for remote spirometric monitoring. In Proceedings of the Thirty-Fourth Southeastern Symposium on System Theory (2002) 53–56.
19. Dolgov A.B., Zane R.: Low-Power Wireless Medical Sensor Platform, In 28th Annual International Conference of the IEEE Engineering in Medicine and Biology Society (2006) 2067–2070.
20. Ruqiang Yan, Robert X. Gao: An efficient approach to machine health diagnosis based on harmonic wavelet packet transform Robotics and Computer-Integrated Manufacturing 21 (2005) 291–301.
21. Chang-Shing Lee, Mei-Hui Wang: Ontology-based intelligent healthcare agent and its application to respiratory waveform recognition Expert Systems with Applications 33 (2007) 606–619.
22. Sokwoo Rhee, Boo-Ho Yang, Kuowei Chang and Hamhiko H. Asada: The Ring Sensor: A New Ambulatory Wearable Sensor for Twenty-Four Hour Patient Monitoring, In Proceedings of the 20th Annual International Conference of the IEEE Engineering in Medicine and Biology Society 20, 4 (1998) 1906–1909.
23. Li Huaming, Tan Jindong: Body Sensor Network Based Context Aware QRS Detection, In Pervasive Health Conference and Workshops (2006) 1–8.
24. Jacques Demongeot, Gilles Virone, Florence Duchêne, Gila Benchetrit, Thierry Hervé, Norbert Noury, Vincent Rialle: Multi-sensors acquisition, data fusion, knowledge mining and alarm triggering in health smart homes for elderly people, C. R. Biologies 325 (2002) 673–682.

25. Aleksandar Milenkovic, Chris Otto, Emil Jovanov: Wireless sensor networks for personal health monitoring: Issues and an implementation, Computer Communications 29 (2006) 2521–2533.
26. Hsueh-Ting Chu, Chir-Chang Huang, Zhi-Hui Lian, Tsai J.J.P: A ubiquitous warning system for asthma-inducement, In IEEE International Conference on Sensor Networks, Ubiquitous, and Trustworthy Computing (2006) 186–191.
27. Charalampos Doukas, Ilias Maglogiannis, Philippos Tragas, Dimitris Liapis, Gregory Yovanof: A Patient Fall Detection System based on Support Vector Machines, In Proc. of 4th IFIP Conference on Artificial Intelligence Applications & Innovations (2007) 147–156.
28. C. Doukas, I. Maglogiannis, G. Kormentzas: Advanced Telemedicine Services through Context-aware Medical Networks, In International IEEE EMBS Special Topic Conference on Information Technology Applications in Biomedicine (2006).
29. C. Doukas, T. Pliakas, I. Maglogiannis: Advanced Scalable Medical Video Transmission based on H.264 Temporal and Spatial Compression, Presented at 2007 IEEE Africon Conference (2007).
30. Vince Stanford: Using Pervasive Computing to Deliver Elder Care, IEEE Pervasive Computing 1 (2002) 10–13.
31. Lakshmi Narasimhan V., Irfan M., Yefremov M.: MedNet: A pervasive patient information network with decision support, In 6th International Workshop on Enterprise Networking and Computing in Healthcare Industry (2004) 96–101.
32. Alex Mihailidis, Brent Carmichael and Jennifer Boger: The Use of Computer Vision in an Intelligent Environment to Support Aging-in-Place, Safety, and Independence in the Home, IEEE Transactions On Information Technology In Biomedicine 8, 3 (2004) 238–247.
33. Tadj Chakib, Hina Manolo Dulva, Ramdane-Cherif Amar, Ngantchaha Ghislain: The LATIS Pervasive Patient Subsystem: Towards a Pervasive Healthcare System, In ISCIT '06. International Symposium on Communications and Information Technologies (2006) 851–856.
34. Jennifer Munnelly, Siobh'an Clarke: ALPH: a domain-specific language for crosscutting pervasive healthcare concerns, In Proceedings of the 2nd workshop on Domain specific aspect languages (2007) 4.
35. Bottazzi D., Corradi A., Montanari R.: Context-aware middleware solutions for anytime and anywhere emergency assistance to elderly people, IEEE Communications Magazine 44, 4 (2006) 82–90.
36. Dong-Oh Kang, Hyung-Jik Lee, Eun-Jung Ko, Kyuchang Kang and Jeunwoo Lee: A Wearable Context Aware System for Ubiquitous Healthcare, In 28th Annual International Conference of the IEEE Engineering in Medicine and Biology Society (2006) 5192–5195.
37. Jakob E. Bardram: Applications of context-aware computing in hospital work: examples and design principles, Proceedings of the 2004 ACM symposium on Applied computing (2004) 1574–1579.
38. Kim Hwa-Jong, Jo Heui-Sug: A Context-Aware Traveler Healthcare Service (THS) System, In Pervasive Health Conference and Workshops (2006) 1–3.
39. Eun-Jung Ko, Hyung-Jik Lee, Jeon-Woo Lee: Ontology-Based Context-Aware Service Engine for U-HealthCare, In The 8th International Conference of : Advanced Communication Technology (2006) 632–637.

40. Choudhri A., Kagal L., Joshi A., Finin T., Yesha Y.: PatientService: electronic patient record redaction and delivery in pervasive environments, In 5th International Workshop on Enterprise Networking and Computing in Healthcare Industry (2003) 41–47.
41. Upkar Varshney: Pervasive Healthcare, IEEE Computer Magazine 36 12 (2003) 138–140.
42. Birnbaum, J.: Pervasive information systems, Communications of the ACM 40, 2 (1997) 40–41.
43. Vasileios Zeimpekis, George M. Giaglis, George Lekakos: A taxonomy of indoor and outdoor positioning techniques for mobile location services, ACM SIGecom Exchanges 3, 4 (2003) 19–27.
44. Lee Shih-wei, Cheng Shao-you, Hsu Jane Yung-jen, Huang Polly, You Chuang-wen: Emergency Care Management with Location-Aware Services, In Pervasive Health Conference and Workshops (2006) 1–6.
45. Ekahau LBS, http://www.ekahau.com (available at http://www.ekahau.com, accessed on September 26, 2005).
46. Bahl P and Padmanabhan V.N: RADAR: An In-Building RF-based User Location and Tracking System, INFOCOM IEEE Press (2000) 775–784.
47. Castro P, Chiu P, Kremenek T. and Muntz R.: A Probabilistic Room Location Service for Wireless Networked Environments, Proceedings of the 3rd international conference on Ubiquitous Computing – UBICOMP (2001) 18–34.
48. Kavi Kumar Khedo: Context-Aware Systems for Mobile and Ubiquitous Networks, International Conference on Networking, International Conference on Systems and International Conference on Mobile Communications and Learning Technologies (2006) 123.
49. John Fox, Martin Beveridge, David Glasspool: Understanding intelligent agents: analysis and synthesis, AI Communications – IOS Press 16, 3 (2003) 139–152.
50. Jun-Hai Zhai, Su-Fang Zhang, Xi-Zhao Wang: An Overview of Pattern Classification Methodologies, In Proceedings of the Fifth International Conference on Machine Learning and Cybernetics (2006) 3222–3227.
51. Enderle J., Blanchard S., Bronzino J.: Introduction to Biomedical Engineering. Second edition. Burlington MA: Elsevier Academic Press Series (2005).

6

An Agent Middleware for Ubiquitous Computing in Healthcare

Marcela D. Rodríguez[1] and Jesús Favela[2]

[1] Facultad de Ingeniería, UABC, Mexicali, México
marcerod@uabc.mx
[2] Ciencias de la Computación, CICESE, Ensenada, México
favela@cicese.mx

Summary. Healthcare environments are characterized by the need for coordination and collaboration among specialists with different areas of expertise, the integration of data from many devices or artifacts and the mobility of hospital staff, patients, documents, and equipment. Ubiquitous computing (ubicomp) enable us to meet these characteristics of medical environment. Ubiquitous computing environments are spaces where computational artifacts are invisible, become present whenever we need them, are adaptive to mobile users, can be enabled by simple and effortless interactions, and act autonomously to support users' activities. We have proposed using software agents to implement these characteristics of a ubiquitous computing system with the aim of enhancing medical activities. Then, we created the SALSA middleware to facilitate the implementation of these agents for ubiquitous computing systems for healthcare environments. In our approach, autonomous agents can represent users, act as proxies to devices and information resources, or wrap a complex system functionality. The SALSA middleware enables developers to create autonomous agents that react to the contextual elements of the medical environment and that communicate with other agents, users and services available in the environment. We used the SALSA middleware for creating the Context-aware Hospital Information System. This chapter presents the SALSA middleware and how it facilitates the development of ubiquitous computing system for healthcare, in which the main systems components were conceived as autonomous agents.

6.1 Introduction

Medical activities in healthcare environments, such as hospitals, are characterized by the need for coordination and collaboration among specialists with different areas of expertise, the integration of data from many devices or artifacts and the mobility of hospital staff, patients, documents, and equipment. Hospital staff demands to promptly extract useful pieces of data from different artifacts to perform their work. The right information has to be in the right place, whenever it is needed by whoever needs it, in whatever representation they need it. With ubiquitous computing (ubicomp)

M.D. Rodríguez and J. Favela: *An Agent Middleware for Ubiquitous Computing in Healthcare*, Studies in Computational Intelligence (SCI) **107**, 117–149 (2008)
www.springerlink.com

technology is feasible to meet these medical environment needs. Ubiquitous computing environments are spaces where computational artifacts are invisible, become present whenever we need them, are adaptive to mobile users, can be enabled by simple and effortless interactions, and act autonomously to support users' activities. We have proposed using software agents to implement these characteristics of a ubiquitous computing system with the aim of enhancing medical activities.

Agent technology has been used to create systems with a specific focus on improving the management of clinical information by reporting the patients' status to the doctor' devices; by enabling the construction of unified medical repositories, or by merging organizational knowledge from various hospitals. However, these systems do not address the challenges related to the implementation of ubiquitous computing environments, such as taking into account the context of users for presenting and adapting the clinical information, neither do they address the need to access the medical information from multiple and heterogeneous computing devices. We have used autonomous agents for dealing with these challenges and created a middleware, named SALSA, to facilitate the implementation of these agents for ubiquitous computing systems for healthcare environments. The SALSA middleware enables developers to create autonomous agents that react to the contextual elements of the medical environment, communicate agents with other agents, users and services available in the environment; communicate different types of medical information; and implement agents that represent users, act as proxies to devices and information resources, or wrap a complex system functionality.

In the next section, we present the characteristics of healthcare environments; we introduce the area of ubiquitous computing and the concept of autonomous agents. Section 6.2 presents the advantages of using autonomous agents for creating ubiquitous computing systems from three points of view: Software Engineering, Distributed Systems and Human-Computer Interaction. In Section 6.3 we present several Multi-agents systems created for supporting medical activities. Section 6.4 describes how ubiquitous computing can enhance medical practices. Section 6.5 presents the design issues regarding the functionality of autonomous agents for creating ubiquitous computing systems. Based on these design issues, was developed the SALSA Middleware which is described in Section 6.6. To illustrate the programming facilities of SALSA, Section 6.7 describes how the Context-aware Hospital Information System was created with SALSA. Finally, Section 6.8 presents our conclusions of using SALSA for the development of ubiquitous computing systems for healthcare settings.

6.1.1 Characteristics of Healthcare Environments

Information management and communication in a hospital setting is characterized by a high degree of collaborative work, mobility, and the integration of data from many devices or artifacts [1]. Exchanges of information are intense, and demands that participants promptly extract useful pieces of data from the artifacts to perform their job. In contrast with other settings such a control rooms [2], information in hospitals is not generally concentrated in a single place but distributed among a collection of artifacts in different locations. For instance, patients' records are maintained and used in coordination with data on whiteboards, computers, or binders located in rooms, labs, common areas or offices. Following Bossen we might say that for practical purposes the whole hospital becomes the information space and it is by "navigating" this space that hospital's staff can get the data to perform effectively [3]. Given the high distribution of information together with the intensive nature of the work, it is clear that tremendous coordination efforts are required from all members of the hospital staff to properly manage the information to attend and take care of patients. The right information has to be in the right place, whenever it is needed by whoever needs it, in whatever format (representation) they need it. Hence the characteristics of artifacts containing information play a fundamental role to achieve this coordination. For instance, patient's records are easily moved from place to place and filled, checked, read and consulted in many locations like nurses' room, analysis labs, or the actual bed where the patient is being attended; nurses, physicians and other workers interact with those records and use them to support their work or to transmit instructions to be followed by others. To have the patient's records at the right place is in part what makes them successful in supporting coordination, as well as the fact that the information contained in them is clear, complete, accurate, and updated. Unfortunately those conditions are not always achieved. Documents get lost, instructions are not clear, or the data is not complete to support decisions.

Physicians, who are in a continuous learning process through their daily practice, are motivated to seek information to reduce the uncertainty of the route they ought to follow for the patient's treatment when faced with a complex clinical case [4,5]. Hospitals provide medical guides to be consulted by the physicians. However, given their current workloads, they seldom have the time to search for information on the local medical guide or in medical digital libraries. On the other hand, doctors often use information from previous clinical cases in their decision-making. For this, they might rely on their own experience or consult other colleagues who are more experienced in a given subject, or just to have a second opinion. Physicians, however, seldom consult the clinical records of previous patients, to a large extent because they are difficult to locate, or because the data that could be used to retrieve them, such as the patient's name or the date of a given case, are difficult to recall. The development of hospital information systems that provide access to electronic patient records is a step in the direction of providing accurate and timely information to hospital staff in support for adequate decision-making.

Providing adequate support for managing information in hospital settings requires technological designs that are based on a proper assimilation of the context where the hospital's staff performs their job. Ubiquitous computing technology enables us to meet with these medical environment requirements.

6.1.2 Ubiquitous Computing

Beyond the era of personal computing, ubiquitous computing begins with the vision of decentralizing computing power: The computer is omnipresent becoming a part of everyday life and an inevigtable component when performing a variety of private and business related tasks [6]. Devices of many forms and sizes enable users to exchange and retrieve information they need quickly, efficiently, and effortlessly from everywhere at any time. This was the vision of Mark Weiser in 1991 which led to diverse unresolved issues that must be addressed before ubiquitous computing truly reaches its goal of improving our everyday lives [7]. Ubiquitous computing involves a new way of thinking about computers, one that takes into account the human world and allows computers to vanish into the background. The vision of a future ubiquitous computing landscape is dominated by the pervasiveness of a vast manifold of heterogeneous computing devices, the autonomy of their programmed behavior, the dynamicity and context-awareness of services and applications they offer, the ad-hoc interoperability of services and the different modes of user interaction upon those services [8]. Today a variety of terms –like Ubiquitous Computing (ubicomp), Pervasive Computing, Calm Computing, Invisible Computing, Ambient Intelligence (AmI), Sentient Computing and Post-PC Computing – refer to new paradigms for interaction among users and mobile and embedded computing devices [9]. Thus, ubiquitous computing is the attempt to modify the traditional human-computer interaction paradigm not only by distributing computers, of all scales, into the environment surrounding users, but by augmenting work practices, knowledge sharing, and communication of users. For this, computers should be able to use implicit situational information, or context, to provide useful services and relevant information whenever users need them [10].

Context-aware computing refers to an application's ability to adapt to changing circumstances and respond based on the context of use. A system is context-aware if it uses context to provide relevant information and/or services to the user, where relevancy depends on the user's task. Dey defined context as "any information that can be used to characterize the situation of an entity, which can be a person, place, or object that is considered relevant between a user and the application, including the user and application themselves" [10]. Among the main types of contextual information considered relevant are identity, time, activity, and location which are known as primary context [10, 11]. This information answers the questions of who, when, what, and where, which can be used to identify whether a specific piece of information is relevant to establish context. Thus, the ubiquitous computing environment should be aware of the user's context to provide information and services whenever users need them, in a proactive fashion and anticipating user's needs. Furthermore, the services provided by the environment have to be accessible to diverse and non-specialist users through simple and effortless interactions. For this, human computer interaction promises to support more sophisticated and natural input and output, to enable users to perform potentially complex tasks more quickly, with greater accuracy, and to improve user satisfaction.

From the previous explanation it can be stated that ubiquitous computing environments are characterized by:

1) the distribution of their devices and services,
2) the high mobility of users,
3) the need to opportunistically access information, services and devices available in the environment,
4) and finally, the implicit and natural interactions of users with the ubiquitous computing environment.

Ubiquitous computing environments require software components that enable the above characteristics. These software components need to seamlessly establish connections and communicate among themselves in a transparent way to provide the services required by the users; the software components should be reactive to the environment and the users' context in order to enable them to opportunistically access pervasive computing resources. For this, the components need to be perceptive to context changes which are highly dynamic due the mobility of users; through adaptive components the environment can learn from the user's interaction in order to adapt its behavior to the users' needs; and finally the components need to act autonomously freeing users to explicitly access the ubiquitous computing resources and decide how to act in order to enhance the users' activities. Thus ubiquitous computing environments are characterized by the collaboration, reactivity, adaptability and autonomy of their software components and in this sense, they share many characteristics with agents. For this reason, we propose using autonomous agents as the software components or main constructs to deal with the challenges in realizing the ubiquitous computing vision for hospitals.

6.1.3 Autonomous Agents

A software agent is a software entity that acts on behalf of someone to carry out a particular task which has been delegated to it. To do this, an agent might be able to infer users' preferences and/or needs by taking into account the peculiarities of users and situation. This definition is based on the notion of agenthood as an ascription made by some person [12]. Other researchers provide a definition of a software agent based on a description of the attributes that an agent may need to act on behalf of someone or something else. Under this approach, each agent might possess a greater or lesser degree of attributes which have to be consistent with the requirements of a particular problem. Some of these attributes are the following: autonomy (to act on their own), re-activity (to respond to changes in the environment), pro-activity (to reach goals), cooperation (with other agents to efficiently and effectively solve tasks), adaptation (to learn from experience) and mobility (to migrate to new places) [12, 13]. For some researchers, particularly those working in Artificial Intelligence (AI), the term "agent" has a stronger meaning than the one presented above. By agent they mean a computer system that in addition to the properties identified above, is conceptualized using terms that are usually applied to humans. Thus, it is quite common in AI to characterize an agent using mentalist notions, such as knowledge, beliefs, desires, intentions or obligations [13]. As the aim of our work is to determine if autonomous agents are an appropriate metaphor for designing and implementing ubiquitous computing systems, the following section presents an analyses of the advantages of using autonomous agents from the perspective of different areas involved in the building of ubiquitous computing systems, such as Software Engineering, Distributed Systems and Human-Computer Interaction.

6.2 Advantages of Using Software Agents for Building Ubiquitous Computing Systems

Software agents have been introduced in many fields of computer science. This makes the term elusive, since some authors emphasize their distributed nature while others think about agents from the perspective of being able to exhibit intelligent behavior. Since ubiquitous computing is a multidisciplinary field, it can take advantage of the use of agents from these different perspectives. We describe these perspectives of software agents and their relevance to the design of ubiquitous computing systems.

6.2.1 Software Engineering and the Agent-oriented Approach

From the software engineering perspective, an agent is seen as a computer system situated in some environment and capable of flexible, autonomous action in that environment in order to meet its design objectives [14]. The role of software engineering is to provide structures and techniques that make it easier to handle complexity. One approach for doing this is to adopt an agent-oriented approach which means decomposing a problem into multiple, autonomous software components that can act and interact in flexible ways to achieve their objectives. Autonomous agents are software components that offer greater flexibility and adaptability than traditional components [15]. In the rest of this document, the term "components" will be used to refer to the main building blocks that form part of a ubiquitous computing system.

6.2.2 Distributed Systems and Multi-agent Systems

From the Distributed Systems stance, the technology of autonomous agents appears appropriate for building systems in which data, control, expertise, or resources are distributed; agents provide a natural metaphor for delivering system functionality [16]. Agents and multi-agent systems have been used as a metaphor to model complex distributed processes. While the area of multi-agent systems addresses distributed tasks, distributed systems support distributed information and processes. In short, multi-agent systems are often distributed systems, and distributed systems are platforms to support multi-agent systems. One characteristic of ubiquitous computing systems is that they should provide services and information whenever users need them. For this, implementing a ubiquitous computing environment as a multi-agent system hides the fact that devices, services and information are disseminated all over the physical environment and makes it possible to create an environment with autonomous components that provide largely invisible support for tasks performed by users, for which the components may require interacting to achieve their objectives. However, in a ubiquitous computing environment it is impossible to a priori know about all potential interactions that may occur at unpredictable times, for unpredictable reasons, between unpredictable components. As agents are components with the ability to initiate and respond to interactions in a flexible manner [17], the agent oriented approach can be the natural way to deal with unpredictable associations and interactions among ubiquitous computing systems' components.

6.2.3 Agents in Human-Computer Interaction

Finally, autonomous agents have been used to change the way people interact with computers which has been referred to as indirect management [18]. In this approach, the agent is a personal assistant that gradually becomes more effective as it learns about the user's interests [19]. Thus, from the Human-Computer Interaction (HCI) viewpoint, autonomous agents can be used to implement a complementary style of interaction [19]. Agents can also radically change the style of human-computer interaction and enhance collaboration in ubiquitous computing environments. The metaphor used is that of a personal assistant who is collaborating with the user in the same work environment. Autonomous agents can assist users in a variety of different ways: they hide the complexity of difficult tasks, they perform tasks on the user's behalf, they can train or teach the user, they help different users collaborate, and they monitor events and procedures. One of the major research directions for Human-Computer Interaction (HCI) has been exploring the novel forms of interaction that can achieve Mark Weiser's vision of naturally integrating computer technology with our daily activities. In this sense, autonomous agents can seamlessly assist users in their interactions with the ubiquitous computing environment. For this, autonomous agents can learn of the users' interactions to infer their preferences and continuously be aware of their contexts in order to be responsiveness to their activities.

6.3 Multi-agent Systems in Healthcare

Agent technology has been used to create systems with a specific focus on improving the management of clinical information within a hospital. For instance, PalliaSys is a multiagent system that collects information about the status of palliative patients and reports it to a doctor. This system enables physicians to consult medical information through different communication technologies, such as mobile phones, PDAs and computers [20]. In [21] an adaptable agent-based system is proposed to aid the medical staff in analyzing the data of diabetic patients which could be previously downloaded from the patient's PDA. In [22] is presented an agent-mediated Organ Transplant Management Application (OTMA) which is provenance-awareness. In this system it was used autonomous agents to enable users to trace how particular results were reached. With OTMA, users (physicians) can extract valuable information to validate steps in a medical process or audit the system over time; for instance, the transplant coordinator can ask OTMA questions related to either a given patient (donor or recipient) or a given organ's fate.

Other research projects have focused on providing support for the management of clinical information that may be distributed among the different hospitals and departments within a hospital. In [23] a multi-agent system is presented that physicians may use to access multiple and heterogeneous medical data sources available at the hospital, in a transparent way. This system enables the proactive construction of unified medical repositories which may contain a wide range of data type, such as video, images, and text. A multi-agent community works autonomously, gathering data from the operational systems, and applying procedures for transforming the data which is then written to a patient record repository. In [24] the use of agents along with grid technology is proposed to merge organizational knowledge from various hospitals. While agents deal with the management of information, such as retrieving and presenting information, grid technology copes with issues of security, such as authentication and authorization services. In [25] the concept of ubiquitous healthcare is introduced that refers to the disposition of any type of health service such that individual consumers can access them through mobile computing devices. This work presents the OnkoNet initiative which proposes developing a multi-agent system for cancer treatments. This system will enable authorized persons/institutions to store, maintain, retrieve and access medical data by using local and mobile devices in order to integrate all patients' information related to diagnosis, therapy and care. Other work proposes to use mobile-agent technology to cope with the security-enhanced gathering of inter-institutional and distributed medical data [26].

Agents have also been used for dealing with other challenges in providing better healthcare services, such as monitoring the state of a patient, providing assistance services to remote patients, and the care of disabled and senior people. These projects selected agents as the main system's components that exhibit dynamic changes and autonomous behavior. For instance, the e-Tools project uses sensors, wireless communications devices and agent technology to provide supportive services to people with disabilities. One such e-Tool is an electric-powered wheelchair in which a multi-agent system autonomously controls its behavior, monitors the state of the patient, interacts with him/her through an interface that provides assistance in navigation, and sends messages indicating the state of the patient to the PDA of the patient's caregivers and relatives [27]. The AINGERU project proposes a multi-agent system for offering tele-assistance services to elderly people. This system consists of agents running on the patient's PDA, in charge of monitoring the patient's health condition and communicating with other agents residing in the healthcare center which perform other tasks, such as appointment negotiation [28].

Most of the projects presented support the management of patient information by means of the use of software agents that have well defined objectives and that must collaborate among themselves to support different activities related to the management of medical information. Thus, through a multi-agent system these information management tasks are transparent to the users. To do this, these systems provide agents at different system's layers. For instance, all of them provide agents at the user interface layer, that interprets the user's request or that present the information to them. Then, agents at a higher layer are in charge of extracting this information and passing it to the interface agents in order to be presented to the user. The use of agents enabled these projects to cope with the distribution and heterogeneity of clinical information. In spite of the fact that some of the above projects introduce the concept of AmI or ubiquitous computing for healthcare, these systems do not address other challenges related to the implementation of ubiquitous computing environments, such as taking into account the context of users for presenting and adapting the clinical information, neither do they address the need to access the medical information from multiple and heterogeneous computing devices. However, providing systems such as the one previously presented is a step towards creating a ubiquitous healthcare computing system. An infrastructure that supports the integration and retrieval of clinical information facilitates the introduction of pervasive and context-aware systems that enable the opportunistic access of medical information.

In our approach, we have explored the use of autonomous agents for designing ubiquitous computing systems for healthcare settings, and for making the design decisions for a middleware that facilitates the development of these autonomous agents.

6.4 Context-aware and Ubiquitous Computing Technology to Enhance Medical Practices

Ubiquitous computing technology, that includes devices such as handhelds computers and large public displays, can provide timely access to medical information and services thru a context-aware system. A ubiquitous and context-aware computing environment can enhance the medical activities of the mobile hospital staff by directly addressing those contextual elements which characterize them.

A ubiquitous computing system can also be able to provide timely access to medical knowledge thru context-aware information retrieval. It is evident that in the health-care domain, vast quantities of medical information are now available through the web and can easily lead to information overload [29]. One way to overcome such a problem is to provide an environment that proactively retrieves and presents information based on the hospital professionals' context [30]. Context-aware computing technology is a key element to construct this new generation of Web retrieval systems by sensing the changes in the users' activities, to predict users' interests and then, retrieve information based on them. Ubiquitous and context-aware computing technology may provide support to healthcare professionals for opportunistically acquiring, managing, and sharing knowledge, which are issues faced everyday by hospital workers.

The following are the desirable features to be addressed through ubiquitous computing systems in order to support the characteristics of healthcare environments described in Section 6.1.1.

6.4.1 Context-aware Communication and Activity Coordination

There are four critical contextual elements that a context-aware system has to consider in supporting the hospital's activity coordination and information management [31]:

1. *Location.* Where hospital staff members are at a particular time determines in part the type of information they require. For example, access to a patient's medical records is most relevant when the doctor or nurse is with that patient.
2. *Delivery timing.* Communication exchanges in a hospital tend to be time sensitive, which means that a message might be relevant for only a certain period. For example, a doctor might leave a message that describes recommendations for treatment to any nurse on the next shift.
3. *Role reliance.* In hospitals, parties who might be strangers or rarely meet must communicate with each other. A user often addresses messages not to particular individuals but to "the nurse on the afternoon shift," or "the next doctor to visit the patient." Thus, the system must be able to recognize roles as well as particular individuals.
4. *Artifact location and state.* An artifact, particularly a device, can have many states. The state of devices (temperature reading) and other artifacts (availability of lab results) can be important triggers for appropriate actions, including information exchanges. Medical staff might need to communicate directly with documents or devices. For example, a doctor might want to display the patient's lab analysis on her office desktop as soon as results become available.

6.4.2 User's Location and Authentication

Hospitals are characterized by the mobility of the professionals that work there and that of the artifacts they use, such as clinical records or medical equipment, and even that of the patients, who are moved from one hospital area to another as required. When a doctor examines a patient, he needs to move to obtain the patient's clinical records and other documents. Hospital workers also need to move to locate information displayed in whiteboards. For instance, the schedule of patient's operations for the current day is displayed on the whiteboard in the office of the chief surgeon, and the activities and working area assigned to nurses are advertised in different boards throughout the hospital. Boards help to communicate information regarding patients' condition and location, and hospital staff often visit the boards to find this information. Thus, hospital workers require access to information from anywhere within the hospital. For instance, a public display should be able to recognize the user as he approaches it and give him access to relevant clinical data without cumbersome login procedures.

6.4.3 Content Adaptation and Personalization based on Contextual Information

Contextual information such as, location, role, and identity should be taken into account to adapt and personalize the presentation of information to the user. For instance, when a physician is in front of public display, the pervasive environment should display the messages addressed to him and enable him to visualize the patients' records he is examining. Thus, information overload is prevented by personalizing the display to provide immediate access to the clinical records of those patients assigned to the doctor [32].

6.4.4 Information Transfer between Heterogeneous Devices

In the hospital, users frequently transfer information from public spaces to personal spaces. For instance, the chief nurse might leave a note on a public board in order to advertise the date of the next meeting; then, another nurse would write this information into her personal agenda. A few physicians actually carry PDA's and reported using them to record information displayed on whiteboards or corkboards. A pervasive environment furnished with devices of all scales, should support the simple and safe transfer of information between devices of different scales. Some of these devices are public, such as large displays, while others are personal, such as PDAs. For instance, a doctor may want to transfer information from his PDA to a public display in order to discuss it with a colleague; and when the doctor approaches the board and is authenticated, the display will use information stored in the user's PDA to personalize the information and applications running in the public display.

6.4.5 Context-aware Retrieval of Medical Information

The electronic patient record offers the opportunity to retrieve relevant medical cases with little effort from the user. To retrieve this information, the pervasive environment has to take into account the type of clinical problem. The recommended clinical cases have to be ranked by similarity with the current case. For instance, it may be more relevant for the physician to consult first how she solved previous cases akin to this, and after that, find out the treatment or diagnosis given by other clinicians to similar problems. The environment may also opportunistically display medical guides relevant to the patient's diagnosis as supporting information for doctors or even locate and establish contact with a specialist who might be available. In the scenario, the display presents the hospital's medical guide relevant to the case they are discussing and links to previous cases that were estimated to be relevant. Based on the description of the diagnosis, the system presents the hospital's medical guide related with this particular case [33].

6.5 Design Issues of Autonomous Agents for Ubicomp

From the above desirable features to be addressed through ubiquitous computing to support the characteristics of healthcare environments, several design issues arose regarding the functionality of autonomous agents for creating ubicomp systems.

- *Autonomous agents are reactive to the contextual elements of the environment.* As explained in the previous section, these contextual elements are: location, delivery time, users' role, and location and state of artifacts and users that agents may need to monitor for opportunistically providing information and services to users. For instance, an autonomous agent can be aware of changes to medical information to be aware of when a patient's medical analyses are available and then notify it to the doctor. Another agent can monitor the environment to make sure that the contextual requirements are satisfied before delivering a message. For this, agents need mechanisms to perceive, recognize and disseminate different types of context information: role, location (of users and devices), state (of documents, services, devices, and users) and time.
- *Autonomous agents can be decisions makers.* We identified the need for third-party decision makers to decide how to act based on the perceived context. Autonomous agents would review context and make decisions about what activities to do, when to do them, and what type of information to communicate to whom.
- *Autonomous agents can represent users, act as proxies to devices or information resources of the environment, or to wrap a complex system's functionality.* In a hospital, the staff requires access to information resources such as the hospital information system from which a doctor accesses a

patient's clinical records. For this, a doctor may interact with her personal agent on the PDA that will request, on her behalf, medical information from an agent acting as proxy to the hospital information server. Agents representing devices, such as the public display, can be aware of the presence of other agents and users available in the environment. These agents enable users and other agents to use the devices; for instance, presenting information on the public display. Finally, agents can be wrappers of complex system's functionality that must be hidden from the users.

- *Autonomous agents should be able to communicate with other agents, or directly to users and services.* For this, agents need a platform of communication that enables them to convey information to other agents, users, and information resources by using the same protocol of communication. This platform and protocol of communication should enable agents to seamlessly interact with users in order to enhance their interaction with the ubicomp environment.
- *Autonomous agents need mechanisms for authentication.* Autonomous agents representing devices or services need mechanisms for authenticating users and agents that want to access them. For instance, not all users are allowed to access the hospital information system or present information on the public display. The physician agent on the PDA may need to know a priori the agent acting as proxy to the public displays available on the environment. An autonomous agent such as this, that represents a public display, needs mechanisms for authenticating users that require accessing it. Thus, only authorized personnel may access these devices or services. And the same can be applied to agents. For instance, the agent acting as a proxy to public display needs to know in advance which other agents may require publishing information on them, or request the personalization of information for a user.
- *Autonomous agents need to communicate different types of messages.* Agents need a communication language that enables them to convey messages for requesting information from devices or services (i.e. requesting medical information from the hospital information system) and responding to such requests, notifying information to users and devices (i.e. notifying that the lab results are available to the user), and requesting from another agent the execution of an action (i.e. personalizing the public display for the user).
- *Autonomous agents may have a reasoning algorithm as complex as the logic of its functionality.* An autonomous agent needs to be aware of information regarding the environment in order to generate its actions. For this, agents may need a reasoning algorithm which may include a simple set of rules or conditions, i.e. to verify that a set of conditions are met in order to deliver a message; or a more complex reasoning algorithm, i.e. for estimating the user's location, or for indexing and retrieving medical cases to be presented on a public display.

6.6 The SALSA Middleware

To facilitate the development of autonomous agents with the characteristics mentioned in the previous section, the Simple Agent Library for Smart Ambients (SALSA) was created. This section presents these requirements and the design and implementation of the middleware.

6.6.1 The SALSA Functional Requirements

Based on the design issues for autonomous agents for ubicomp systems, the following functional requirements for an agent middleware were identified. In our approach, an agent of a ubicomp environment has specific goals, and to achieve them, they have to monitor the context of the environment, and autonomously decide how to act. This lead to the first requirement for the agent middleware for ubiquitous computing system:

- *To implement autonomous agents as decision makers, the middleware should provide mechanisms for implementing the agents' components for perceiving, reasoning, and acting.* An agent should include a perception module to gather information from environment sensors and devices (e.g. to estimate the users location), directly from users (through an interface), and other agents; a reasoning module governs the agent's actions, including deciding what to perceive next; and finally, the agent executes the appropriate action, which may include: sending a notification message to a user or requesting a service from a device.
- *The middleware should provide higher-level mechanisms to enable agents to perceive context information from other agents, directly from the devices or services, or from the users.* Considering that ubiquitous computing environments are highly dynamic, mainly due the fact that the user's context may change unpredictably, the agent's perception component should be able to perceive context information at unpredictable times. The middleware should provide an agent communication language flexible enough to enable programmers to specify the type of context information that will be perceived by the agents of a ubicomp system. Thus, the agent communication language should enable agents to identify the type of information perceived and the target of the information. Once an agent received information, the reasoning component of an autonomous agent has to analyze it to decide how to act.
- *The middleware should be flexible enough to enable developers to endow agents with any reasoning algorithm.* The middleware should provide abstractions that permit not only the implementation of any kind of reasoning algorithm, but also enables developers to easily modify or update the agent's reasoning requiring little or no modifications to the other agent's components.

- *The middleware should provide a communication platform that enables agents to convey information to other agents, users, devices and services by using the same protocol and communication channel.* The actions of autonomous agents may require them to communicate with other agents by interchanging different types of messages for conveying the intention of the interaction and the information content. Agents may also need to communicate with users in order to notify and present information to them. For this, the communication platform should enable users to be aware of the presence of other users and agents that offer relevant services for their activities, but they should be unconscious of other agents with whom they do not need to interact explicitly or that hide a complex functionality. Finally, it should enable agents to negotiate services with other agents, or request them to execute an action. The messages conveyed among agents can be of the following types: a request of information, response to a request, request to execute an action or service, notification that the action was executed, notification of information (that was not previously requested), notification of the presence of an agent (representing a user or a service), and notification of information perceived from a device or sensor. The communication language should be flexible enough to allow programmers to specify the content of each of these messages and the programming language of the middleware should facilitate the creation of these messages.
- *Autonomous agents need mechanisms for registering and authenticating agents.* Autonomous agents need to know what agents have permission to request their services. The middleware should provide an infrastructure of services that enables the naming, registration, authentication, and location of agents representing users, devices and services.

Based on the above requirements, the Simple Agent Library for Smart Ambients (SALSA) was implemented to enable developers to create the software entities of a ubiquitous computing environment with which users need to seamlessly interact. The following Section presents the design of SALSA to address the above requirements.

6.6.2 Design of SALSA

The design of SALSA includes defining: the agent's life cycle which implements the agent's behavior; an expressive language that enables agents to communicate with other agents; and the architecture which consists of a set of services and a library of abstract classes to implement autonomous agents [34].

Agent's Life Cycle

Since it was identified that a SALSA agent should have components for perceiving, reasoning and acting which may involve communicating with other

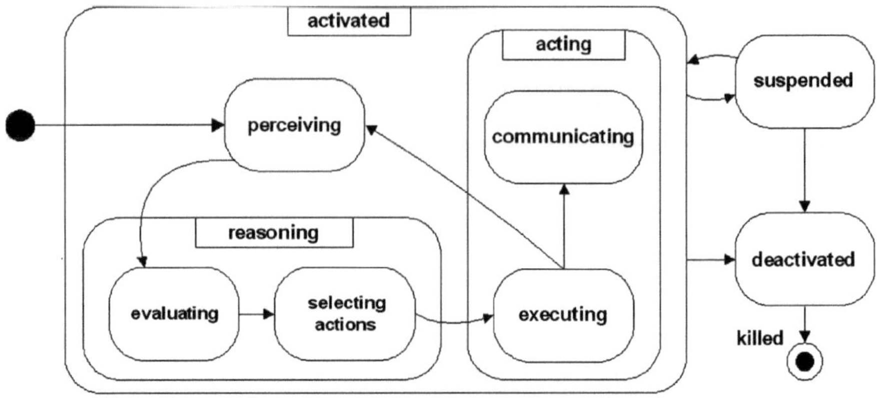

Fig. 6.1. The life-cycle of an agent

agents, the life cycle of agents in a ubicomp environment was defined. As showed in Figure 6.1 the agent's life cycle includes the following states:

- *Activated.* This is the initial state of an agent when it is created. This is a super-state that contains different sub-states that an activated agent can present.
- *Perceiving.* It is the initial sub-state. An agent acquires contextual information from its environment in different ways. For example, an agent may receive information from a user or another agent representing a service; or agents may perceive information directly from devices or sensors. An agent may get into this state if its action plan requires it. That is, it moves from the acting state to the perceiving state.
- *Reasoning.* The agent evaluates the perceived information, which may require applying a simple or complex reasoning algorithm to interpret or transform this information into derived contextual information.
- *Executing.* Based on the results of the reasoning component, the agent executes an action that may involve: communicating with other agents; moving agent's code to another platform, continuing perceiving information, or terminating its execution.
- *Communicating.* The agent interacts with one or more agents in order to provide the information that is necessary to reach its goals. An agent can enter into this state if it is dictated by its action plan or because the agent needs to transmit specific knowledge.
- *Suspended.* An agent in this state is alive but it is not performing any activity. It is waiting to be reactivated. For example, if an agent is waiting for information that it has requested from another agent, then it changes from the communicating state to the suspended state, and when contacted by another agent, its state returns to communicating.
- *Deactivated.* If the agent has met its goal, then it is deactivated and killed.

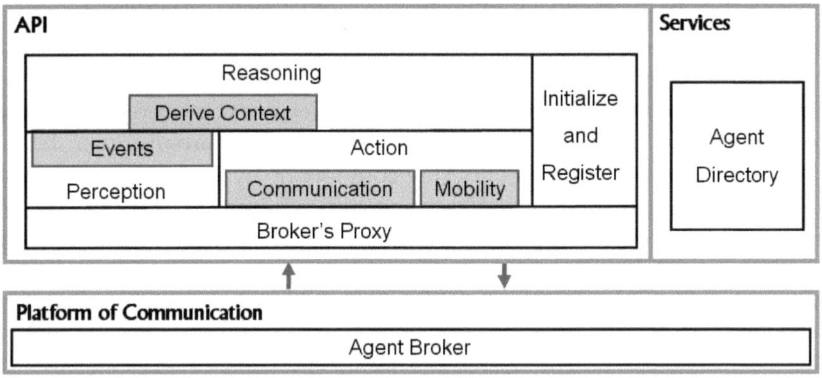

Fig. 6.2. SALSA's Architecture

Architecture of the SALSA Middleware

As illustrated in Figure 6.2, the SALSA middleware consists of the following layers:

Communication Platform

The communication channel among agents and users is a Broker component which is responsible for coordinating communication, and enables the configuration of the environment in a manner that is transparent for users since they do not know the location of the agents even though they can be aware of the presence of some of these agents.

Thus, an Agent Broker is the component that should handle the communication among the ubiquitous devices, services and users, which are represented by agents. SALSA provides a protocol of communication which consists of an expressive language that enables the exchange of different types of objects between agents (such as perceived information, requests for services), between agents and users (such as events generated by the user's actions), and between agents and services (such as the state of a service). This information will be sent or perceived by the agent through a proxy to the Broker, which is an agent's component. The Broker's Proxy and the set of messages that can be communicated among agents are created by developers by using the SALSA API.

API (Application Programming Interface)

The SALSA API is a class framework designed for facilitating the implementation of the agents' components and the use of the services provided by the SALSA middleware. Thus, it is the SALSA API that enables developers to implement the agent's components for perceiving, reasoning and acting, and to control the agent's life cycle. The Perception component gathers context information from the environment's sensors and devices, from the users through a graphical user interface, and from other agents through the Broker's Proxy. The perceived information generates events which are captured by the Reasoning component, which governs the agent's actions. The programmer, based on the logic of the agent, implements this component by using a reasoning algorithm, such as a simple conditional-action rule, a neural network or case based reasoning. The Action component contains the action plan to follow based on the agent's reasoning. It also includes sub-components that allow the agent Communication, and Mobility in order to update its reasoning component, and to Derive Context information based on information perceived by the agent.

Services

The SALSA middleware provides an Agent Directory service which is accessible through the Initialize and Register module of the SALSA API. It provides a set of classes that allows programmers to register the agent's attributes in one or more Agent Directories, and enables agents to look for services provided by other agents.

SALSA Class Framework

The SALSA class framework provides a set of classes to facilitate the implementation of the internal architecture of an agent and control its life cycle. The SALSA API was initially implemented in Java, which enabled agents to be executed on any computing platform. However, it was observed that this version of SALSA does not enable agents to access the native libraries of Widows CE, therefore a sub-set of the SALSA API was implemented in C#, called micro-SALSA (mSALSA), which enables developers to create the components of the agents and use the SALSA communication protocol. Developers have the option of programming in any of these languages and take advantage of the programming facilities offered by each of them. The complete set of classes provided by SALSA are depicted in Figure 6.3 and explained in the following sections.

Agent perception

Two types of perception were identified for SALSA agents: active and passive. In active perception, an agent decides when to request or gather information from another agent or entity in the environment such as a sensor. In passive perception, the agent receives data without requesting it. The Passive Perception was implemented based on the Observer design pattern [35]. This type of agent perception starts when a user, device or other agent sends data to an agent through the Agent Broker. In this case an agent has the role of observing the environment and acting according to the information received. Figure 6.4

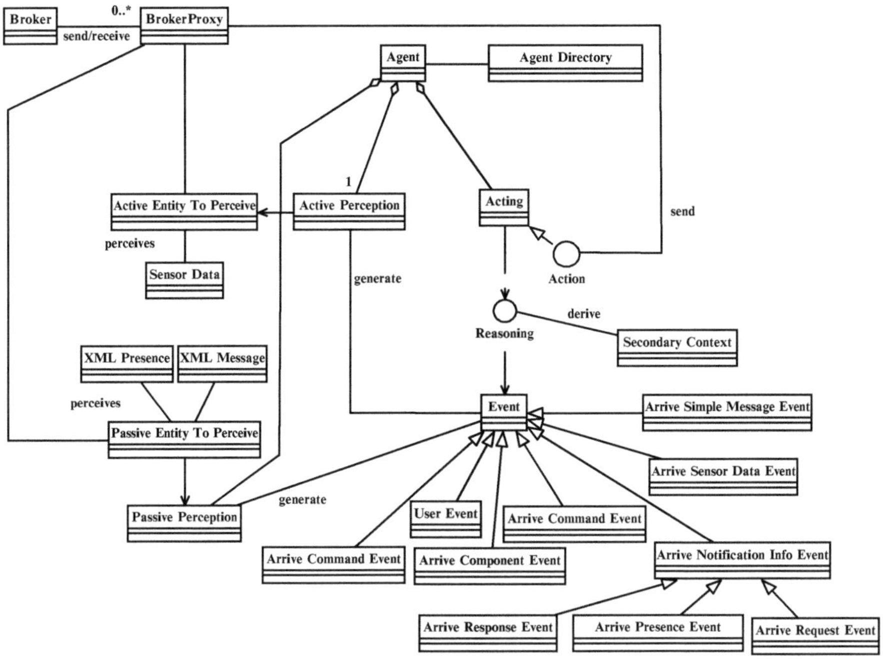

Fig. 6.3. Class Library of SALSA

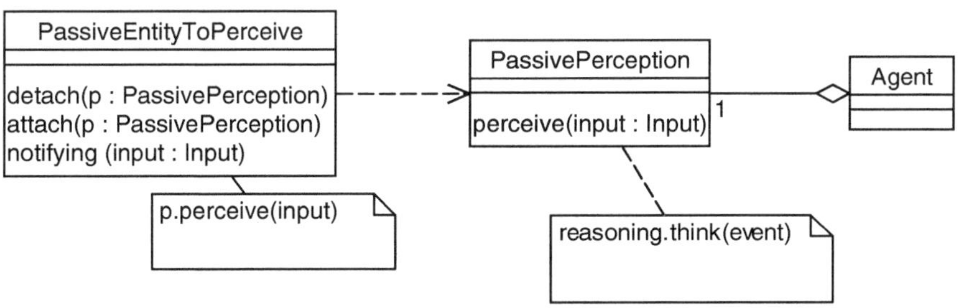

Fig. 6.4. Passive Perception of a SALSA Agent

shows the main classes for implementing this type of perception. The PassiveEntityToPerceive class represents the subject to be observed by the agent; and the PassivePerception class captures the information sent by the subject. For the active perception, an agent decides on its own when to sense an environment entity, and requests this information from another agent, or directly from a sensor's entity. This type of perception implements the Adapter design pattern. Figure 6.5 shows that the classes for implementing active perception are ActiveEntityToPerceive, which has the role of an Adaptee according to the Adapter design pattern. This class represents the environment entity that obtains data from a sensor or device. An agent decides when to perceive

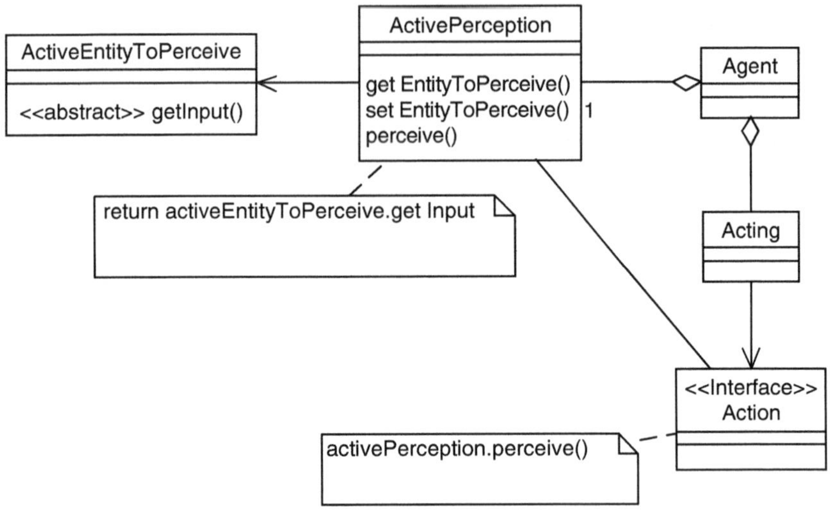

Fig. 6.5. Active Perception of SALSA agents

information by invoking the method passivePerception.perceive() from the Action object. Then ActivePerception, which has the role of Adapter, invokes the ActiveEntityToPerceive object, that is the interface to the sensor, in order to get data from a sensor or device (activeEntityToPerceive.getInput()).

When any of the perception components receive information, a SALSA event is generated indicating the type of information to the reasoning component, as described in Table 6.1. In addition to this, a SALSA event also contains the perceived data, which can be an XML message received through the Agent Broker, or an object containing the data that was read directly from a sensor's interface (i.e, ArriveSensorDataEvent). Table 6.1 shows in column 2 the events produced when information is perceived by an agent. The third column explains the type of information that was received and how the event may be produced. The only active perception supported by SALSA, is when the agent perceives data directly from a sensor or device. The passive perception of a SALSA agent, in which data is received through its IM client, is due to another agent that sends information by using the communication methods of the SALSA API which are presented in column 1.

Agent reasoning

The information perceived by an agent is subtracted from the event by the reasoning component in order to be analyzed. The programmer, based on the logic of the agent, implements this component by using an appropriate reasoning algorithm, such as production rules, a neural network or case base reasoning. The Reasoning class contains the abstract method think() that should be implemented by the developer. Its implementation depends on the complexity of the agent's behavior. The reasoning component can use the

Table 6.1. Description of the SALSA events generated when information is perceived

1. Method used by an agent for sending information	2. Event generated when an agent receives information	3. Description of the event
`sendRequest()`	`ArriveRequestEvent`	A request for information arrives from an agent
`sendResponse()`	`ArriveResponseEvent`	Information that was previously requested by this agent arrives
`sendCommandRequest()`	`ArriveCommandEvent`	An agent is requesting to execute a functionality provided by this agent, such as a service
`sendNotificationInfo()`	`ArriveNotification InfoEvent`	Information that was not previously requested arrives
`sendPresence()`	`ArrivePresenceEvent`	A presence message arrives indicating a change of state of others agents and users
`sendDataSensor()`	`ArriveSensorData Event`	Data perceived from a sensor arrives. It can be an XML message or a SensorData object wrapping information perceived directly from a sensor.
`sendMessage()`	`ArriveSimpleMessage Event`	A non-SALSA message which is defined by the programmer arrives.

facilities of SALSA to derive context information from the primary context information perceived by an agent. For this, SALSA provides the class DeriveContext which uses an XSL file as a filter that contains a set of rules to deduce secondary context from the data perceived by the agent. The set of rules of the XSL filter should be defined by the developer. Using these SALSA facilities, developers need only indicate, to the DeriveContext class, the primary contextual variables and the name of the XSL file. Thus, when an event is passed to the reasoning component, its derive context component is in charge of: detecting the type of event, extracting the data contained in the event, and verifying if the data is an expected contextual variable in order to be analyzed by the filter to check if some of the conditions have been met. Then, the derive context component returns an XML message to the agent's reasoning in order to indicate the inferred situation.

Agent action

To implement the action component, the framework provides the Action class with an abstract method that a developer should overwrite to specify how the agent must react. From, the action component, the agent can invoke the communication methods provided by SALSA in order to collaborate with other agents. These methods are presented in column 1 of Table 6.1. The acting component also enables the agent mobility. It was implemented based on the pattern Rc2s (request a component to a server), which enables an agent to update its reasoning component by getting a copy of the reasoning algorithm from other agent residing on a server [36].

Agent communication

The messages sent among agents through the Agent Broker, are encoded using XML (eXtensible Markup Language). The aim of the SALSA development framework is to use a friendly agent language taking advantage of XML to encode any kind of message. For defining the types of messages that can be communicated among SALSA agents, the Extensible Messaging and Presence Protocol (XMPP) of the IM server (www.jabber.org) was extended. SALSA provides developers with an API that facilitates the composing, sending, and receiving of messages between agents. However, the code for every content message type of the communicative act is left to the programmer, because it depends on the intent of the message generated by each agent in the ubiquitous environment. The SALSA API for implementing the communication among agents consists of several methods that form the message that will be communicated. The SALSA communication protocol enables agents to collaborate to reach a common goal, such as adapting and personalizing information for a user. This collaboration may involve one or more of the following actions:

- *Negotiating for a service.* In this case, an agent (A) requires a service from another agent (B). For instance, if agent A requests agent B to execute a service or a specific action with a sendCommandRequest(), agent B could respond by notifying agent A that the action was successfully executed or notifying that it can provide such a service by using the sendNotificationInfo(); or with the method sendResponseInfo() agent B could provide information returned by the requested service.
- *Requesting information.* An agent (A) requires information from another agent (B). As illustrated in Figure 6.6, agent A request information by using sendRequest(); and agent B can respond by sending the requested information to agent A with a sendResponse(); or by sending a notification that it can not provide this information through a sendNotificationInfo().
- *Notifying information perceived from a sensor or device.* Agents that act as proxies to devices or sensors, get information from them and may require communicating with other agents in the environment to be processed. The information can be communicated by using the sendDataSensor() method.

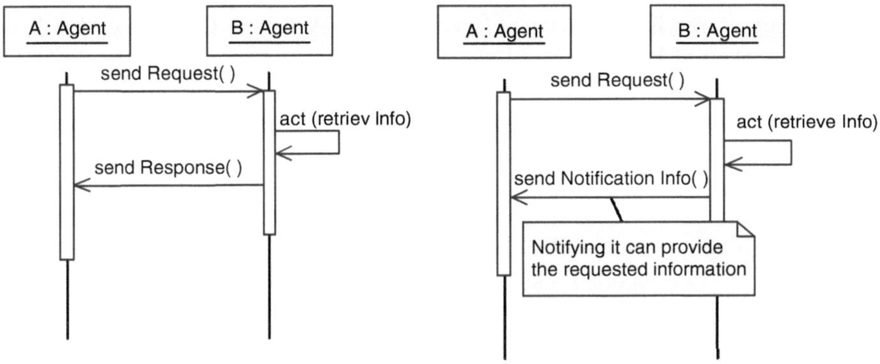

Fig. 6.6. SALSA's communication methods for requesting information

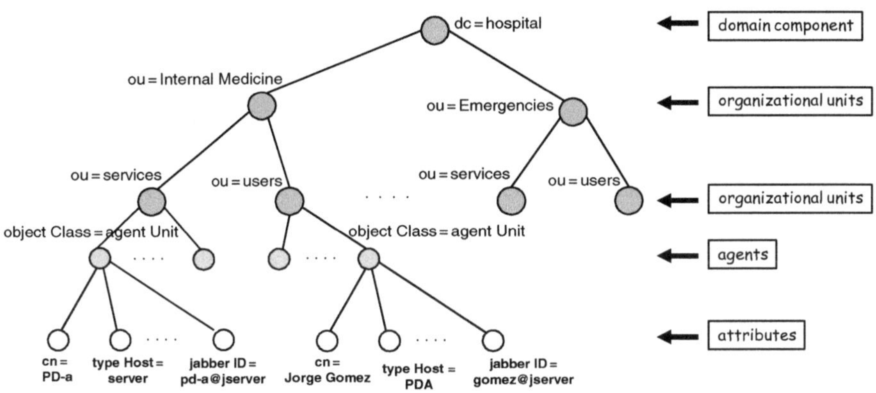

Fig. 6.7. LDAP structure for the SALSA Agent Directory

- *Notifying the presence and status of agents.* An agent notifies a change of presence or status to other agents subscribed to its presence. This enables agents to be aware of the available services of the ubicomp environment. Agents also received the presence of the users in the ubicomp environment.

Agent initialization and registration

SALSA provides a set of services that allow programmers to register and look for new agents added to the ubicomp environment in an Agent Directory. The implementation of the Agent Directory consists of a server that implements the Lightweight Directory Access Protocol (LDAP); and a SALSA agent (AD-proxy agent) acting as proxy to the Agent Directory.

The LDAP information model is based on entries. An entry is a collection of attributes that has a globally-unique Distinguished Name (DN). The DN is used to refer to the entry unambiguously. Each of the entry's attributes has a type and one or more values. The types are typically mnemonic strings, like "cn" for common name. As illustrated in Figure 6.7 entries are arranged in a hierarchical tree-like structure. For the SALSA Agent Directory, it reflects the organizational boundaries of the hospital setting, represented by the top of the tree. Below it are entries representing other areas of the hospital (i.e. Emergency). In the next level are entries representing organizational units, which are the users (i.e. physicians, nurses) and services/devices (i.e. public display) of the ubicomp environment. In the last level are the agents that represent users or services/devices; for instance, PD-a is an agent representing the public display. And finally the leaves of the tree represent the attributes of these agents (i.e. agent location, device or user that it represents).

The SALSA API provides the facilities to register agents in the LDAP directory and for making specialized searches of agents. Thus, agents can communicate with a proxy to the Agent Directory (AD-proxy agent) by using the communication protocol provided by SALSA.

The following Section illustrates how SALSA facilitates the development of a ubicomp system for a hospital environment.

6.7 Creation of a Ubicomp System for a Hospital Setting

With SALSA we built the context-aware hospital information system (CHIS) with the aim to support the activities of the hospital staff [31, 32]. CHIS is a handheld-based system that enables users to locate relevant documents, such as patient's records and laboratory results; locate patients and colleagues; and locate and track the availability of devices such as medical equipment, and other computational resources such as public displays. The following scenario illustrates how we envisioned that CHIS will enable hospital staff to access medical information through public displays:

While Dr. Garcia is checking the patient in bed 234, his PDA alerts him that a new message has arrived. His handheld displays a hospital floor map indicating to him that the X-ray results of patient in bed 225 are available. Before Dr. Garcia visits this patient, he approaches the nearest public display that detects the physician's presence and provides him with a personalized view of the Hospital Information System. In particular, it shows a personalized floor map highlighting recent additions to clinical records of patients he is in charge of, messages addressed to him, and the services most relevant to his current work activities. Dr. Garcia selects the message on bed 225, which opens windows displaying the patient's medical record, the X-ray image recently taken and the hospital's medical guide related with this case. While Dr. Garcia is analyzing the X-ray image, he notices in the map, that a resident physician is nearby and calls him up to show him this interesting clinical case. The resident physician notices that this is indeed a special case and decides to make a short note on his handheld computer by linking both the X-ray image and the medical guide. He can later on use these links to study the case in more detail or discuss it with other colleagues from any computer within the hospital.

6.7.1 Architecture of CHIS

Figure 6.8 presents the design of the system architecture illustrating the main nodes in which the system's components are executing. These components are SALSA agents communicating through the Agent Broker (an IM server), as specified by the SALSA communication infrastructure.

The Location-aware client resides in the handheld computer which notifies the user's location to other users and agents, provides mobile users with information relevant to their location, and communicates with other members of the hospital staff. Its interface is based on the IM paradigm, through which users are notified of the availability of other users and their location. The location-estimation agent (LE-a) also resides in the handheld with the purpose of obtaining the user's position (X,Y coordinates), and informs it to the location-aware client. By using the mobility attribute of agents, the LE-a on the PDA can update its reasoning component by getting the reasoning component from the server on which resides the LE-a that holds a trained neural network for a specific building's floor.

The Agent Directory provides information of the agents available in the environment. For instance, the LE-a can know in which server the agent containing the trained neural network resides by communicating with the agent acting as proxy to the Agent Directory (AD-a). The hospital information system agent (HIS-a) acts as proxy of the HIS that manages and stores the patient's clinical records and other data relevant to the hospital. This agent provides access to information contained in the HIS, and monitors its changes. The Context-aware agent (Ca-a) is the system's component that sends the messages that depend on contextual variables for their delivery, such as the recipients, location and role. In the display server node, several agents reside

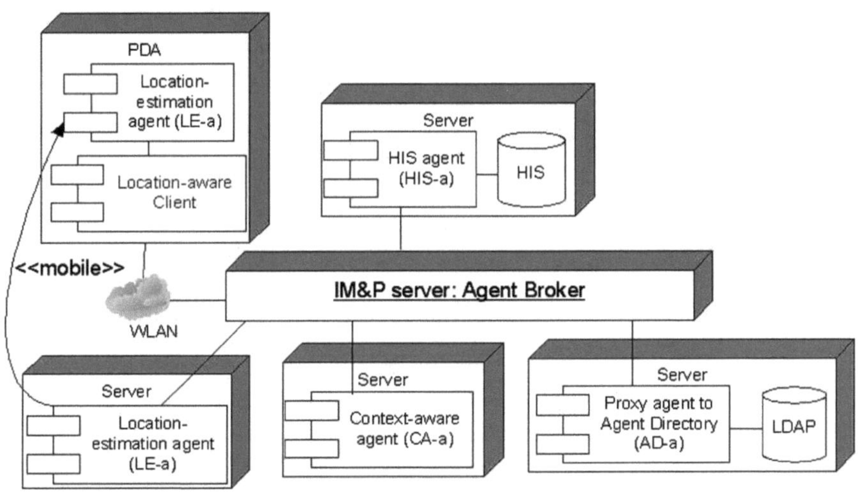

Fig. 6.8. Architecture of the context-aware hospital information system

offering several services for the medical personnel. These services were implemented as SALSA agents. Thus, the responsibility of the Public Display agent (PD-a) is to act as a proxy to a public display available at the hospital. This agent enables users to access the public display and have control over the applications displayed. The responsibility of presenting a personalized map of the hospital floor was delegated to the map agent (Map-a). It displays a map of the hospital floor that indicates the location of the hospital staff, available services, and highlights the beds of patients assigned to the current physician using the display. The Map-a also shows messages addressed to the user, i.e. messages related to his patients that may indicates additions to their electronic records. Finally, the knowledge management agent (KM-a) is responsible for displaying the hospital medical guide and previous cases relevant to the case being consulted on the public display.

6.7.2 Implementation of CHIS

This section revisits the scenario presented in Section 6.7 to explain the functionality and implementation of the context-aware hospital information system. Figure 6.9 depicts a sequence diagram illustrating how the autonomous agents of CHIS interact by using the SALSA communication protocol (the SALSA methods are in bold font style on the diagram). In this scenario, the HI System-a (HIS-a) perceives a change on the hospital information system and notifies it to Dr. Garcia by sending a message (sendNotificationInfo) indicating that the X-ray results of patient on bed 225 are available. When the location-aware client receives this message, it will act by updating its instant messaging interface. Dr. Garcia approaches the near-

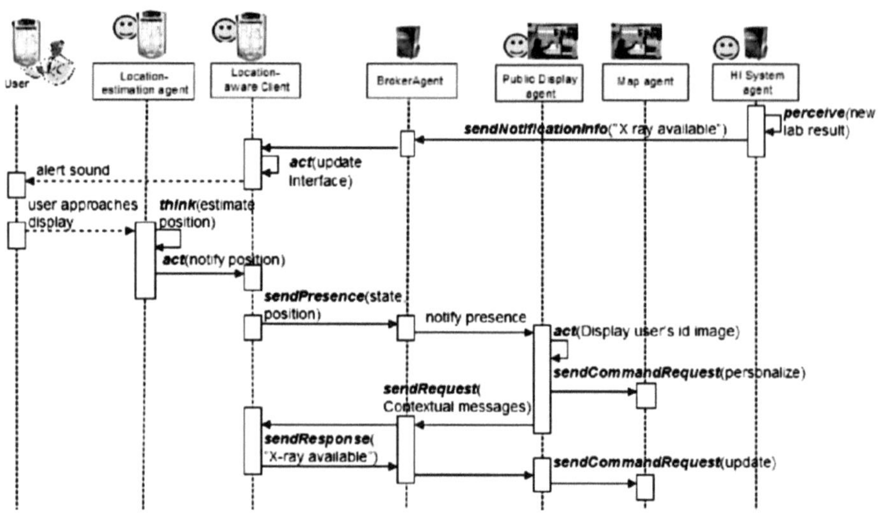

Fig. 6.9. Implementation of CHIS using the SALSA development framework

est public display when finished with her current patient and before visiting patient 225. The doctor's location, which is constantly being tracked by the location-estimation agent on her PDA, is notified (sendPresence) to all users and agents in the environment by the Location-aware client. The Public Display agent (PD-a) acts by displaying the user's photograph, indicating with this that the user has been logged into the system. Then, the PD-a requests (sendCommandRequest) that the Map agent (Map-a) personalize the map application for Dr. Garcia. Finally, the PD-a also requests (sendRequest) the contextual messages recently received by the location-aware client, and display them on the floor map. Thus, the physician can continue accessing the records of his patients and other medical information by interacting with the public display.

Implementation of the Location-estimation Agent of CHIS

To illustrate how an autonomous agent is implemented with SALSA, this section describes the functionality and implementation of the Location-estimation agent of CHIS [37]. Figure 6.10 presents a sequence diagram with a detailed description of the interactions carried out to estimate the user's location. Thus, when the physician Dr. Diaz visits his patient, the Location-estimation agent (LE-a) perceives that the Signal to Noise Ratio (SNR) to the access points change (perceive(SNR)). Then, the LE-a estimates the user's location based on its trained neural network (think(estimate user's position)). Thus, the agent obtains the user's position (X,Y coordinates) which is communicated to the location aware client (sendDataSensor()). The location aware client translates the X,Y coordinates to an ID of the place in which the

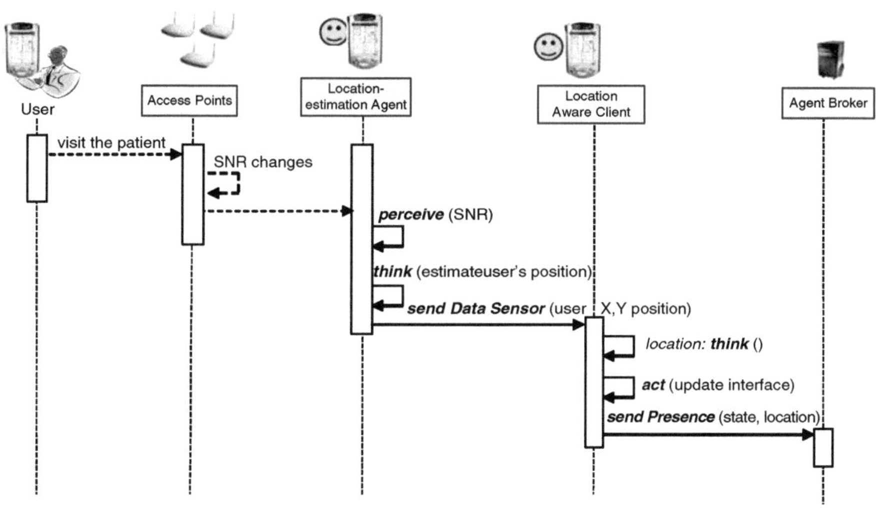

Fig. 6.10. Location-estimation agent interacting with the agents of CHIS

user is located (i.e. bed number, room). Thus, the reasoning component maps the user's X,Y coordinates to an area identifier (location: think()) and finally, its acting component communicates the user's location to the rest of the system's agents and users (sendPresence(state,location)). This functionality of LE-a is wrapped in its components for perceiving, reasoning and acting which were implemented by extending the SALSA classes as explained in the following sections:

Perception Component

The agent's perception module receives the SNR (Signal to Noise Ratio) through the PassiveEntityToPerceive object, which represents the memory of the wireless network (WLAN) card. The developer implemented this interface to read data from the WLAN card, wrap the data in an Input object, and then notify it to the PassivePerception component of the LE-a. When the SNR value is changed, the PassivePerception object generates an arriveSensorDataEvent which is passed to the reasoning component.

Figure 6.11a) shows the pseudo code for implementing the perception component of the LE-a using the SALSA classes. Element (1) of the LE-a is the entity for perceiving information. This is the WirelessCardInterface that contains the code for reading the SNR from the wireless LAN card. This class has an embedded a PassiveEntityToPerceive object (pp) which has a reference to the LE-a. Thus, when a new SNR is read, it is passed to the passive perception component (2) by invoking the method pp.notifying(). Thus, developers need to implement just the interface that reads the data from a device/sensor and to use the SALSA classes to connect the interface with the perception component, which is automatically activated when an instance of the Agent class is created.

```
import SALSA.*;           (1)
public class WirelessCardInterface{

    PassiveEntityToPerceive pp;

    public WirelessCardInterface(Agent LE_a){
       pp=new PassiveEntityToPerceive();
       pp.attach(LE_a.passivePerception);
    }

     protected void read_SNR() {
      // Code to get the SNR
         . . .
      //Creates an instance of the LE-a
  (2) pp.notifying(new Input(snr));
    }
}
```

a)

```
import SALSA.*;           (3)
class ReasoningLE_a extends SALSA.Reasoning{

  public void think(EventObject ev){
    SALSA.Events.Event event = (SALSA.Events.Event) ev;
        //if the SNR changed
    if (event.getType() == event.arriveSensorDataEvent) {
      coordinates = estimatesLocation(ev.input);

        //Invokes the action component
      agent.acting.act(new CommunicateNewLocation());
    }

        //if the new neural network for that floor was obtained
    else if (event.getType() == event.ArriveComponentEvent){
      agent.acting.act(new IntegrateComponent());
    }
  . . . .
```

b)

Fig. 6.11. Code for implementing the entity for perceiving information from the WLAN card. b) Code of the reasoning component

Reasoning component

As illustrated in Figure 6.11b), the ReasoningLE class (3) is specialized from the Reasoning abstract class of SALSA. Its think method was overwritten to process the perceived input and then, to indicate to the agent what action should be executed. If the received SALSA event was of type arriveSensorDataEvent, it indicates that a new estimation of the user's location has to be calculated. Then, the estimatesLocation() method is invoked, which implements the trained Neural Network. Providing an abstract class to implement the reasoning component enables programmers to easily update or replace its logic with another algorithm that may be more efficient.

Action component

When a new user's location is estimated, the reasoning component decides to communicate it to the location-aware client which is also executing in the handheld computer. To do this, the execute() method of the abstract class Action was overwritten to invoke the SALSA method sendDataSensor().

Creation of the agent

Finally, once the Perception, Reasoning, and Action components of the agent were implemented, the main body of the agent had to be created. This was done by extending the SALSA Agent class. Thus, when an instance of this agent is created, its components are activated and the life cycle of the agent begins.

6.8 Conclusions

Ubiquitous computing (ubicomp) enables us to fulfill the medical environment needs. A ubiquitous computing environment is characterized by the distribution, reactivity, collaboration and adaptation of their artifacts, thus sharing these characteristics with autonomous agents. This provided us with the motivation to explore the use of agents as an abstraction tool for the design and implementation of ubiquitous computing systems for hospitals. We used autonomous agents as a technique to model and design ubiquitous computing systems for the healthcare domain since they provide a natural and elegant means to manage the system's complexities and hospital characteristics. We identified the design issues of autonomous agents for ubicomp that were the foundation for creating the SALSA middleware that provides the mechanisms to facilitate the development of ubicomp systems for healthcare environments. Thus, we have presented how the SALSA middleware facilitates the implementation of ubiquitous computing systems for hospital settings in which autonomous agents are the proactive components that enable users to seamlessly and opportunistically interact with the users, devices and services of the environment. To illustrate the facilities provided by SALSA we presented the Context-aware Hospital Information System (CHIS) whose main components are agents that respond autonomously in accordance with the context surrounding the activities performed at the hospital.

The communication channel among agents and users is an Agent Broker (its implementation is an Instant Messaging Server) which is responsible for coordinating the communication among agents. As the architecture of SALSA is based on the instant messaging (IM) paradigm, it allows a standardized form of interaction among users and services represented by autonomous agents. In the same form, users are aware of the presence of other users, they are also aware of the presence and state of the environment's services and devices. The scalability of a system implemented with SALSA is enabled by the IM server used as an Agent Broker, since it scales to a high volume of streaming XML connections serving hundreds of thousands of simultaneous users and agents. By using SALSA, developers may easily integrate any reasoning mechanism; or change the current reasoning algorithm for other, without modifying the code of the rest of the agent's components. For instance, we may change the neural network of the Location-estimation agent of CHIS by a nearest neighbor algorithm without altering the perception and acting component. With SALSA, different types of agents can be created, such as personal agents and service agents that may have attributes of autonomy, mobility, reactivity and collaboration. SALSA agents have well-defined interfaces to interact with their environment, and mechanisms to encapsulate its implementation. For this reason, these agents may be considered as units of independent deployment or components, which may be re-used or integrated to any SALSA ubiquitous system. For instance, the location-estimation agent may be integrated to a different environment than a hospital by just training its neural network for this new physical environment. To implement autonomous agents as decision makers, the SALSA middleware provides a library of classes for implementing and handling the execution model of agents, which consists of the components for perceiving information, reasoning, and acting. Due to the fact that the ubicomp environment is highly dynamic, an agent can perceive context information at unpredictable times from other agents, from the devices or services, or from the users. Agents can perceive information through the Agent Broker or directly from devices or sensors. The programmer, based on the logic of the agent, implements the reasoning component by using any reasoning algorithm. SALSA provides abstractions to enable developers to easily modify or update the agent's reasoning requiring little or no modifications to the other agent's components. The action component implements the action plan to follow based on the agent's reasoning. It also includes subcomponents that allow the agent's communication and mobility in order to update its reasoning component, and to derive context information based on information perceived by the agent. The actions of autonomous agents may require that they communicate with other agents and users. The SALSA communication protocol allows agents to negotiate services with other agents, request them to execute an action and communicate with users in order to notify or present information to them. Finally, SALSA enables the naming and registration of agents in an Agent Directory (AD). This is a service which is accessible through an agent acting as a proxy to the AD.

SALSA is an agent middleware to facilitate the implementation and evolution of ubiquitous computing systems in which autonomous agents are the proactive components that enable users to seamlessly and opportunistically interact with the healthcare environment.

References

1. Reddy, M. and Dourish, P.: A Finger on the Pulse: Temporal Rhythms and Information Seeking in Medical Work. Computer Supported Cooperative Work (CSCW). New Orleans, Louisiana, USA. Nov. 16–20. ACM Press (2002) 344–353
2. Theureau, J., Filippi, G.: Analysing cooperative work in a urban traffic control room for the design of a coordination support system. In Workplace Studies: Recovering Work Practice and Informing System Design. Cambridge Press (2000) 68–91
3. Bossen, C.: The Parameters of Common Information Spaces: the Heterogenity of Cooperative Work at a Hospital Ward. In the ACM Conference on Computer Supported Cooperative Work (CSCW). New Orleans, Louisiana, USA. 16–20 November (2002) 176–185
4. Casebeer, L.L., Strasser, S.M., Spettell, C., Wall, M.T., Weissman, N., Ray, M.N., and Allison, J.J.: Designing Tailored Web-Based Instruction to Improve Physicians' Preventive Practices. Journal of Medical Internet Research, Vol. 5, No. 3 (2003)
5. Schoen, D.A.: The reflective practitioner: how professionals think in action. New York: Basic Books (1983)
6. Hansmann, U., Merk, L., Nicklous, M.S., and Stober, T.: Pervasive Computing Handbook. Springer-Verlag (2001)
7. Weiser, M.: The Computer for the Twenty-First Century. Scientific American, Vol. 265, No. 3 (1991) 94–104
8. Fersha, A.: Context-aware: Bridging Physical and Virtual Worlds. In Conf. on Reliable Software Technologies – Ada-Europe. Vienna, Austria. June 17–21. LNCS, Vol. 2361, Springer-Verlag, (2002) 51–64
9. Banavar, G. and Bernstein, A.: Software Infrastructure and Design Challenges. Communications of the ACM. Vol. 45, No 12 (2002) 92–96
10. Dey, A.K.: Understanding and Using Context. Personal and Ubiquitous Computing. Springer-Verlag. London, UK. (2001) 4–7
11. Schilit, B.N. and Theimer, M.M.: Disseminating active map information to mobile hosts. IEEE Network, Vol. 8, No. 5: (1994) 22–32
12. Bradshaw, J.: Software Agents. AAAI Press/MIT Press: (1997) 3–49
13. Wooldridge, M. and Jennings, N.: Intelligent Agents: Theory and Practice. Knowledge Engineering Review, Cambridge University Press, Vol. 10, No. 2 (1995) 115–152
14. Wooldridge, M.: Agent-based software engineering. IEE Proc. Software Engineering, Vol. 144, No. 1 (1997) 26–3

15. Griss, M.L. and Pour, G.: Accelerating Development with Agent Components. IEEE Computer (2001) 37–43
16. Wooldridge, M.J. and Jennings, N.R.: Software Engineering with Agents: Pitfalls and Pratfalls. IEEE Internet Computing. (1999) 20–27
17. Jennings, N.R.: An Agent-based Approach for Building Complex Software Systems. Communications of the ACM. Vol. 44, No. 4 (2001) 35–41
18. Kay, A.: User Interface: A personal view. In B. Laurel (ed.): The Art of Human-Computer Interface Design. Addison-Wesley, Reading, Mass (1990) 190
19. Maes, P.: Agents that Reduce Work and Information Overload. Communications of the ACM. Vol. 37, No. 7 (1994) 30–40
20. Moreno, A., Valls, A., and Riaño, D.: Medical Applications of Multi-Agent Systems. ECAI Workshop on Agents Applied in Health Care. Valencia, Spain. Aug. (2004) 22–27
21. Greenwood, S., Nealon, J.L., and Marshall, P.: Agent-Based User Interface Adaptivity in a Medical Decision Support System. Applications of Software Agent Technology in the Health Care Domain. Whitestein Series in Software Agent Technologies, Birkhäuser Springer-Verlag, Basel, (2003) 35–48
22. Kifor, T., László Z.V., Vázquez-Salceda, J., Alvarez, S., Willmontt, S., Miles, S., Moreau, L.: Provenance in Agent-Mediated Healthcare Systems. IEEE Intelligent Systems. Published by IEEE Computer Society. Nov.–Dec. (2006) 38–46.
23. Castro-Oliveira, I., Belo, O., and Cunha, J.P. Agents Working on the Integration of Heterogeneous Information Sources in Distributed Healthcare Environments. In Proceedings of 7th Ibero-American Conference on AI, 15th Brazilian Symposium on AI, IBERAMINA-SBIA. Atibaia, SP, Brazil. Nov. 19–22. Springer-Verlag. (2000) 136–145
24. Singh, S., Ikhwan-Ismail, B., Haron, F., and Yong, C.H.: Architecture of Agent-based Healthcare Intelligent Assistant on Grid Environment. In Proceedings of the International Conference on Parallel and Distributed Computing, Applications and Technologies (PDCAT). Singapore. December 8–10. LNCS Vol. 3320, Springer-Verlag (2004) 58–61
25. Kirn, S. Ubiquitous Healthcare: The OnkoNet Mobile Agents Architecture. In Proceedings of International Conference NetObjectDays (NODe). Erfurt, Germany. October 7–10. LNCS Vol. 2591, Springer-Verlag. (2003) 265–277
26. Vieira-Marques, P., Cruz-Correia, R., Robles, S., Cucurull, J., Navarro, G., Marti, R.: Secure Integration of Distributed Medical Data Using Mobile Agents. IEEE Intelligent Systems. Published by IEEE Computer Society. Nov-Dec (2006) 47–53
27. Cortés, U., Annicchiarico, R., Vázquez-Salceda, J., Urdiales, C., Cañamero, L., López, M., Sánchez-Marré, M., and Caltagirone, C.: Assistive technologies for the disabled and for the new generation of senior citizens: the e-Tools architecture. AI Communications, IOS Press, Vol. 16 (2003) 193–207
28. Tablado, A., Illarramendi, A., Bermúdez, J., and Goñi, A.: Intelligent Monitoring of Elderly People. In Proceedings of the 4th. Annual IEEE Conference on Information Technology Applications in Biomedicine Buckingham, UK. (2003) 78–81
29. Budzik, J. and Hammond, K.: User Interactions with Every Applications as Context for Just-in-time Information Access. In Proceedings of Intelligent User Interfaces 2000. New Orleans, LA, USA January 9–12. ACM Press. (2000) 44–51

30. Brown, P.J. and Jones, G.J.F.: "Context-aware Retrieval: Exploring a New Environment for Information Retrieval and Information Filtering". Personal and Ubiquitous Computing, Vol. 5 (2001) 253–263
31. Muñoz, M.A., Rodriguez, M., Favela, J., Martinez-García, A., Gonzalez., V.M.: Context-aware mobile communication in hospitals. IEEE Computer. Vol. 36, No. 9 (2003) 38–46
32. Favela, J., Rodríguez, M., Preciado, A., and González, V.M.: Integrating Context-aware Public Displays into a Mobile Hospital Information System. IEEE Transactions on Information Technology in Biomedicine. Vol. 8, No. 3 (2004) 279–286
33. Rodríguez, M. and Preciado, A.: An Agent Based System for the Contextual Retrieval of Medical Information. In proceedings of AWIC 2004, LNAI Vol. 3034, Springer-Verlag Berlin Heidelberg (2004) 64–73
34. Rodríguez, M.D., Favela, J., Preciado, A. and Vizcaíno, A.: Agent-based ambient intelligence for healthcare. AI Communications IOS Press (2005) 1–16
35. Breemen, A.J.N.v.: Integrating Agents in Software Applications. In Proceedings of the Agent Technology Workshops LNAI 2692, Springer-Verlag (2003) 343–354
36. Koukoumpetsos, K. and Antonopoulos, N.: Mobility Patterns: An Alternative Approach to Mobility Management. In Proceedings of the 6th World Multi-Conference on Systemics, Cybernetics and Informatics (SCI), Orlando, Florida, USA. 14–18 July (2002)
37. Rodriguez, M, Favela, J., Martínez, E., and Muñoz, M.: Location-aware Access to Hospital Information and Services. IEEE Trans. on IT in Biomed. Vol. 8, No. 4 (2004) 448–455

7

Detection and Classification of Microcalcification Clusters in Mammograms using Evolutionary Neural Networks

Rolando R. Hernández-Cisneros and Hugo Terashima-Marín, and Santiago E. Conant-Pablos

Center for Intelligent Systems, Tecnológico de Monterrey, Campus Monterrey
Ave. Eugenio Garza Sada 2501 Sur, Monterrey, Nuevo León 64849 Mexico
{a00766380, terashima, sconant}@itesm.mx

Summary. Breast cancer is one of the main causes of death in women and early diagnosis is an important means to reduce the mortality rate. The presence of microcalcification clusters are primary indicators of early stages of malignant types of breast cancer and its detection is important to prevent the disease. This chapter presents a procedure for the classification of microcalcification clusters in mammograms using sequential difference of gaussian filters (DoG) and three evolutionary artificial neural networks (EANNs) compared against a feedforward artificial neural network (ANN) trained with backpropagation. It is shown that the use of genetic algorithms (GAs) for finding the optimal weight set for an ANN, finding an adequate initial weight set before starting a backpropagation training algorithm and designing its architecture and tuning its parameters, results mainly in improvements in overall accuracy, sensitivity and specificity of an ANN, compared with other networks trained with simple backpropagation.

7.1 Introduction

Cancer is a term used to refer to a group of diseases where a group of cells of the body grow, change and multiply out of control. Usually, each type of cancer is named after the body part where it originated. When this erratic and uncontrolled proliferation of cells occurs in the breast tissues, it is known as breast cancer.

Breast cancer is the fifth cause of death caused by cancer worldwide, after lung cancer, stomach cancer, liver cancer and colon cancer. During 2005, breast cancer caused approximately 502,000 deaths in the world. Among women, breast cancer is the type of cancer that causes the largest number or deaths worldwide, followed by lung, stomach, colorectal and cervical cancers [71].

The highest survival rates for breast cancer occur when it is detected in its earlier stages, when it usually appears in mammograms as very small specks

R.R. Hernández-Cisneros et al.: *Detection and Classification of Microcalcification Clusters in Mammograms using Evolutionary Neural Networks*, Studies in Computational Intelligence (SCI) **107**, 151–180 (2008)
www.springerlink.com

of calcium known as microcalcifications. This survival rate decreases as cancer progresses undetected forming a mass or lump, called a tumor (extra tissue formed by rapidly dividing cells). Tumors can be either malignant (cancerous) or benign (non-cancerous). Breast malignant tumors penetrate and destroy healthy breast tissues. Eventually, a group of cells from a tumor may break away and spread to other parts of the body. These groups of cells spreading to another region are called metastases. Survival rates when breast cancer is discovered and begins to be treated in these latest stages are low.

In this chapter, it is presented a procedure for detecting microcalcification clusters in mammograms and classifying them into two classes: benign (usually presence of tiny benign cysts) or malignant (possible presence of early breast cancer). This procedure is mainly based in difference of gaussian (DoG) filters for the detection of suspicious objects in a mammogram, and artificial intelligence techniques like genetic algorithms (GA) and artificial neural networks (ANN) for the classification of such objects into microcalcifications or non-microcalcifications, and later for classifying the detected microcalcification clusters into benign or malignant.

This chapter is organized as follows. In this section, an overview of breast cancer, artificial intelligence techniques and previous work on detection and classification of microcalcifications are presented. In the second section, the proposed procedure along with its theoretical framework are discussed. The third section deals with the experiments and the main results of this work. Finally, in the fourth section, the conclusions are presented.

7.1.1 Breast Cancer

The breast is composed of two main types of tissues: glandular tissues and stromal (supporting) tissues. Glandular tissues include the lobules (milk-producing glands) and the ducts (the milk passages). Stromal tissues consist of all the fatty and fibrous connective tissues of the breast. Additionally, the breast is also made up of lymphatic tissue-immune system tissue whose function is to remove cellular fluids and waste. In Figure 7.1, the stages of breast cancer are shown. Initially, cancer cells are confined to the part of the breast where it originated, and in these stages, it is referred as non-invasive or *in situ*. Ductal carcinoma *in situ* (DCIS), shown in Figure 7.1(b), is the most common form of non-invasive breast cancer (90%). Lobular carcinoma *in situ* (LCIS) is less common and considered a marker for increased breast cancer risk. In time, cancer cells may break from the duct or lobular walls and invade the surrounding fatty and connective tissues of the breast. When this happens, breast cancer is referred as invasive (not necessarily metastasic), as shown in Figure 7.1(c). The previously mentioned types of breast cancer are now referred as infiltrating ductal carcinoma (IDC) and infiltrating lobular carcinoma (ILC) respectively. Finally, at some point they invade through the basement membrane of the duct or lobule and ultimately metastasize to distant organs, as presented in Figure 7.1(d).

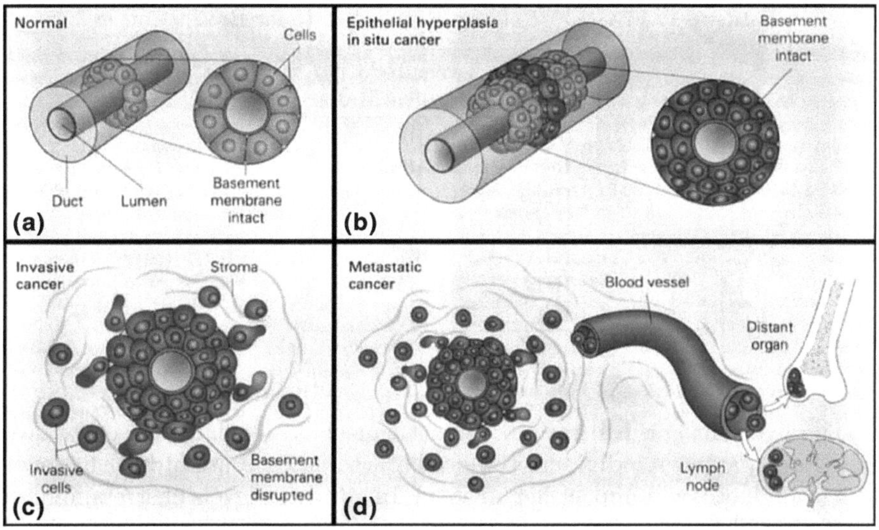

Fig. 7.1. Stages of Breast Cancer [8] (source: http://carcin.oxfordjournals.org/)

In order to assess the size and location of a patient's cancer, physicians use a process called staging. Identifying the cancer stage is one of the most important factors in selecting treatment options. There are several tests that may be performed to help to determine the stage of the breast cancer, like clinical breast exams, biopsy, and some imaging tests such as a chest x-ray, mammogram, bone scan, CT scan, and MRI scan. A woman's overall health is evaluated using blood tests, which are also useful to detect if the cancer has metastasized to other parts of the body.

Breast cancer is staged using the TNM system, which is included in the American Joint Committee on Cancer (AJCC) Staging Manual [23]. These stages are:

- Stage 0 - Carcinoma *in situ*.
- Stage I - Tumor (T) does not involve axillary lymph nodes (N).
- Stage IIA - T 2-5 cm, N negative, or T $<$ 2 cm and N positive.
- Stage IIB T $>$ 5 cm, N negative, or T 2-5 cm and N positive ($<$4 axillary nodes).
- Stage IIIA T $>$ 5 cm, N positive, or T 2-5 cm with 4 or more axillary nodes
- Stage IIIB T has penetrated chest wall or skin, and may have spread to $<$10 axillary N
- Stage IIIC T has $>$10 axillary N, 1 or more supraclavicular or infraclavicular N, or internal mammary N.
- Stage IV Distant metastasis (M)

Table 7.1. Five-year Relative Survival Rate for Breast Cancer

Stage	5-year Relative Survival Rate
0	100%
I	100%
IIA	92%
IIB	81%
IIIA	67%
IIIB	54%
IV	20%

The five-year survival rate for breast cancer is calculated based on averages. Each patient's individual tumor characteristics, state of health, genetic background, etc. will impact her survival. In addition, levels of stress, immune function, will to live, and other unmeasurable factors also play a significant role in a patient's survival. The survival rates for each stage of breast cancer are shown in Table 7.1 [1].

It can be deduced that the key to surviving breast cancer is early detection and treatment. In Stage 0, the cancer is "*in situ*" ("in place"), it is contained and has not spread beyond the ducts or lobules where it originated. As shown in Table 7.1, when breast cancer is detected and treated since stage 0, the five-year survival rate is close to 100%. The early detection of breast cancer helps reduce the need for therapeutic treatment and minimizes pain and suffering, allowing women to continue leading happy, productive lives.

Ductal carcinoma *in situ* (DCIS) and lobular carcinoma *in situ* (LCIS) are the two types of breast cancer in stage 0. DCIS is the most frequent of the stage 0 breast cancers, accounting for 80% of the cases, against 20% of the LCIS. DCIS may be detected on mammogram as tiny specks of calcium (known as microcalcifications) 80% of the time. Less commonly DCIS can present itself as a mass with calcifications (15% of the time); and even less likely as a mass without calcifications (less than 5% of the time).

7.1.2 Mammography

Mammography is a special type of x-ray imaging used to create detailed images of the breast. Mammography uses low dose x-ray; high contrast, high-resolution film; and an x-ray system designed specifically for imaging the breasts. Successful treatment of breast cancer depends on early diagnosis. Mammography plays a major role in early detection of breast cancers. According to the US Food and Drug Administration (FDA), mammography can find 85 to 90 percent of breast cancers in women over 50 and can discover a lump up to two years before it can be felt. The benefits of mammography far outweigh the risks and inconvenience.

Mammography can show changes in the breast well before a woman or her physician can feel them. Once a lump is discovered, mammography can be a key in evaluating the lump to determine if it is cancerous or not. If a breast abnormality is found or confirmed with mammography, additional breast imaging tests such as ultrasound (sonography) or a breast biopsy may be performed. A biopsy involves taking a sample(s) of breast tissue and examining it under a microscope to determine whether it contains cancer cells. Many times, mammography or ultrasound is used to help the radiologist or surgeon guide the needle to the correct area in the breast during biopsy.

There are two types of mammography exams, screening and diagnostic:

- Screening mammography is an x-ray examination of the breasts in a woman who is asymptomatic (has no complaints or symptoms of breast cancer). The goal of screening mammography is to detect cancer when it is still too small to be felt by a woman or her physician. Early detection of small breast cancers by screening mammography greatly improves a woman's chances for successful treatment. Screening mammography is recommended every one to two years for women once they reach 40 years of age and every year once they reach 50 years of age. In some instances, physicians may recommend beginning screening mammography before age 40 (i.e. if the woman has a strong family history of breast cancer). Screening mammography is available at a number of clinics and locations. For screening mammography each breast is imaged separately, typically from above (cranial-caudal view, CC) and from an oblique or angled view (mediolateral-oblique, MLO).
- Diagnostic mammography is an x-ray examination of the breast in a woman who either has a breast complaint (for example, a breast lump or nipple discharge is found during self-exam) or has had an abnormality found during screening mammography. Diagnostic mammography is more involved and time-consuming than screening mammography and is used to determine exact size and location of breast abnormalities and to image the surrounding tissue and lymph nodes. Typically, several additional views of the breast are imaged and interpreted during diagnostic mammography, including views from each side (lateromedial, LM: from the outside towards the center and mediolateral view, ML: from the center of the chest out), exaggerated cranial-caudal, magnification views, spot compression, and others. Thus, diagnostic mammography is more expensive than screening mammography. Women with breast implants or a personal history of breast cancer will usually require the additional views used in diagnostic mammography.

Mammography is currently the only exam approved by the U.S. Food and Drug Administration (FDA) to screen for breast cancer in women who do not show any signs or symptoms of the disease. Mammography can detected approximately 85% of breast cancers. If a screening mammography indicates an abnormality, women will most likely be recommended for further breast imaging (i.e., with spot view mammography, ultrasound or other imaging tests). If further imaging confirms or reveals an abnormality, the woman may be referred for biopsy to determine whether she has breast cancer.

However, while screening mammography can detect most breast cancers, it can miss up to 15% of cancers. These cancers may not be detected on a mammogram film, because of [20]:

- Low differentiation between the appearance of the cancerous tissue compared against the normal parenchymal tissue, specially when the predominant tissue in the breast is very dense.
- Varied morphology of the findings, many of them not related with the cancer.
- Similarities between the morphologies of the findings.
- Possible deficiencies in the mammogram acquisition process.
- Visual fatigue of the radiologist.

The sensitivity may be improved having each mammogram checked by two or more radiologists. It has been proved that double diagnosis improves sensitivity in at most 15% [12,16]. While one radiologist could fail to detect cancer in a small fraction of cases, another one could detect them. Nevertheless, double reading makes the process inefficient from the practical viewpoint, because the small number of specialists available at a given medical institution and their reduced individual productivity. A viable alternative is replacing one of the radiologists by a computer system, giving a second opinion [2,67].

7.1.3 Automatic Detection and Classification of Microcalcifications

Microcalcifications are tiny specks of mineral deposits (calcium), which can be scattered through the mammary gland, or can appear forming clusters. When a specialist detects microcalcifications in a mammogram, he or she observes some features of the particles themselves, and the patterns they present, in order to decide if the specks are of concern and further investigatory techniques or more regular screening are needed. A computer system can be used as a support for the specialists, helping them to make better decisions.

Several authors have tried to solve the problem of automatic detection of microcalcifications in digital mammograms [6,7,11,13,37,38,42,45–47,69,73]. This is not an easy problem to solve, because there are many difficulties caused mainly by the low contrast between microcalcifications and its surroundings, specially when the normal tissue is very dense. Additionally, microcalcifications may be very small, specially in their first stages of formation, making the observation very difficult.

Other authors have dealt with the problem of detecting microcalcification clusters [21, 51, 54, 61, 76]. In this case, the objective is to identify individual microcalcifications first, in order to use a clustering algorithm for grouping those microcalcifications.

For the detection of possible microcalcifications in mammograms, several methods have been used, like fractal models [7, 45], adaptive algorithms [68], mathematical morphology [6, 77], image differences [50, 59], artificial neural networks [76], laplacian of gaussians [19], support vector machines [5, 17], etc. For the classification of microcalcifications, methods like artificial neural networks [56], radial basis function (RBF) networks [34], kernel bayer classifiers [10], support vector machines [5], etc. have been applied.

In the following subsections, we describe the methods we use in more detail:

Difference of Gaussians (DoG) Filters

The method selected for this work for the detection of potential microcalcifications was the difference of gaussian filters (DoG). A gaussian filter is obtained from a gaussian distribution. When it is applied to an image, it eliminates high frequency noise, acting as a smoothing filter. A 2-D Gaussian distribution is defined by Equation 7.1:

$$G(x, y) = ke^{(x^2+y^2)/2\sigma^2} \tag{7.1}$$

where k is the height of the function and σ is the standard deviation.

A DoG filter is a band-pass filter, constructed from two simple gaussian filters. These two smoothing filters must have different variances. By subtracting two images obtained by the application of separate gaussian filters, DoG image containing only a desired range of frequencies is obtained. The DoG is obtained by subtracting two gaussian function, as shown in Equation 7.2.

$$DoG(x, y) = k_1 e^{(x^2+y^2)/2\sigma_1^2} - k_2 e^{(x^2+y^2)/2\sigma_2^2} \tag{7.2}$$

The parameters of a DoG must be adapted in order to enhance its detection performance. In other words, the detection capacity of a DoG filter depends of an adequate choice of the standard deviations of each gaussian filter that constitute it. When a DoG filter is applied to an image, a set of regions containing local maxima and minima is obtained. A binarization process allows retrieving only the local maxima, and a segmentation process extracts the regions of interest. DoG filters are adequate for the noise-invariant and size-specific detection of spots, resulting in a DoG image. This DoG image represents the microcalcifications if a thresholding operation is applied to it. We developed a procedure that applies a sequence of Difference of Gaussian Filters, in order to maximize the amount of detected probable microcalcifications (signals) in the mammogram, which are later classified in order to detect if they are real microcalcifications or not. Finally, microcalcification clusters are identified and also classified into malignant and benign.

DoG filters has been used in [14, 48, 52, 58].

Artificial Neural Networks

An artificial neural network (ANN), often just called simply a "neural network" (NN), is a massively parallel distributed processor made up of simple processing units, which has a natural propensity for storing experiential knowledge and making it available for use [28]. The original inspiration for the technique was from examination of the central nervous system and the neurons (and their axons, dendrites and synapses) which constitute one of its most significant information processing elements. It resembles the human brain in two respects:

- Knowledge is acquired through a learning process.
- Synaptic weights are used to store the knowledge.

An ANN has several benefits:

- *Nonlinearity*: A neural network made up of nonlinear neurons has a natural ability to realize (approximate) nonlinear inputoutput functions.
- *Universal approximation*: A neural network can approximate input-output functions (both static and dynamic) to any desired degree of accuracy, given an adequate computational complexity.
- *Adaptivity*: With the synaptic weights of a neural network being adjustable, the network can adapt to its operating environment and track statistical variations.
- *Fault tolerance*: A neural network has the potential to be fault-tolerant, or capable of robust performance, in the sense its performance degrades gradually under adverse operating conditions.
- *Neurobiological analogy*: Neurobiologists look to neural networks as a research tool for the interpretation of neurobiological phenomena. By the same token, engineers look to the human brain for new ideas to solve difficult problems.

According to its architecture, ANNs can be classified in:

- *Single-layer feedforward networks*, which consist of an input layer of source nodes and a single layer of processing units (neurons).
- *Multi-layer feedforward networks*, which contain one or more layers of hidden neurons that are inaccessible from both the input and output sides of the network. In a feedforward network, regardless of its type, signals propagate through the network in a forward direction only.
- *Recurrent networks*, Recurrent networks, which distinguish themselves from feedforward networks in that they contain one or more feedback loops that can be of a local or global kind. The application of feedback provides the basis for short-term memory, and provides a powerful basis for the design of nonlinear dynamical models.

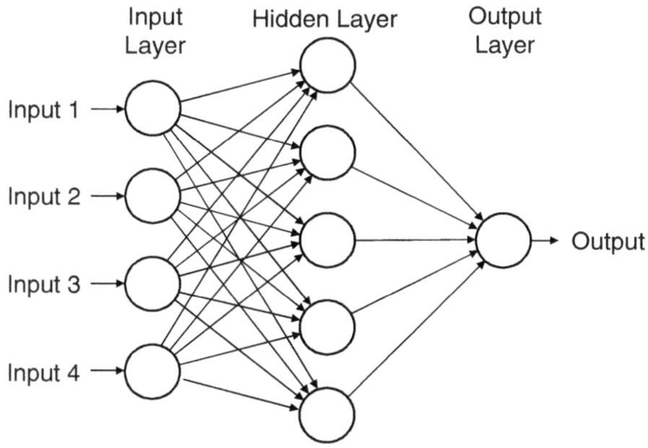

Fig. 7.2. Architecture of a Multi-layer Feedforward Neural Network

In Figure 7.2, the architecture of a multi-layer feedforward neural network (which will be referred as ANN for the remainder of this chapter, for reasons of simplicity) is shown. ANNs are considered to be very powerful classifiers compared to classical algorithms such as the nearest neighbour method. The algorithms used in neural network applications are capable of finding a good classifier based on a limited and in general a small number of training examples. This capability, also referred to as generalization, is of interest from a pattern recognition point of view since a large set of parameters is estimated using a relatively small data set.

Artificial neural networks (ANNs) have been successfully used for classification purposes in medical applications [55, 57, 64], including the classification of microcalcifications in digital mammograms [4, 7, 26, 39, 54, 62, 70, 72, 78]. Unfortunately, for an ANN to be successful in a particular domain, its architecture, training algorithm and the domain variables selected as inputs must be adequately chosen. Designing an ANN architecture is a trial-and-error process; several parameters must be tuned according to the training data when a training algorithm is chosen and, finally, a classification problem could involve too many variables (features), most of them not relevant at all for the classification process itself.

Genetic Algorithms

A Genetic algorithm (GA) is a search algorithm based on the mechanics of natural selection and natural genetics [22]. GAs were developed by John Holland and his colleagues at the university of Michigan in the early 1970s, and became more popular particularly with the publication of his 1975 book [33]. GAs are categorized as global search heuristics, and are a particular class of evolutionary algorithms (also known as evolutionary computation) that use techniques inspired by evolutionary biology such as inheritance, mutation, selection, and crossover (also called recombination).

GAs are implemented as a computer simulation in which a population of abstract representations (called chromosomes, the genotype or the genome) of candidate solutions (called individuals, creatures, or phenotypes) to an optimization problem evolves toward better solutions. Traditionally, solutions are represented in binary as strings of 0s and 1s, but other encodings are also possible. The evolution usually starts from a population of randomly generated individuals and happens in generations. In each generation, the fitness of every individual in the population is evaluated, multiple individuals are stochastically selected from the current population (based on their fitness), and modified (recombined and possibly randomly mutated) to form a new population. The new population is then used in the next iteration of the algorithm. Commonly, the algorithm terminates when either a maximum number of generations has been produced, or a satisfactory fitness level has been reached for the population. If the algorithm has terminated due to a maximum number of generations, a satisfactory solution may or may not have been reached. GAs have been applied successfully in many field, like biogenetics, computer science, engineering, economics, chemistry, manufacturing, mathematics, physics, etc.

A typical GA requires two things to be defined:

- a genetic representation of the solution domain,
- a fitness function to evaluate the solution domain.

A solution is commonly represented as an array of bits. Arrays of other types (integer, real numbers, etc.) and structures can be used in essentially the same way. The main property that makes these genetic representations convenient is that their parts are easily aligned due to their fixed size, that facilitates simple crossover operation. Variable length representations may also be used, but crossover implementation is more complex in this case. The fitness function is defined over the genetic representation and measures the quality of the represented solution.

The pseudo-code of a simple GA is the following:

1. Choose initial population
2. Evaluate the fitness of each individual in the population
3. Repeat
4. a) Select best-ranking individuals to reproduce
   b) Breed new generation through crossover and mutation (genetic operations) and give birth to offspring
   c) Evaluate the individual fitnesses of the offspring
   d) Replace worst ranked part of population with offspring
5. Until <terminating condition>

The population size depends on the nature of the problem, but typically contains several hundreds or thousands of possible solutions. Traditionally, the initial population is generated randomly, covering the entire range of possible solutions (the search space). Occasionally, the solutions may be "seeded" in areas where optimal solutions are likely to be found. During each successive generation, a proportion of the existing population is selected to breed a new generation. Individual solutions are selected through a fitness-based process, where fitter solutions (as measured by a fitness function) are typically more likely to be selected. Popular and well-studied selection methods include roulette wheel selection and tournament selection.

The next step is to generate a second generation population of solutions from those selected through genetic operators: crossover (also called recombination), and/or mutation. For each new solution to be produced, a pair of "parent" solutions is selected for breeding from the pool selected previously. By producing a "child" solution using the above methods of crossover and mutation, a new solution is created which typically shares many of the characteristics of its "parents". New parents are selected for each child, and the process continues until a new population of solutions of appropriate size is generated. These processes ultimately result in the next generation population of chromosomes that is different from the initial generation. Generally the average fitness will have increased by this procedure for the population, since only the best organisms from the first generation are selected for breeding, along with a small proportion of less fit solutions.

This generational process is repeated until a termination condition has been reached. Common terminating conditions are

- A solution is found that satisfies minimum criteria
- A fixed number of generations is reached
- The allocated budget (computation time/money) is reached
- The highest ranking solution's fitness is reaching or has reached a plateau such that successive iterations no longer produce better results
- Manual inspection
- Combinations of the above.

Evolutionary Neural Networks

Genetic algorithms (GAs) may be used to address the inherent problems presented by the ANNs mentioned previously, helping to obtain more accurate ANNs with better generalization abilities. Evolutionary artificial neural networks (EANNs) refer to a special class of ANNs in which evolution is another fundamental form of adaptation in addition to learning [74].

A distinctive feature of EANNs is their adaptability to a dynamic environment. EANNs are able to adapt to an environment as well as changes in the environment. These two forms of adaptation, evolution and learning in EANNs, make their adaptation to a dynamic environment much more effective and efficient. In a broader sense, EANNs can be regarded as a general framework for adaptive systems, systems that can change their architectures and learning rules appropriately without human intervention.

GAs can interact with ANNs at roughly three different levels: connection weights, architectures, and learning rules. The evolution of connection weights introduces an adaptive and global approach to training, especially where gradient-based training algorithms often experience great difficulties. The evolution of architectures enables ANNs to adapt their topologies to different tasks without human intervention and thus provides an approach to automatic ANN design as both ANN connection weights and structures can be evolved. The evolution of learning rules can be regarded as a process of "learning to learn" in ANNs where the adaptation of learning rules is achieved through evolution. It can also be regarded as an adaptive process of automatic discovery of novel learning rules [75].

EANNs that evolve connection weights overcome the shortcomings of the common gradient-descent-based training algorithms, by formulating the training process as the evolution of connection weights in the environment determined by the architecture and the learning task. GAs can then be used effectively in the evolution to find a near-optimal set of connection weights globally without computing gradient information. The fitness of an ANN can be defined according to different needs. Two important factors which commonly appear in the fitness (or error) function are the error between target and actual outputs and the complexity of the ANN. Unlike the case in gradient-descent-based training algorithms, fitness (or error) function does not have to be differentiable or even continuous since GAs do not depend on gradient information. Because GAs can treat large, complex, non-differentiable, and multimodal spaces, considerable research and application has been conducted on the evolution of connection weights.

In the evolution of connection weights, the architecture of the EANN is assumed to be predefined and fixed. The architecture design of an ANN is crucial for it successful application, because the architecture has a significant impact in the ANN performance. Traditionally, ANN architecture design is a job for human experts, who define the topology of the ANN based on their experience and a trial-and-error process. There is no a systematic way to design a near-optimal architecture for a given task. Design of the optimal architecture for an ANN has been formulated as a search problem in the architecture space where each point represents an architecture. Given some performance (optimality) criteria (lowest training error, lowest network complexity, etc.) about architectures, the performance level of all architectures forms a discrete surface in the space. The optimal architecture design is equivalent to finding the highest point on this surface, and GAs are adequate for this task.

Exhaustive reviews about EANNs have been presented by Yao [75] and Balakrishnan and Honavar [3]. More specifically, Fogel et al. [18] presented one of the first works about EANNs for screening features from mammograms. In this chapter, we present an automated procedure for feature extraction and training data set construction for training an ANN is proposed. It is also described the use of GAs for 1) finding the optimal weight set for an ANN, 2) finding an adequate initial weight set for an ANN before starting a backpropagation training algorithm and 3) designing the architecture and tuning some parameters of an ANN. All of these methods are applied to the classification of microcalcifications and microcalcification clusters in digital mammograms, expecting to improve the accuracy of an ordinary feedforward ANN performing this task. Some of our previous work on this subject is presented in [29–32, 53].

7.2 Methodology

The mammograms used in this project were provided by the Mammographic Image Analysis Society (MIAS) [66]. The MIAS database contains 322 images with resolutions of 50 microns/pixel and 200 microns/pixel. Only 118 in the database contain some abnormality (66 are benign and 52 are malignant) and the other 204 are diagnosed as normal. The abnormalities found in these mammograms are microcalcifications (25 cases), circumscribed masses (20 cases), spiculated masses (21 cases), ill-defined masses (15 cases), architectural distortions (20 cases) and asymmetries (17 cases). In this work, the images with a resolution of 200 microns/pixel were used. The data has been reviewed by a consultant radiologist and all the abnormalities have been identified and marked. The truth data consists of the location of the abnormality and the radius of a circle which encloses it. From the 25 images containing microcalcifications, 13 cases are diagnosed as malignant and 12 as benign. Several related works have used this same database [35, 44], some of them specifically for detecting individual microcalcifications [24, 41, 49, 60] and some others for detecting clusters [15, 27, 43, 65].

The general procedure receives a digital mammogram as an input, and it is conformed by five stages: pre-processing, detection of potential microcalcifications (signals), classification of signals into real microcalcifications, detection of microcalcification clusters and classification of microcalcification clusters into benign and malignant. The diagram of the proposed procedure is shown in Figure 7.3. As end-products of this process, we obtain two ANNs for classifying microcalcifications and microcalcifications clusters respectively, which in this case, are products of the evolutionary approaches that are proposed.

7.2.1 Pre-processing

During the mammogram acquisition process, and during the digitalization of the X-ray plaque, some noise can be added unintentionally to the images. Furthermore, only about 40% of each mammogram corresponds to the actual mammary gland. The remainder of the image is the background, that may also contain marks or labels that identify the mammogram, not relevant to the computer system. The pre-processing stage has the aim of eliminating those elements in the images that could interfere in the process of identifying microcalcifications. A secondary goal is to reduce the work area only to the relevant region that exactlycontains the breast.

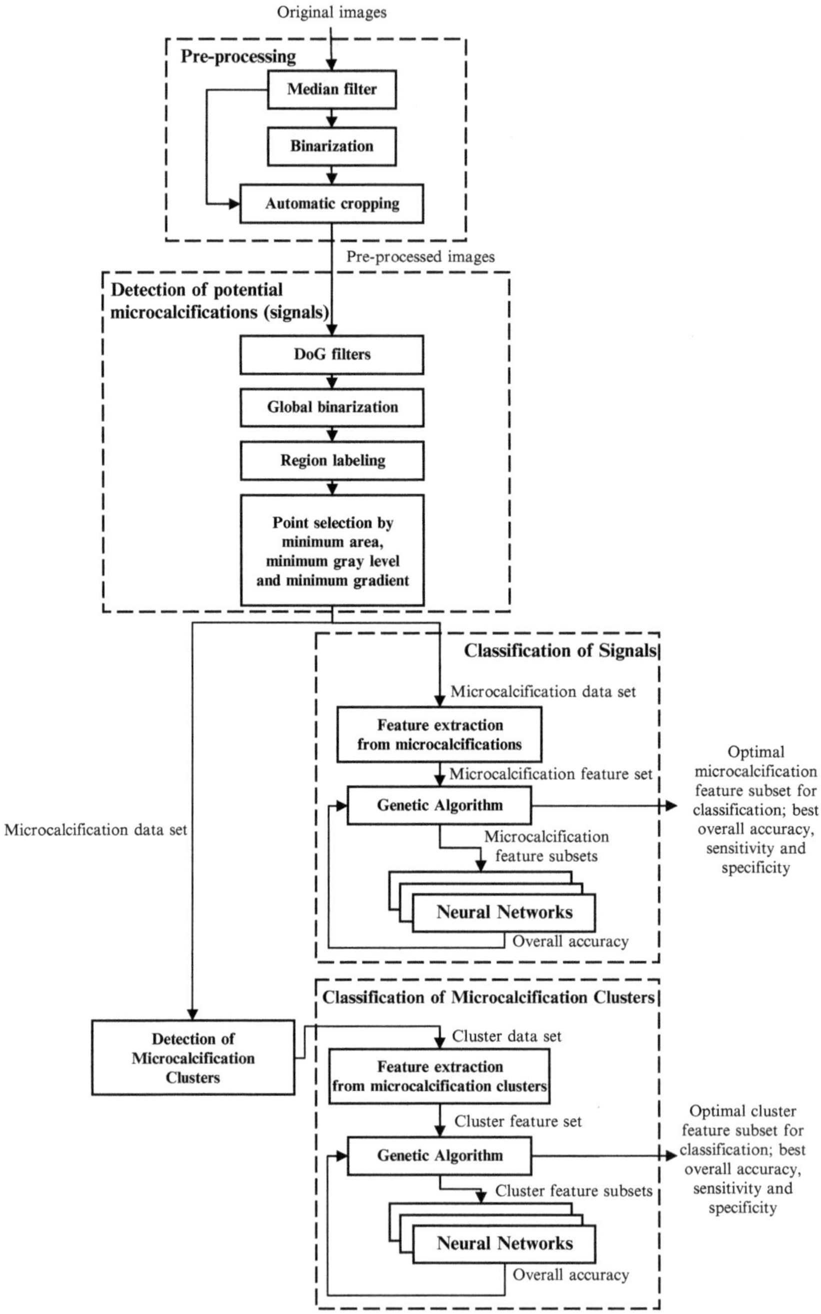

Fig. 7.3. Diagram of the proposed procedure

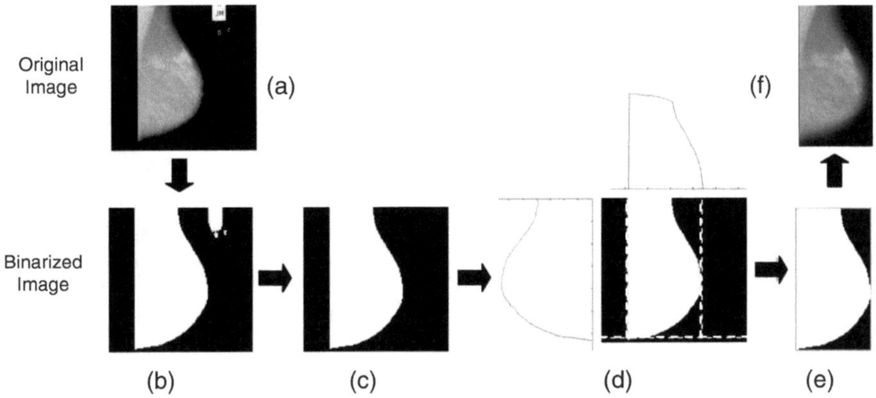

Fig. 7.4. The Pre-processing Stage: **(a)** original image, **(b)** binarized image, **(c)** binarized image without isolated regions, **(d)** determination of the boundaries for trimming, **(e)** trimmed binarized image and **(f)** trimmed original image

The procedure receives the original images as input. First, a median filter is applied in order to eliminate the background noise, keeping the significant features of the images. A median filter is a non-linear filter frequently used to eliminate high frequency noise without deleting significant features of the image. A 3x3 mask was used, centering it in each pixel of the image, replacing the value of the central pixel with the median of the surrounding nine pixels covered by the mask. The size of this mask was chosen empirically, trying to avoid the loss od local details.

Next, binary images are created from each filtered image. The purpose of the binary images is to help an automatic cropping procedure to delete the background marks and the isolated regions, so the image will contain only the region of interest. The cropping procedure first eliminates isolated elements that are not connected with the group of pixels corresponding to the breast, and then makes adequate vertical and horizontal cuts based on the sums of pixels by rows and columns in the binary image. Figure 7.4 depicts the pre-processing stage.

7.2.2 Detection of Potential Microcalcification (Signals)

The main objective of this stage is to detect the mass centers of the potential microcalcifications in the image (signals). The optimized difference of two gaussian filters (DoG) is used for enhancing those regions containing bright points. The resultant image after applying a DoG filter is globally binarized, using an empirically determined threshold. In Figure 7.5, an example of the application of a DoG filter is shown. A region-labeling algorithm allows the identification of each one of the points (defined as high-contrast regions detected after the application of the DoG filters, that cannot be considered microcalcifications yet). Then, a segmentation algorithm extracts small 9x9

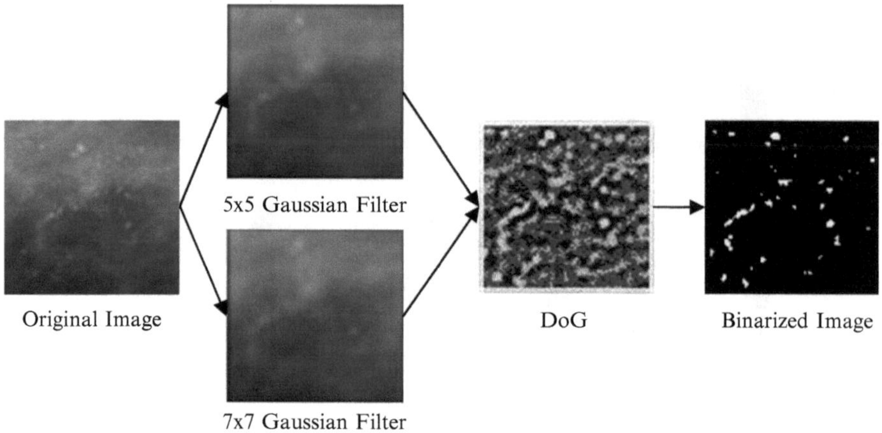

Fig. 7.5. Example of the application of a DoG filter (5×5, 7×7)

windows each, containing the region of interest whose centroid corresponds to the centroid of each point. In order to detect the greater possible amount of points, six gaussian filters of sizes 5×5, 7×7, 9×9, 11×11, 13×13 and 15×15 are combined, two at a time, to construct 15 DoG filters that are applied sequentially. Each one of the 15 DoG filters was applied 51 times, varying the binarization threshold in the interval [0, 5] by increments of 0.1. The points obtained by applying each filter are added to the points obtained by the previous one, deleting the repeated points. The same procedure is repeated with the points obtained by the remaining DoG filters. All of these points are passed later to three selection procedures.

These three selection methods are applied in order to transform a point into a signal (potential microcalcification). The first method performs selection according to the object area, choosing only the points with an area between a predefined minimum and a maximum. For this work, a minimum area of 1 pixel (0.0314 mm^2) and a maximum of 77 pixels (3.08 mm^2) were considered. The second method performs selection according to the gray level of the points. Studying the mean gray levels of pixels surrounding real identified microcalcifications, it was found they have values in the interval [102, 237] with a mean of 164. For this study, we set the minimum gray level for points to be selected to 100. Finally, the third selection method uses the gray gradient (or absolute contrast, the difference between the mean gray level of the point and the mean gray level of the background). Again, studying the mean gray gradient of point surrounding real identified microcalcifications, it was found they have values in the interval [3, 56] with a mean of 9.66. For this study, we set the minimum gray gradient for points to be selected to 3, the minimum vale of the interval. The result of these three selection processes is a list of signals (potential microcalcifications) represented by their centroids.

7.2.3 Classification of Signals into Real Microcalcifications

The objective of this stage is to identify if an obtained signal corresponds to an individual microcalcification or not. A set of features are extracted from the signal, related to their contrast and shape. From each signal, 47 features are extracted, related to:

- *Signal contrast*: Features related to the gray level of the pixels that are part of the signal (7 features).
- *Background contrast*: Features related to the gray level of the pixels that form the background in the window containing the signal (7 features).
- *Relative contrast*: Features that relate the mean gray level of the signal with the mean gray level of the background (3 features).
- *Shape features*: Features that describe the shape of the signal (20 features).
- *Contour sequence moments*: Moments of shape, mean and standard deviation extracted from the distance to the signal centroid (6 features).
- *Invariant geometric moments:* The first four invariants of Hu [36] (4 features).

A summary of the features extracted from the signals is presented in Table 7.2.

There is not an a priori criterion to determine what features should be used for classification purposes, so the features pass through two feature selection processes [40]: the first one attempts to delete the features that present

Table 7.2. Summary of features extracted from the signals (potential microcalcifications)

Signal contrast	Maximum gray level, minimum gray level, median gray level, mean gray level, standard deviation of the gray level, gray level skewness, gray level kurtosis.
Background contrast	Background maximum gray level, background minimum gray level, background median gray level, background mean gray level, standard deviation of the background gray level, background gray level skewness, background gray level kurtosis.
Relative contrast	Absolute contrast, relative contrast, proportional contrast.
Shape features	Area, convex area, background area, perimeter, maximum diameter, minimum diameter, equivalent circular diameter, fiber length, fiber width, curl, circularity, roundness, elongation1, elongation2, eccentricity, aspect ratio, compactness1, compactness2, compactness3, solidity.
Contour sequence moments	CSM1, CSM2, CSM3, CSM4, mean radii, standard deviation of radii.
Invariant geometric moments	IM1, IM2, IM3, IM4.

high correlation with other features, and the second one uses a derivation of the forward sequential search algorithm, which is a sub-optimal search algorithm. The algorithm decides what feature must be added depending of the information gain that it provides, finally resulting in a subset of features that minimize the error of the classifier (which in this case was a conventional feed-forward ANN). After these processes were applied, only three features were selected and used for classification: absolute contrast (the difference between the mean gray levels of the signal and its background), standard deviation of the gray level of the pixels that form the signal and the third moment of contour sequence. Moments of contour sequence are calculated using the signal centroid and the pixels in its perimeter, and are invariant to translation, rotation and scale transformations [25].

In order to process signals and accurately classify the real microcalcifications, we decided to use ANNs as classifiers. Because of the problems with ANNs already mentioned, we decided also to use GAs for evolving populations of ANNs, in three different ways, some of them suggested by Cantú-Paz and Kamath [9]. The first approach uses GAs for searching the optimal set of weights of the ANN. In this approach, the GA is used only for searching the weights, the architecture is fixed prior to the experiment. The second approach is very similar to the previous one, but instead of evaluating the network immediately after the initial weight set which is represented in each chromosome of the GA, is assigned, a backpropagation training starts from this initial weight set, hoping to reach an optimum quickly [63]. The last approach is not concerned with evolving weights. Instead, a GA is used to evolve a part of the architecture and other features of the ANN. The number of nodes in the hidden layer is very important parameter, because too few or to many nodes can affect the learning and generalization capabilities of the ANN. In this case, each chromosome encodes the learning rate, a lower and upper limits for the weights before starting the backpropagation training, and the number of nodes of the hidden layer.

At the end of this stage, we obtain three ready-to-use ANNs, each one taken from the last generation of the GAs used in each one of the approaches. These ANNs have the best performances in terms of overall accuracy (fraction of well classified objects, including microcalcifications and other elements in the image that are not microcalcifications).

7.2.4 Detection of Microcalcification Clusters

During this stage, the microcalcification clusters are identified. The detection and posterior consideration of every microcalcification cluster in the images may produce better results in a subsequent classification process, as we showed in [53].

Some authors define a microcalcification cluster as a group of three or more microcalcifications occupying a space lesser than 1 cm^2 [21,54,61], while others state that it is a group of two or more microcalcifications [76]. In this work, only the first definition is considered. We consider that every cluster fits inside a circle that contains a square with an area of 1 cm^2, that is, q circle with a radius of 0.7 cm. This radius, translated to pixels considering the resolution of 200 microns per pixel, is about 100 pixels in lenght.

This procedure receives a list of the microcalcifications obtained in the previous stage as input, and then produces a list of cluster features extracted and selected from each cluster. An algorithm for locating microcalcification cluster regions where the quantity of microcalcifications per cm^2 (density) is higher, was developed. This algorithm keeps adding microcalcifications to their closest clusters at a reasonable distance until there are no more microcalcifications left or if the remaining ones are too distant for being considered as part of a cluster. Every detected cluster is then labeled.

7.2.5 Classification of Microcalcification Clusters into Benign and Malignant

This stage has the objective of classifying each cluster in one of two classes: benign or malignant. This information is provided by the MIAS database.

From every microcalcification cluster detected in the mammograms in the previous stage, a cluster feature set is extracted. The feature set is constituted by 30 features, related to:

- *Cluster shape*: Features related to the convex polygon that contains all the microcalcifications of a cluster, and from the radii that connect each microcalcification to the cluster centroid (14 features).
- *Microcalcification area*: Features obtained from the area of the microcalcifications in the cluster (6 features).
- *Microcalcification contrast*: Features obtained from the mean gray level of the microcalcifications in the cluster (10 features).

These features are shown in Table 7.3.

The same two feature selection procedures mentioned earlier are also performed in this stage. Only three cluster features were selected for the classification process: minimum diameter, minimum radius and mean radius of the clusters. The minimum diameter is the maximum distance that can exist between two microcalcifications within a cluster in such a way that the line connecting them is perpendicular to the maximum diameter, defined as the maximum distance between two microcalcifications in a cluster. The minimum radius is the shortest of the radii connecting each microcalcification to the centroid of the cluster and the mean radius is the mean of these radii.

In order to process microcalcification clusters and accurately classify them into benign or malignant, we decided again to use ANNs as classifiers. We use GAs for evolving populations of ANNs, in the same three different approaches we used before for classifying signals. The first approach uses GAs for searching the optimal set of weights of the ANN. The second approach uses a GA

Table 7.3. Summary of features extracted from the microcalcification clusters

Cluster shape	Number of calcifications, convex perimeter, convex area, compactness, microcalcification density, total radius, maximum radius, minimum radius, mean radius, standard deviation of radii, maximum diameter, minimum diameter, mean of the distances between microcalcifications, standard deviation of the distances between microcalcifications.
Microcalcification Area	Total area of microcalcifications, mean area of microcalcifications, standard deviation of the area of microcalcifications, maximum area of the microcalcifications, minimum area of the microcalcifications, relative area.
Microcalcification Contrast	Total gray mean level of microcalcifications, mean of the mean gray levels of microcalcifications, standard deviation of the mean gray levels of microcalcifications, maximum mean gray level of microcalcifications, minimum mean gray level of microcalcifications, total absolute contrast, mean absolute contrast, standard deviation of the absolute contrast, maximum absolute contrast, minimum absolute contrast.

for defining initial weight sets, from which a backpropagation training algorithm is started, hoping to reach an optimum quickly. The third approach uses a GA for evolving the architecture and other features of the ANN as it was shown in a previous stage, when signals were classified. Again, each chromosome encodes the learning rate, a lower and upper limits for the weights before starting the backpropagation training, and the number of nodes of the hidden layer. For comparison, a conventional feedforward ANN is used also.

At the end of this stage, we obtain three ready-to-use ANNs, each one taken from the last generation of the GAs used in each of the approaches. These ANNs have the best performances in terms of overall accuracy (fraction of well classified clusters).

7.3 Experiments and Results

In this section, the experiments performed and the results obtained in every phase of the process are presented and discussed in detail.

7.3.1 From Pre-processing to Feature Extraction

Only 22 images were finally used for this study. In the second phase, six gaussian filters of sizes 5×5, 7×7, 9×9, 11×11, 13×13 and 15×15 were combined, two at a time, to construct 15 DoG filters that were applied sequentially. Each one of the 15 DoG filters was applied 51 times, varying the binarization threshold in the interval [0,5] by increments of 0.1. The points obtained by applying each filter were added to the points obtained by the previous one, deleting the repeated points. The same procedure was repeated with the points obtained by the remaining DoG filters. These points passed through the three selection methods for selecting signals (potential microcalcifications), according to region area, gray level and the gray gradient. The result was a list of 1,242,179 signals (potential microcalcifications) represented by their centroids.

The additional data included with the MIAS database define, with centroids and radii, the areas in the mammograms where microcalcifications are located. With these data and the support of expert radiologists, all the signals located in these 22 mammograms were preclassified into microcalcifications, and non-microcalcifications. From the 1,242,179 signals, only 4,612 (0.37%) were microcalcifications, and the remaining 1,237,567 (99.63%) were not. Because of this imbalanced distribution of elements in each class, an exploratory sampling was performed. Several sampling with different proportions of each class were tested and finally we decided to use a sample of 10,000 signals, including 2,500 real microcalcifications in it (25%).

After the 47 microcalcification features were extracted from each signal, the feature selection processes reduced the relevant features to only three: absolute contrast, standard deviation of the gray level and the third moment of contour sequence. Finally, a transactional database was obtained, containing 10,000 signals (2500 of them being real microcalcifications randomly distributed) and three features describing each signal.

7.3.2 Classification of Signals into Microcalcifications

In the third stage, a conventional feedforward ANN and three evolutionary ANNs were developed for the classification of signals into real microcalcifications.

The feedforward ANN had an architecture of three inputs, seven neurons in the hidden layer and one output. All the units had the sigmoid hyperbolic tangent function as the transfer function. The data (input and targets) were scaled in the range $[-1, 1]$ and divided into ten non-overlapping splits, each one with 90% of the data for training and the remaining 10% for testing. A ten-fold crossvalidation trial was performed; that is, the ANN was trained ten times, each time using a different split on the data and the means and standard deviations of the overall performance, sensitivity and specificity were reported. These results are shown in Table 7.4 on the row "BP".

For the three EANNs used to evolve signal classifiers, all of their GAs used a population of 50 individuals. We used simple GAs, with gray encoding, stochastic universal sampling selection, double-point crossover, fitness based reinsertion and a generational gap of 0.9. For all the GAs, the probability of crossover was 0.7 and the probability of mutation was $1/l$, where l is the length of the chromosome. The initial population of each GA was always initialized uniformly at random. All the ANNs involved in the EANNs are feedforward networks with one hidden layer. All neurons have biases with a constant input

Table 7.4. Mean (%) and standard deviation of the sensitivity, specificity and overall accuracy of simple backpropagation and different evolutionary methods for the classification of signals into real microcalcifications

	Sensitivity		Specificity		Overall	
Method	Mean	Std. Dev.	Mean	Std. Dev.	Mean	Std. Dev.
BP	75.68	0.044	81.36	0.010	80.51	0.013
WEIGHTS	72.44	0.027	84.32	0.013	82.37	0.011
WEIGHTS+BP	75.81	0.021	86.76	0.025	84.68	0.006
PARAMETERS	73.19	0.177	84.67	0.035	83.12	0.028

of 1.0. The ANNs are fully connected, and the transfer functions of every unit is the sigmoid hyperbolic tangent function. The data (input and targets) were normalized to the interval $[-1, 1]$. For the targets, a value of "-1" means "non-microcalcification" and a value of "1" means "microcalcification". When backpropagation was used, the training stopped after reaching a termination criteria of 20 epochs, trying also to find individual with fast convergence.

For the first approach, where a GA was used to find the ANNs weights, the population consisted of 50 individuals, each one with a length of $l = 720$ bits and representing 36 weights (including biases) with a precision of 20 bits. There were two crossover points, and the mutation rate was 0.00139. The GA ran for 50 generations. The results of this approach are shown in Table 7.4 on the row "WEIGHTS". In the second approach, where a backpropagation training algorithm is run using the weights represented by the individuals in the GA to initialize the ANN, the population consisted of 50 individual also, each one with a length of $l = 720$ bits and representing 36 weights (including biases) with a precision of 20 bits. There were two crossover points, and the mutation rate was 0.00139 ($1/l$). In this case, each ANN was briefly trained using 20 epochs of backpropagation, with a learning rate of 0.1. The GA ran for 50 generations. The results of this approach are shown in Table 7.4 on the row "WEIGHTS+BP".

Finally, in the third approach, where a GA was used to find the size of the hidden layer, the learning rate for the backpropagation algorithm and the range of initial weights before training, the population consisted of 50 individuals, each one with a length of $l = 18$ bits. The first four bits of the chromosome coded the learning rate in the range [0,1], the next five bits coded the lower value for the initial weights in the range [-10,0], the next five bits coded the upper value for the initial weights in the range [0,10] and the last four bits coded the number of neurons in the hidden layer, in the range [1,15] (if the value was 0, it was changed to 1). There was only one crossover point, and the mutation rate was 0.055555 ($1/l$). In this case, each ANN was built according to the parameters coded in the chromosome, and trained briefly with 20 epochs of backpropagation, in order to favor the ANNs that learned quickly. The results of this approach are shown also in Table 7.4, on the row "PARAMETERS".

We performed several two-tailed Students t-tests at a level of significance of 5% in order to compare the mean of each method with the means of the other ones in terms of sensitivity, specificity and overall accuracy. We found that for specificity and overall accuracy, evolutionary methods are significantly better than the simple backpropagation method for the classification of individual microcalcifications. No difference was found in terms of sensitivity, except that simple backpropagation was significantly better than the method that evolves weights.

We can notice too that, among the studied EANNs, the one that evolves a set of initial weights and is complemented with backpropagation training is the one that gives better results. We found that in fact, again in terms of specificity and overall accuracy, the method of weight evolution complemented with backpropagation is significantly the best of the methods we studied. Nevertheless, in terms of sensitivity, this method is only significantly better than the method that evolves weights.

7.3.3 Microcalcification Clusters Detection and Classification

The process of cluster detection and the subsequent feature extraction phase generates another transactional database, this time containing the information of every microcalcification cluster detected in the images. A total of 40 clusters were detected in the 22 mammograms from the MIAS database that were used in this study. According to MIAS additional data and the advice of expert radiologists, 10 clusters are benign and 30 are malignant. The number of features extracted from them is 30, but after the two feature selection processes already discussed in previous sections, the number of relevant features we considered relevant was three: minimum diameter, minimum radius and mean radius of the clusters.

As in the stage of signal classification, a conventional feedforward ANN and three evolutionary ANNs were developed for the classification of clusters into benign and malignant. The four algorithms we use in this step are basically the same ones we used before, except that they receive as input the transactional database containing features about microcalcifications clusters instead of features about signals. Again, the means of the overall performance, sensitivity and specificity for each one of these four approaches are reported and shown in Table 7.5.

We also performed several two-tailed Students t-tests at a level of significance of 5% in order to compare the mean of each method for cluster classification with the means of the other ones in terms of sensitivity, specificity and overall accuracy. We found that the performance of evolutionary methods is significantly different and better than the performance of the simple backpropagation method, except in one case. Again, the method that evolves

Table 7.5. Mean (%) and standard deviation of the sensitivity, specificity and overall accuracy of simple backpropagation and different evolutionary methods for the classification of microcalcification clusters

	Sensitivity		Specificity		Overall	
Method	Mean	Std. Dev.	Mean	Std. Dev.	Mean	Std. Dev.
BP	55.97	0.072	86.80	0.032	76.75	0.032
WEIGHTS	72.00	0.059	92.09	0.038	86.35	0.031
WEIGHTS+BP	89.34	0.035	95.86	0.025	93.88	0.027
PARAMETERS	63.90	0.163	85.74	0.067	80.50	0.043

initial weights, complemented with backpropagation, is the one that gives the best results.

7.4 Conclusions

This chapter has presented a comparison of simple backpropagation training and three methods for combining GAs and ANNs, applied to the classification of signals into real microcalcifications and microcalcification clusters into benign and malignant, on mammograms containing microcalcifications from the MIAS database. Our experimentation suggests that evolutionary methods are significantly better than the simple backpropagation method for the classification of individual microcalcifications, in terms of specificity and overall accuracy. No difference was found in terms of sensitivity, except that simple backpropagation was significantly better than the method that only evolves weights. In the case of the classification of microcalcification clusters, we observed that the performance of evolutionary methods is significantly better than the performance of the simple backpropagation method, except in one case. Again, the method that evolves initial weights, complemented with backpropagation, is the one that gives the best results.

As future work, it would be useful to include and process other mammography databases, in order to have more examples and produce transactional feature databases more balanced and complete, and test also how different resolutions could affect system effectiveness. The size of the gaussian filters could be adapted depending on the size of the microcalcifications to be detected and the resolution of images. The correspondence between the spatial frequency of the image and the relation σ_1/σ_2 has to be thoroughly studied. Different new features could be extracted from the microcalcifications in the images and tested also.

In this study, simple GAs and ANNs were used, and more sophisticated versions of these methods could produce better results. The use of real valued chromosomes, chromosomes with indirect representation (metaheuristics, NN construction rules, etc.), use of EANNs for feature selection, etc. are other approaches that could give different results. The inclusion of simple backpropagation training in the EANNs have consequences of longer computation times, so alternatives to backpropagation should be tested in order to reduce time costs.

Acknowledgments

This research was supported by the Instituto Tecnológico y de Estudios Superiores de Monterrey (ITESM) under the Research Chair CAT-010 and the National Council of Science and Technology of Mexico (CONACYT) under grant 41515.

References

1. American Cancer Society (ACS): Cancer facts and figures 2007. American Cancer Society, Inc., Clifton Road, NE, Atlanta, GA (2007).
2. Anttinen, I., Pamilo, M., Soiva, M., Roiha, M.: Double reading of mammography screening films: one radiologist or two? Clin. Radiol. **48** (1993) 414–421.
3. Balakrishnan, K., Honavar, V.: Evolutionary design of neural architectures. A preliminary taxonomy and guide to literature. Technical Report CS TR 95-01, Department of Computer Sciences, Iowa State University (1995).
4. Bankman, I. N., Tsai, J., Kim, D. W. et al.: Detection of microcalcification clusters using neural networks. In Proceedings of the 16th Annual International Conference of the IEEE Engineering in Medicine and Biology Society, Volume **16** (1994) 590–591.
5. Bazzani, A., Bollini, D., Brancaccio, R. et al.: System for automatic detection of clustered microcalcifications in digital mammograms. International Journal of Modern Physics, **11**(5) (2000) 901–912.
6. Betal, D., Roberts, N., Whitehouse, G. H.: Segmentation and numerical analysis of microcalcifications on mammograms using mathematical morphology. The British Journal of Radiology, **70** (1997) 903–917.
7. Bocchi, L., Coppini, G., Nori, J., Valli, G.: Detection of single and clustered microcalcifications in mammograms using fractal models and neural networks. Med. Eng. Phys, **26**(4) (2004) 303–312.
8. Bowcock, A. M.: Breast cancer: Molecular genetics, pathogenesis, and therapeutics (Contemporary cancer research). (1st Edition). Humana Press (1999) 582 pp.
9. Cantú-Paz, E., Kamath, C.: Evolving neural networks for the classification of galaxies. In Proceedings of the Genetic and Evolutionary Computation Conference, GECCO 2002, San Francisco, CA, USA (2002) 1019–1026.
10. Caputo, B., La Torre, E., Gigante, G. E.: Microcalcification detection using a kernel bayes classifier. in Proceedings of the Third International Symposium on Medical Data Analysis, ISMDA 2002, Rome, Italy, Springer, (2002) 20–31.
11. Cheng, H. D., Lui, Y. M., Freimanis, R. I.: A novel approach to microcalcification detection using fuzzy logic technique. IEEE Transactions on Medical Imaging, **17**(3) (1998) 442–450.

12. Ciatto, S., Del Turo, M. R., Risso, S. et al.: Comparison of standard reading and computer aided detection (CAD) on a national proficiency test of screening mammography. European Journal of Radiology, **45**(2) (2003) 135–138.
13. Comer, M. L., Liu, S., Delp, E. J.: Statistical segmentation of mammograms. In 3rd International Workshop on Digital Mammography, Chicago, IL (1996) 475–478.
14. Dengler, R., Behrens, S., Desaga, J. F.: Segmentation of microcalcifications in mammograms. IEEE Trans. Med. Imag., **12**(4) (1993).
15. Diyana, W. M., Larcher, J., Besar, R.: A comparison of clustered microcalcifications automated detection methods in digital mammograms. IEEE International Conference on Acoustics, Speech and Signal Processing ICASSP 2003, Hong Kong (2003).
16. Elmore, J. G., Miglioretti, D. L., Reisch, L. M. et al.: Screening mammograms by community radiologists: Variability in false-positive rates. Journal of the National Cancer Institute, **94**(18) (2002) 1373–1380.
17. El-Naqa, I., Yang, Y., Wernick, M. N. et al.: A support vector machine approach for detection of microcalcifications. IEEE Transactions on Medical Imaging, **21**(12) (2002) 1552–1563.
18. Fogel, D. B., Wasson III, E. C., Boughton, E. M., Porto, V. W.: Evolving artificial neural networks for screening features from mammograms. Artificial Intelligence in Medicine, Volume **14** (1998) 317–326.
19. Führ, H., Treiber, O., Wanninger, F.: Cluster-oriented detection of microcalcifications in simulated low-dose mammography. Bildverarbeitung für die Medizin (2003) 96–100.
20. Ganott, M. A., Harris, K. M., Klaman, H. M., Keeling, T. L.: Analysis of false-negative cancer cases identified with a mammography audit. The Breast Journal, **5**(3) (1999) 166.
21. Gavrielides, M. A.: A computer aid for the detection of suspicious microcalcification clusters in digitized mammograms. Master's thesis, Duke University (2002).
22. Goldberg, D. E.: Genetic algorithms in search, optimization and machine learning. Kluwer Academic Publishers, Boston, MA (1989).
23. Greene, F. L., Page, D. L., Fleming, I. D. et al.: AJCC Cancer Staging Manual (6th Edition). Springer (2002) 435.
24. Gulsrud, T. O.: Analysis of mammographic microcalcifications using a computationally efficient filter bank. Technical Report, Department of Electrical and Computer Engineering, Stavanger University College (2001).
25. Gupta, L., Srinath, M. D.: Contour sequence moments for the classification of closed planar shapes. Pattern Recognition, **20**(3) (1987) 267–272.
26. Gurcan, M. N., Chan, H.-P., Sahiner, B. et al.: Optimal neural network architecture selection: Improvement in computerized detection of microcalcifications, Academic Radiology **9**(4) (2002) 420–429.
27. Halkiotis, S., Mantas, J., Botsis, T.: Computer-aided detection of clustered microcalcifications in digital mammograms. In 5th European Conference in Systemic Science, Crete (2002).
28. Haykin, S.: Neural networks: A comprehensive foundation. Prentice Hall (1999).
29. Hernández-Cisneros, R. R., Terashima-Marín, H., Conant-Pablos, S. E.: Comparison of class separability, forward sequential search and genetic algorithms

for feature selection in the classification of individual and clustered microcalcifications in digital mammograms. International Conference in Image Analysis and Recognition ICIAR 2007, Springer Verlag, Montreal, Canada (2007) 911–922.

30. Hernández-Cisneros, R. R., Terashima-Marín, H.: Classification of individual and clustered microcalcifications in digital mammograms using evolutionary neural networks, MICAI 2006, Springer Verlag, Apizaco, Tlaxcala, Mexico (2006) 1200–1210.
31. Hernández-Cisneros, R. R., Terashima-Marín, H.: Evolutionary neural networks applied to the classification of microcalcification clusters in digital mammograms. In Proceedings of the 2006 IEEE Congress on Evolutionary Computation, Vancouver, BC, Canada (2006) 2459–2466.
32. Hernández-Cisneros, R. R., Terashima-Marín, H.: Feature selection for the classification of microcalcification clusters in digital mammograms using genetic algorithms. GECCO Workshop on Medical Applications of Genetic and Evolutionary Computation MedGEC 2006, Seattle, USA (2006).
33. Holland, J. H.: Adaptation in natural and artificial systems. University of Michigan Press, Ann Arbor (1975).
34. Hojjatoleslami, A., Sardo, L., Kittler, J.: An RBF based classifier for the detection of microcalcifications in mammograms with outlier rejection capability. International Conference on Neural Networks, Volume **3** (1997) 1379–1384.
35. Hong, B.-W., Brady, M.: Segmentation of mammograms in topographic approach. In IEE International Conference on Visual Information Engineering, Guildford, UK (2003).
36. Hu, M.-K.: Visual pattern recognition by moment invariants. IRE Trans. Information Theory, Vol. **IT-8** (1962) 179–187.
37. Ibrahim, N., Fujita, H., Hara, T., Endo, T.: Automated detection of clustered microcalcifications on mammograms: CAD system application to MIAS database. Physics in Medicine and Biology, **42**(12) (1997) 2577–2589.
38. Kim, J. K., Park, H. W.: Statistical textural features for detection of microcalcifications in digital mammograms. IEEE Transactions on Medical Imaging, **18**(3) (1999) 231–238.
39. Kim, J. K., Park, J. M., Song, S. S., Park, H. W.: Detection of clustered clustered microcalcifications on mammograms using surrounding region dependence method and artificial neural network. J. VLSI Signal Process., Volume **18** (1998) 251–262.
40. Kozlov, A., Koller, D.: Nonuniform dynamic discretization in hybrid networks. In Proceedings of the 13th Annual Conference of Uncertainty in AI (UAI), Providence, Rhode Island, USA (2003) 314–325.
41. Lasztovicza, K., Pataki, B., Székely, N., Tóth, N.: Neural network based microcalcification detection in a mammographic CAD system. In Intelligent Data Acquisition and Advanced Computing Systems: Technology and Applications, IDAACS 2003, Lviv, Ukraine (2003).
42. Lefebvre, F., Benali, H., Gilles, R. et al. A fractal approach to the segmentation of microcalcifications in digital mammograms. Med. Phys., **22**(4) (1995) 381–390.
43. Lemaur, G., Drouiche, K., DeConinck, J.: Highly regular wavelets for the detection of clustered microcalcifications in mammograms. IEEE Transactions on Medical Imaging, **25**(3) (2003) 393–401.

44. Li, S., Hara, T., Hatanaka, Y. et al.: Performance evaluation of a CAD system for detecting masses on mammograms by using the MIAS database. Medical Imaging and Information Science, **18**(3) (2001) 144–153.
45. Li, H., Liu, K. J., Lo, S. C.: Fractal modeling and segmentation for the enhancement of microcalcifications in digital mammograms. IEEE Trans. Med. Imaging, **16**(6) (1997) 785–798.
46. Linguraru, M. G., Brady, J. M., Yam, M.: Detection of microcalcifications using SMF. In 6th International Workshop of Digital Mammography (Lecture Notes in Computer Science), Springer Verlag (2002).
47. Liu, J., Hwang, W., Chen, M.: Estimation of 2-D noisy fractional brownian movement and its applications using wavelets. IEEE Transactions on Image Processing, **9**(8) (2000) 1407.
48. McGarry, G.: Performance of the generalized gaussian distribution for detection of calcifications in mammographic images. Signal Processing Research Centre, Queensland University of Technology, Brisbane, Australia (1999).
49. Melloul, M., Joskowicz, L.: Segmentation of microcalcifications in X-ray mammograms using entropy thresholding. In Computer Assisted Radiology and Surgery, CARS 2002, Springer (2002).
50. Nishikawa, R. M.: Computer aided detection of clustered microcalcifications: An improved method for grouping detected signals. Medical Physics, **20**(6) (1993) 1661–1666.
51. Norhayati, I., Hiroshi, F., Takeshi, H., Tokiko, E. Automated detection of clustered microcalcifications on mammograms: CAD system application to MIAS database. Phys. Med. Biol., **42** (1997) 2577–2589.
52. Ochoa, E. M.: Clustered microcalcification detection using optimized difference of gaussians. Master's Thesis, Air Force Institute of Tech. Wright-Patterson (1996).
53. Oporto-Díaz, S., Hernández-Cisneros, R. R., Terashima-Marín H.: Detection of microcalcification clusters in mammograms using a difference of optimized gaussian filters. In Proceedings of the International Conference in Image Analysis and Recognition ICIAR 2005, Toronto, Canada (2005) 998–1005.
54. Papadopoulossa, A., Fotiadisb, D. I., Likasb, A.: An automatic microcalcification detection system based on a hybrid neural network classifier. Artificial intelligence in Medicine, **25** (2002) 149–167.
55. Papik, K., Molnar, B., Schaefer, R. et al.: Application of neural networks in medicine - a review. Med. Sci. Monit., **4**(3) (1998) 538–546.
56. Patrocinio, A. C., Schiabel, H., Benatti, R. H. et al.: Investigation of clustered microcalcification features for an automated classifier as part of a mammography CAD scheme. Engineering in Medicine and Biology Society. Proceedings of the 22nd Annual International Conference of the IEEE Volume **2** (2000) 1203–1205.
57. Penny, W., Frost, D.: Neural networks in clinical medicine. Med. Decis. Making, **16** (1996) 386–398.
58. Polakowski, W. E., Cournoyer, D. A., Rogers, S. K. et al.: Computer-aided breast cancer detection and diagnosis of masses using difference of gaussians and derivative-based feature saliency. IEEE Transactions on Medical Imaging, **16**(6) (1997) 811–819.
59. Ricketts, I. W., Cairns, A. Y., Folkes, D. et al.: The automated detection of clusters of microcalcifications. In IEE Colloquium: Applications of Image Processing in Mass Health Screening, Digest No. 1992/056, London (1992) 13–15.

60. Sajda, P., Spence, C., Pearson, J.: Learning contextual relationships in mammograms using a hierarchical pyramid neural network. IEEE Transactions on Medical Imaging, **21**(3) (2002) 239–250.
61. Salfity, M. F., Kaufmann, G. H., Granitto, P., Ceccatto, H. A.: Automated detection and classification of clustered microcalcifications using morphological filtering and statistical techniques. In 5th International Workshop on Digital Mammography, Toronto, Canada (2000).
62. Sehad, S., Desarnaud, S., Strauss, A.: Artificial neural classification of clustered microcalcifications on digitized mammograms. In Proceedings of the IEEE International Conference on Systems, Man and Cybernetics, Volume **5** (1997) 4217–4222.
63. Skinner, A., Broughton, J. Q.: Neural networks in computational material science: traning algorithms. Modeling and Simulation in Material Science and Engineering, **3** (1995) 371–390.
64. Sordo, M.: Introduction to neural networks in healthcare [WWW document]. Open Clinical (2002) URL: http://www.openclinical.org/docs/int/neuralnetworks011.pdf
65. Strausz, G., Horváth, G., Pataki, B. et al.: Intelligent solution for mammography image diagnosis. In Engineering Application of Neural Networks Conference EANN 2003, Malaga, Spain (2003).
66. Suckling, J., Parker, J., Dance, D. et al.: The Mammographic Images Analysis Society digital mammogram database. Exerpta Medica International Congress Series, **1069** (1994) 375–378. URL: http://www.wiau.man.ac.uk/services/MIAS/MIASweb.html
67. Thurfjell, E. L., Lernevall, K. A., Taube, A. A. S.: Benefit of independent double reading in a population-based mammography screening program. Radiology, **191** (1994) 241–244.
68. Treiber, O., Wanninger, F., Führ, H. et al.: An adaptive algorithm for the detection of microcalcifications in simulated low-dose mammography. GSF - National Research Center for Environment and Health (2002) 1–24.
69. Ustymowics, M., Nieniewski, M.: Clustering microcalcifications in mammograms by means of morphology based strategy. In Fourth IEEE Benelux Signal Processing Symposium, Hilvarenbeek, Netherlands (2004).
70. Verma, B.: A neural network based technique to locate and classify microcalcifications in digital mammograms. In Proceedings of the IEEE International Conference on Neural Networks, Volume **3** (1998) 1790–1793.
71. World Health Organization: Fact sheet No. 297: Cancer [WWW document]. (2006) URL: http://www.who.int/mediacentre/factsheets/fs297/en/index.html
72. Woods, K., Doss, C., Bowyer, K. et al.: A neural network approach to microcalcification detection. IEEE 1992 Nuclear Science Symposium and Medical Imaging Conference, Orlando, FL (1992) 1273–1275.
73. Wróblewska, A., Boninski, P., Przelaskowski, A., Kazubek, M.: Segmentation and feature extraction for reliable classification of microcalcifications in digital mammograms, Opto Electronics Review, **11**(3) (2003) 227–235.
74. Yao, X.: Evolution of connectionist networks. In Preprints Int. Symp. AI, Reasoning and Creativity, Queensland, Australia, Griffith Univ. (1991) 49–52.
75. Yao, X.: Evolving artificial neural networks. In Proceedings of the IEEE, **87**(9) (1999) 1423–1447.

76. Yu, S., Guan, L.: A CAD system for the automated detection of clustered microcalcifications in digitized mammogram films. IEEE Transactions on Medical Imaging, **19**(2) (1999) 115–126.
77. Zhao, D., Shridhar, M., Daut, D. G.: Morphology on detection of calcifications in mammograms. In IEEE International Conference on Acoustics, Speech and Signal Processing ICASSP 92, Volume **3** (1992) 129–132.
78. Zheng, B., Qian, W., Clarke, L. P.: Digital mammography: mixed feature neural network with spectral entropy decision for detection of microcalcifications. IEEE Trans. Med. Imag., **15**(5) (1996) 589–597.

8

Bayesian Constrained Spectral Method for Segmentation of Noisy Medical Images. Theory and Applications

T. Sołtysiński

Institute of Precision and Biomedical Engineering, Department of Mechatronics, Warsaw University of Technology, Św. Andrzeja Boboli 8, 02-525 Warsaw, Poland
solek@mchtr.pw.edu.pl

Summary. The spectral method of medical images segmentation that is constrained by Bayesian inference on initial edge map detection is introduced and characterized. It is followed by discussion of the accuracy of the method, that depends on the noise that affects the data. Gaussian noise model is constructed and a method for noisy data multiscale wavelet decomposition and denoising is applied. The proposed segmentation method is tested for denoised cardiac ultrasonic data and its performance is compared for different noise clipping values. Further applications for multiple multimodal cases are presented showing the universality of the proposed method that is fixable and adaptable to the number of clinical applications. The brief discussion of the future development of the method is provided.

8.1 Introduction

Medical imaging, and particularly the methods of image recognition, analysis and interpretation is one of the most important fields of present days science. These methods are widely used for research purposes as well as in daily clinical practice. Since the advent of modern computing and graphical presentation of data a number of methods and algorithms for segmentation of medical images, one of the crucial points in automatic or semi-automatic image analysis, has been developed and introduced.

Segmentation is a process that reveals the required structure hidden in the data. The data are often disturbed by a noise what further makes the delineation of contours difficult. Segmentation is realized by finding all the data voxels or pixels which belongs to an object or its boundary. Number of technics is used [1] to achieve such a goal. One group, that is based on investigation of pixel intensity values covers technics like thresholding [2, 3], watershed algorithms [4–6], gradient filters, region growing [7] or level sets method [8–11]. Another approach is based on pattern recognition in an image. There are also methods derived from fuzzy sets theory and membership functions known

T. Sołtysiński: *Bayesian Constrained Spectral Method for Segmentation of Noisy Medical Images. Theory and Applications*, Studies in Computational Intelligence (SCI) **107**, 181–206 (2008)
www.springerlink.com

as fuzzy clustering methods. Different realization of segmentation is done by neural networks which process the data in the parallel distributed manner [12].

Very widely used are the methods adapting deformable models [13–20]. Having the initial model of particular geometrical shape it is further deformed according to the data properties as long as the final shape representing the required contour is found. This procedure is usually realized iteratively and certain criterion is checked at each step to control if the required accuracy is satisfied for currently found object's approximation. If not, the process is repeated. The criterion is usually a kind of cost function and the algorithm search for parameters that minimize it. The deformable model is given in analytical form and it is expressed as a partial differential equation (PDE). Another branch of deformable models are discrete models [21–23]. The great advantage of deformable models applications is their ability to follow the dynamics of a structure. Such applications are useful, for instance, for investigation of cardiac cycle or elastography of organs. The main limitations of these methods due to imprecise description of boundary conditions as well as concave boundaries has been overcome by more advanced methods based on force field called gradient vector flow (GVF) [24, 25]. One of the important feature of application of deformable models is the possibility of direct adaptation of *a priori* knowledge taken, for instance, from numerical anatomical atlases.

Incorporation of a priori knowledge is a complex task and is realized by a number of technics. Again, cost functions may be used to optimize a problem. Another approach is based on statistical analysis. One of such methods is Bayesian inference [26–30]. If the data and the model(s) may be described in terms of probability a new distribution *a posteriori*, containing the updated knowledge about the modified model given the data, may be derived. The inference allows one to find the maximum probability *a posteriori* that describes a modified model given the data and is the best representation of what is looked for. Bayesian inference is one of the state-of-the-art technics currently used for numerous methods of segmentation of medical images.

Another technic that has recently become widely used is multiscale segmentation. Development of number of transformations based on orthogonal and non orthogonal basis functions as well as the increase of computational power at low level costs make this approach especially attractive. These methods also offers a numbers of features not available in single scale methods. Besides the unique opportunity for efficient noise analysis and reduction that is provided by multiscale approaches such methods also enable the researcher or physician to investigate the multi level components of data independently. Multiscale methods covers such applications like denoising of data by wavelet coefficients clipping [31], optimal interpolation and statistical analysis of data [32], segmentation and contour detection based on multiscale measurement of pixel intensities [33], decreasing the time of segmentation [34], morphometric analysis of data [35], overlaying the surfaces on elastic bodies during their modeling [36] and image fusion [37].

The method proposed in this study is somehow combination of the most up-to-date approaches: multiscale decomposition and noise reduction, Bayesian inference and spectral method and offers some unique features difficult or impossible to achieve by other known methods [51].

8.2 Theory of Bayesian-constrained Spectral Method of Segmentation

8.2.1 Materials and Methods

The method proposed here is discussed on the chart shown on Figure 8.1. There are two main branches, the left showing the multiscale decomposition and noise reduction and the right, showing Bayesian-constrained spectral method. The right branch is composed of three main steps that are essential for the method: initial presegmentation realized by simple method like thresholding, Bayesian inference on edge position in the region of interest selected from data and the spectral method to smooth the raw edge map approximation found by the inference. All these steps are further explained in details through the next sections.

Raw Ultrasonic Data

For testing the method the algorithm has been applied to a number of ultrasonographic cardiac images. A centroid was calculated for each scan and then the final analysis of contour was done. The data was collected from a

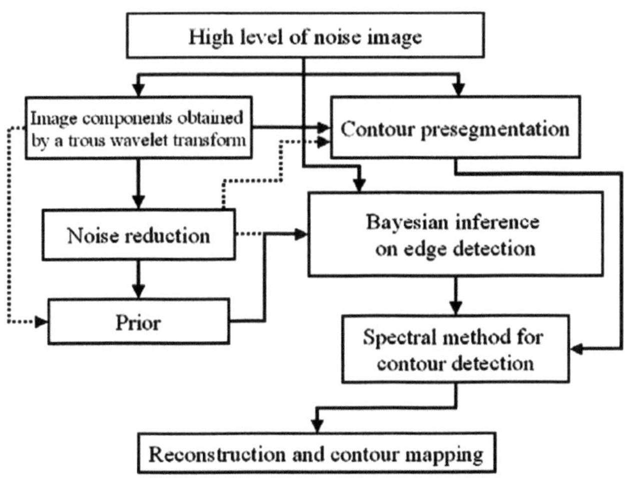

Fig. 8.1. Flow chart showing connections between different steps that may (*dotted lines*) or must be taken (*solid lines*) when the Bayesian constrained spectral method is applied. See text for detailed explanations

healthy volunteer, using an Ultramark ATL scanner equipped with a 3.5 MHz phased array probe. The data was sampled at 20 MHz rate. Throughout this paper one frame of cardiac cycle is used to test the approach (Fig. 8.2). The same raw frame was denoised at different levels.

The proposed method is new approach to image segmentation that combines the speed of spectral method in contour detection [40] and the Bayesian inference that allows for the most probable estimation on initial edge map. The method has been successfully applied to ultrasonic data and CT brain data with aneurysm and is described in details in [38, 39]. The real contour of investigated and segmented organ, see fig. 8.3, right, is extracted in the iterative process of solving the nonlinear partial differential equation (PDE). This step is realized in Fourier space by fast spectral method. PDE is approaching the function, as shown on fig. 8.4, that reveals the real edge of the object and starts from an initially guessed edge map, similar to

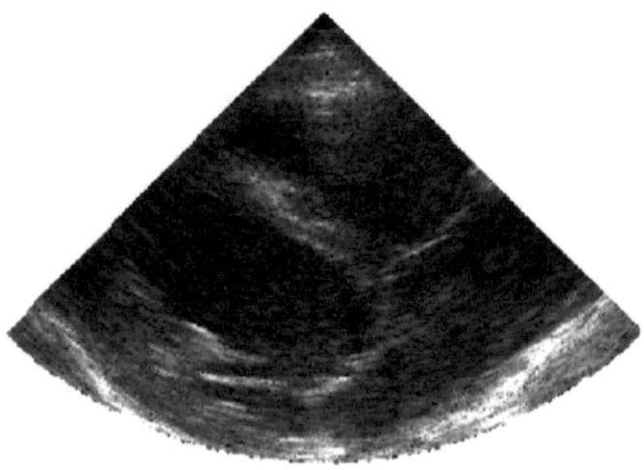

Fig. 8.2. Raw ultrasonic data presenting a frame of cardiac cycle. Left ventricle and mitral valve is clearly visible. The data is affected by typical ultrasonic speckle noise

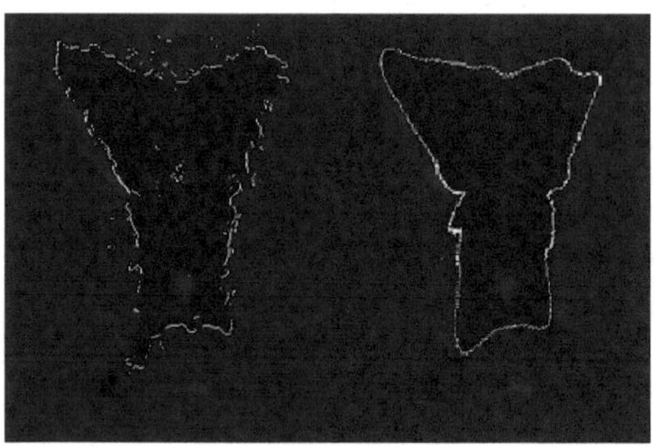

Fig. 8.3. Bayesian inferred edge map of the ventricle in brain with aneurysm in bad quality CT data, on the left. The same ventricle segmented due to the shown edge map by Bayesian constrained spectral method, the right image. Images taken from [38]

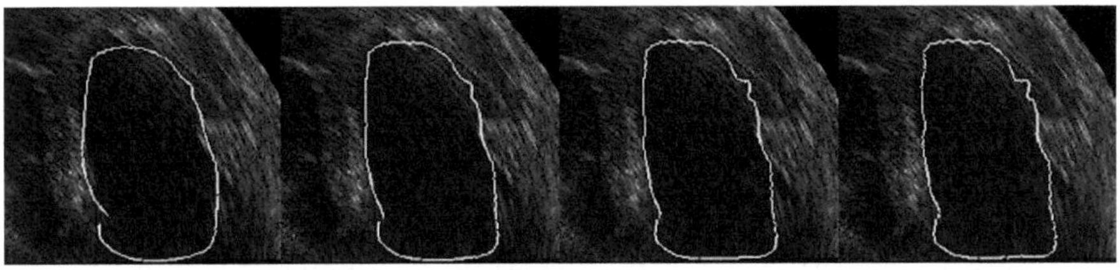

Fig. 8.4. First four steps, from the left, of PDE's iteration leading to the proper segmentation. Starting from the inferred Bayesian edge map the contour is approaching the real shape of the structure. The best approximation is reached after four iterations and shown at the most right frame. Images taken from [39]

the one shown on fig. 8.3, left. This iterative process is controlled by two parameters that describe fidelity of reconstruction: one, μ is steering the PDE and the other is responsible for slight smoothing of the resolved subsequent partial approximations of the final solution.

Contouring may be expressed as partial differential equation (PDE). This is the approach commonly found in methods based on active contours that are iteratively approaching the final contour. Following the work presented in [40] the final contour f may be found by solving the elliptic equation of Helmholtz type

$$\nabla^2 f - \mu(f - g) = 0 \tag{8.1}$$

This equation uses known variable which is initially guessed edge map g. It is solved in spherical coordinates. Moving the g term to right side and relating it to a previously found value of f, called f_n the PDE can be expressed in linearized form

$$\alpha \nabla^2 f_{n+1} - f_{n+1} = g_{f_n} \tag{8.2}$$

Such an equation is further easily solved by the fast spectral method. Applying $\alpha = 1/\mu$ the solution may be controlled by value of μ.

The edge map g is determined by Bayesian inference on edge placement in image data. Let $P(E_i/I)$ denote the required probability of the most appropriate edge in our existing data set. This is the conditional probability as it depends on the contents of I. $P(E_i/I)$ is the probability of the fact that the I's point belongs to the edge class E_i, knowing the value of intensity of this point. Let $P(I/E_i)$ be a probability of how much the value or intensity of a point is depending on edge class E_i. This term serves as a kernel. $P(E_i)$ is simply the probability of existence of the edge class E_i among all other detected edge classes. Edge class is a set of some subsequent pixel intensity values. Then the required probability can be found by solving the Bayes rule:

$$P(E_i/I) = \frac{P(I/E_i)P(E_i)}{P(I)} = \frac{P(I/E_i)P(E_i)}{\sum_i P(I/E_i)P(E_i)} \tag{8.3}$$

$P(I)$ is a sum of all probabilities $P(I/E_i)$ weighted by $P(E_i)$ and thus remaining constant. $P(I)$ is only a normalizing term and can be excluded from further analysis. The standard way of solving Bayes equation is the maximization of the right side over the parameter E_i (maximum likelihood, *ML* step) and then maximization of the found solution over all accessible data (maximum-a-posteriori, *MAP* step). The $P(E_i)$ is a prior and contains a priori knowledge.

In practice the $P(I/E_i)$ (Fig. 8.8) is estimated from the histogram of I along given radius (figure 8.5a) from centroid to a point of circumference of some bounding box selecting the region of interest (ROI). The histogram (figure 8.6) is shrank in such a way that each bin is equal to the edge size assuming that each expected edge covers the same number of intensity levels. Calculating the normalized probability over all edges E_i (figures 8.6 and 8.7), ML step is performed and the most probable edge in I is estimated. Then the MAP is done by searching for maximum over the data itself, and usually the first maximum in $P(I/E_i)$ is detected as an edge. $P(E_i)$ may be a constant value if we assume all edge classes as equally probable or may be distributed uniquely according to the prior knowledge. From $P(E/I)$ the polar edge map, $g(\theta)$ is derived (as shown on figure 8.5b).

The linearized equation 8.2 is solved by a spectral method [40]. Adapting Cheong's method [46] the Laplacian operator ∇^2 on the unit circle is expressed as follows:

$$\nabla^2 \frac{1}{\sin\theta}\frac{\delta}{\delta\theta}\left(\sin\theta\frac{\delta}{\delta\theta}\right) \tag{8.4}$$

Both functions, f and g are defined on the computational grid (θ_i), where $\theta_i = \pi(j+0.5)/J$. J is the number of points along the longitude of unit circle's

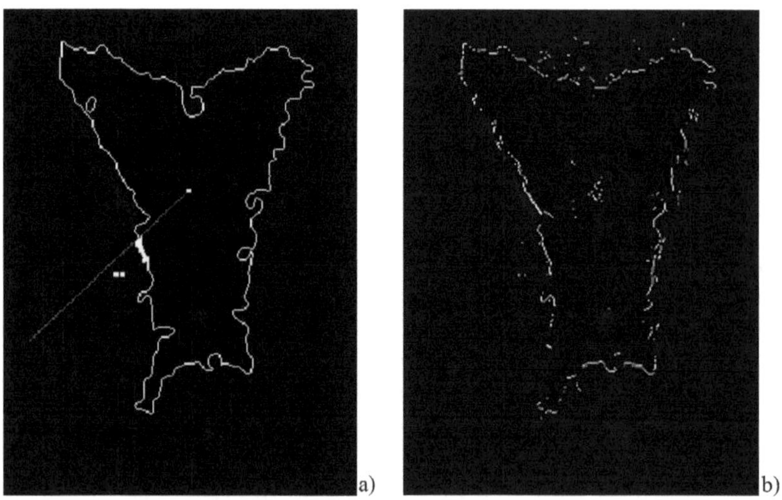

Fig. 8.5. Scanning radius used to select the data for Bayesian analysis, inside the ROI is presegmented contour **(a)**. The edge as it is found by Bayesian inference before spectral method is applied **(b)**

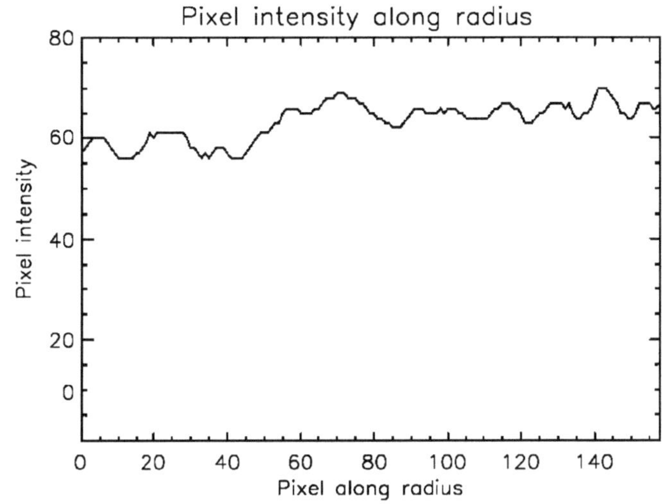

Fig. 8.6. The values of pixels along the radius that are further used for Bayesian inference

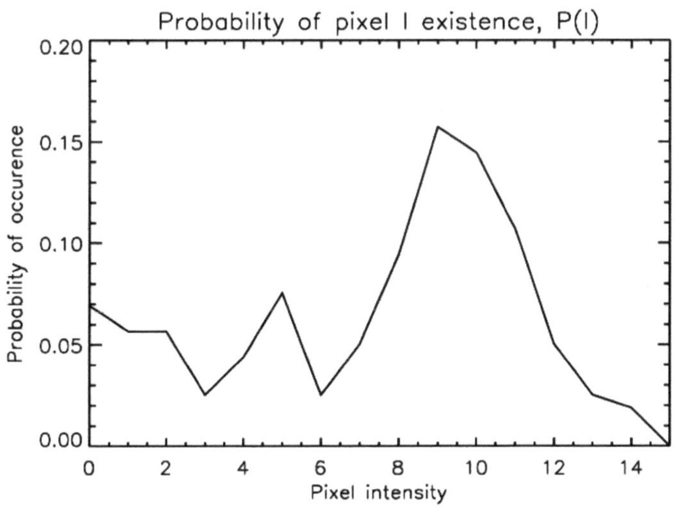

Fig. 8.7. Probability of existence of a pixel of given intensity value in data taken along scanning radius

circumference high enough to engage all points covered by g. Each point in g may be now expressed by its discrete cosine transform (DCT) representation yielding

$$g(\theta_i) = \sum_{n=0}^{J-1} g_n \cos n\theta_i \tag{8.5}$$

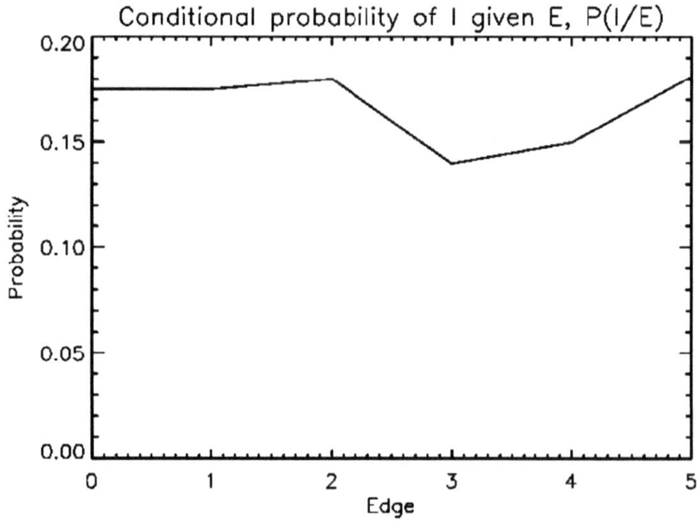

Fig. 8.8. Conditional probability of intensity values I in data given the edge class E. The edge class covers a subset of intensity values within certain range

with g_n being simply the coefficients of discrete cosine transform. Applying equation 8.4 into equation 8.1, it may be written as an ordinary differential equation (ODE):

$$\frac{1}{\sin\theta}\frac{\delta}{\delta\theta}\left(\sin\theta\frac{\delta}{\delta\theta}f(\theta)\right) = \mu\left[f(\theta) - g(\theta)\right] \tag{8.6}$$

which yields an algebraic system of equations in Fourier space:

$$p_{n-2}f_{n-2} - p_n f_n + p_{n+2}f_{n+2} = \mu\left[\frac{1}{4}g_{n-2} - \frac{1}{2}g_n + \frac{1}{4}g_{n+2}\right] \tag{8.7}$$

where

$$p_{n-2} = \frac{(n-1)(n-2)+\mu}{4}, \quad p_n = \frac{n^2+\mu}{2}, \tag{8.8}$$
$$p_{n+2} = \frac{(n+1)(n+2)+\mu}{4}$$

after substitution of eq. 8.5 into eq. 8.6 and expressing f in the same way as g. The index $n = 1, 3, \ldots J-1$ for odd n and $n = 0, 2, \ldots, J-2$ for even n. The system of equation 8.7 may be now expressed as a double matrix equation:

$$\mathbf{B}_e\hat{\mathrm{h}}_e = \mathbf{A}_e\hat{\mathrm{g}}_e, \qquad \mathbf{B}_o\hat{\mathrm{h}}_o = \mathbf{A}_o\hat{\mathrm{g}}_o \tag{8.9}$$

with subscripts e for even and o for odd n, $\hat{h}$ and $\hat{g}$ denote the column vector of expansion coefficients of $f(\theta)$ and $g(\theta)$, respectively. **B** is a tridiagonal matrix containing the left side of equation 8.7 and **A** is tridiagonal matrix with constant coefficients along each diagonal corresponding to right side of eq. 8.7.

Matrices **B** and **A** are of J/2 × J/2 size and contains only tridiagonal components. The f and g are column vectors with cosinus transform coefficients $f_m(\theta)$ and $g_m(\theta)$. The mark $\hat{}$ annotates vector's transposition. Subscripts o and e are for odd and even indexes, respectively.

For odd indexes the equation 8.9 in its full form is expressed as follows:

$$\begin{pmatrix} b_1 & c_1 & & & \\ a_3 & b_3 & c_3 & & \\ & \ddots & \ddots & \ddots & \\ & & a_{J-3} & b_{J-3} & c_{J-3} \\ & & & a_{J-1} & b_{J-1} \end{pmatrix} \begin{pmatrix} f_1 \\ f_2 \\ \vdots \\ f_{J-3} \\ f_{J-1} \end{pmatrix} = \begin{pmatrix} 2 & -1 & & & \\ -1 & 2 & -1 & & \\ & \ddots & \ddots & \ddots & \\ & & -1 & 2 & -1 \\ & & & -1 & 2 \end{pmatrix} \begin{pmatrix} g_1 \\ g_2 \\ \vdots \\ g_{J-3} \\ g_{J-1} \end{pmatrix} \tag{8.10}$$

with coefficients $\mathrm{a_n} = \mathrm{p_{n-2}}$, $\mathrm{b_n} = \mathrm{p_n}$, $\mathrm{c_n} = \mathrm{p_{n+2}}$. Similar equation may be shown for even indexes.

The calculated set of expansion coefficients f_{n+1} serves for the reconstruction of f_i the representation of g on the certain level of approximation i. By smoothing and summing all partial functions f_i, the required smooth approximation to g is recovered revealing the most probable edge map. Figure 8.9 shows the role of μ coefficient.

Application of Bayesian methodology allows for the initial detection of the most probable edge map. The uncertainty in map estimation is due to noise. This uncertainty may be decreased if the noise is removed first.

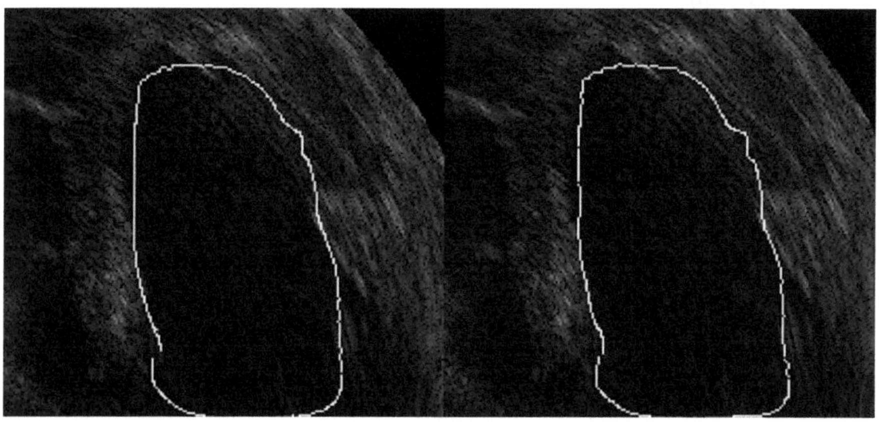

Fig. 8.9. Contour reconstruction for different μ values, (*left*) $\mu = 50$, (*right*) $\mu = 80$

8.3 Noise Model and Denoising of Medical Data by *à trous* Transform

We investigate noise removal from the data by multiscale wavelet analysis. The noisy medical data is decomposed by means of *à trous* algorithm [41, 42, 45] that provides the multiscale components of data. Each component represents details belonging to a particular scale. Those details also are affected by noise that differs between scales. Assuming a noise model, its influence on particular scales may be predicted a priori and efficiently removed by simple cancellation of appropriate coefficients of decomposition and subsequent synthesis [43]. In this work we apply our Bayesian constrained spectral algorithm to the same noisy medical data set with noise reduced at different rates by *à trous* decomposition (see also figure 8.10). It may be summarized as follows:

1. Initialize j, the scale index, to 0, starting with an image $c_{j,k}$ where k ranges over all pixels.
2. Carry out a discrete convolution of the data $c_{j,k}$ using a wavelet filter, yielding $c_{j+1,k}$. The convolution is an interlaced one, where the filter's pixel values have a gap (growing with level j) between them of 2^j pixels, giving rise to the name *à trous* – with holes.
3. From this smoothing it is obtained the discrete wavelet transform, $w_{j+1,k} = c_{j,k} - c_{j+1,k}$.
4. If j is less than the number J of resolution levels wanted, then increment j and return to step 2.

The original image is reconstructed by the summation of all $w_{j,k}$ and the smoothed array $c_{J,k}$, where J is the maximum that j may reach.

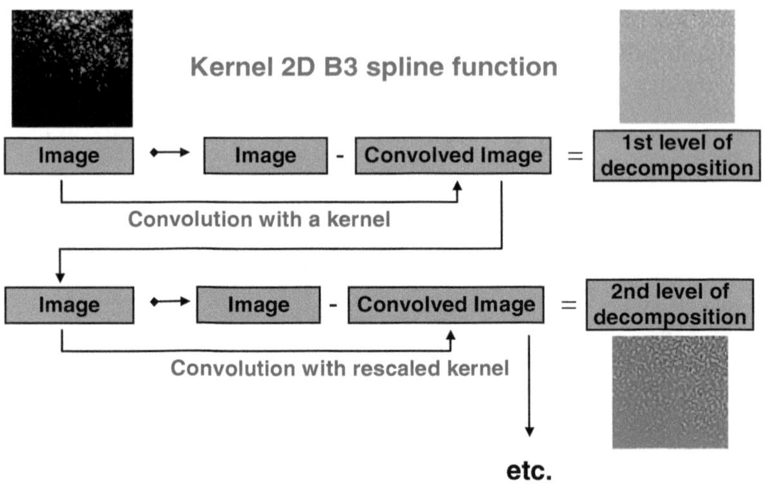

Fig. 8.10. Scheme that describes *à trous* wavelet decomposition algorithm

For the purpose of this study, further in the chapter, the reversed notation is used that, as it is believed, makes the analysis more intuitive and convenient. The smoothed component (originally $c_{J,k}$) has index 0 and all subsequent components, with increasing level of details have growing indexes. Hence, level $w_{1,k}$ (originally $w_{J,k}$) with index 1 has low details but of higher resolution than the base level with index 0, level $w_{2,k}$ contains details with higher resolution than previous level but lower than these ones at next level, etc.

The noise model has been assumed to be Gaussian [44]. This approach is justified when some data's noise is modeled at the first level of approximation. For the ultrasonic speckle noisy data it is valid as long as the data are nonlinearly logarithmically rescaled. Thus all further study of ultrasonic data are performed on logarithmically rescaled data that are further scaled back to linear scale for presentation that seems to be more convenient. The Gaussian model – with zero mean and standard deviation σ_j, where index j corresponds to scale – decomposed by *à trous* transform into its wavelet domain yields the probability density [45]:

$$p(w_{j,l}) = \frac{1}{\sqrt{2\pi}\sigma_j} e^{-w_{j,l}^2/2\sigma_j^2} \tag{8.11}$$

If the noise is stationary it is enough to compare $w_{j,l}$ to $k\sigma_j$, where l is given pixel position in image. If k is equal to 3 then we have standard rejection rate of 3σ. Further analysis is done as follows:

if $|w_{j,l}| \geq k\sigma_j$ then $w_{j,l}$ is significant and not treated as noise
if $|w_{j,l}| < k\sigma_j$ then $w_{j,l}$ is not significant and treated as noise (removed)

To find the accurate values of σ_j it is sufficient to decompose the image containing only the Gaussian noise with $\sigma = 1$. After decomposition each wavelet plane (scale or level) will contain the noise only but with different σ_j^e. Calculation of σ_j^e for each scale independently yields the table:

Scale j	0	1	2	3	4	5	6
σ_j^e	0.005	0.01	0.02	0.041	0.086	0.2	0.889

If for any 2D data, a standard deviation of its Gaussian noise σ_s is estimated, the σ_j may be easily found by simple calculation $\sigma_j = \sigma_s \sigma_j^e$.

Figures 8.11 and 8.12 shows the decomposed, denoised and synthesized data.

Both figures present the data and the noise residuals that are due to Gaussian noise model. Fig. 8.11 is generated for $k = 1\sigma_j$ clipping, while fig. 8.12 has $k = 3$.

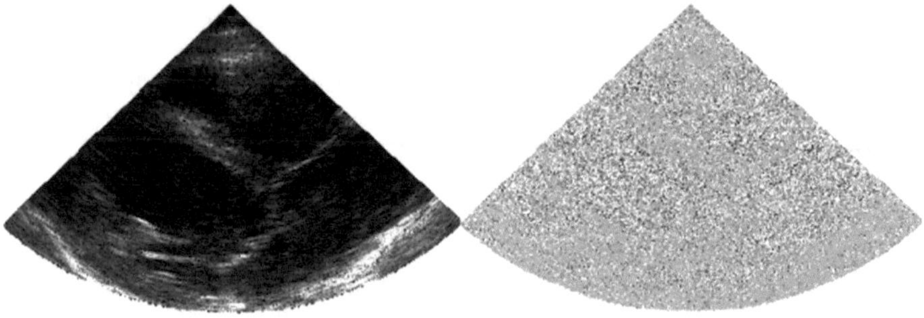

Fig. 8.11. The denoised data from fig. 8.2. On the left there is the frame with noise reduced by *à trous* decomposition, cancellation of wavelet coefficient below $k\sigma$, with $k = 1$, and subsequent synthesis. On the right there is an image of noise residuals, the data removed from the original frame and treated as noise

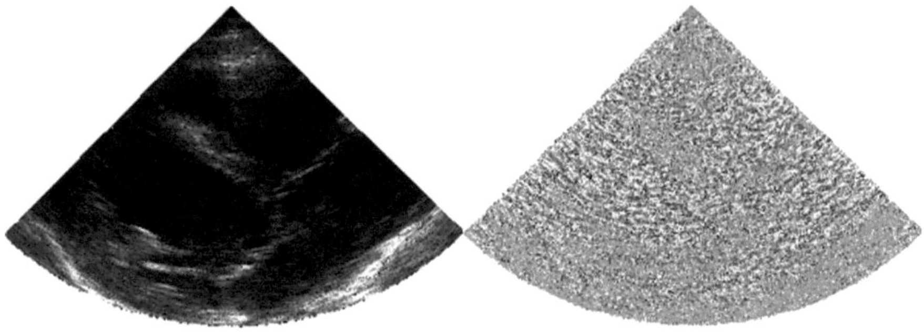

Fig. 8.12. The same as on fig. 8.11 but with noise reduced at $k = 3$

All obtained contours of the same structure are presented for different noise clipping k parameter. Due to limited size of the images only some minor differences are visible (figure 8.13). The contours are also plotted as a radial function of angles, where all the radii are bound to the numerically found centroid of the segmented structure (figure 8.14).

Due to anatomical properties of a heart's inner walls their structure is smooth. However, in ultrasonic imaging and the contour reconstruction by proposed algorithm there are some disturbances from smoothed shape if the noise is dominating. Suppressing the noise increases the smoothness of the structure, i.e. top curve seen on fig. 8.14, and more accurately recovers the real contour.

Denoising of the raw data also improves the Bayesian inference on edge map estimation. The residuals shown on figure 8.15 are obtained after noise removal and shows the significant difference between raw edge map, top curve of figure 8.15, and denoised edge map. The latter is more accurate as the inference is not confused by noise introducing accidental points that are falsely recognized as a structure.

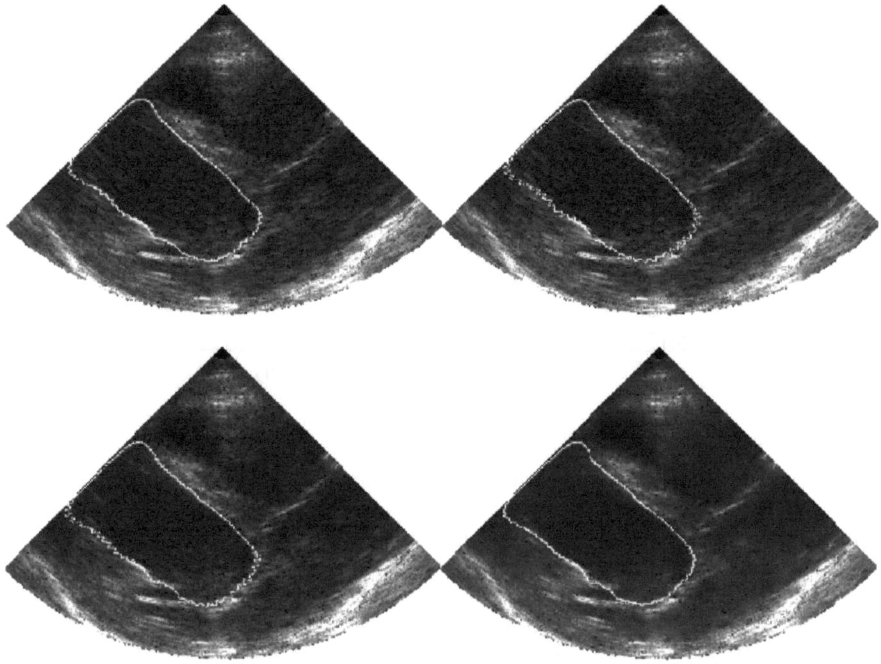

Fig. 8.13. From top left there is the segmented raw data, top right and at the bottom there are the contours obtained on denoised data, with $k = 1$, top right, $k = 3$, bottom left and $k = 6$, bottom right

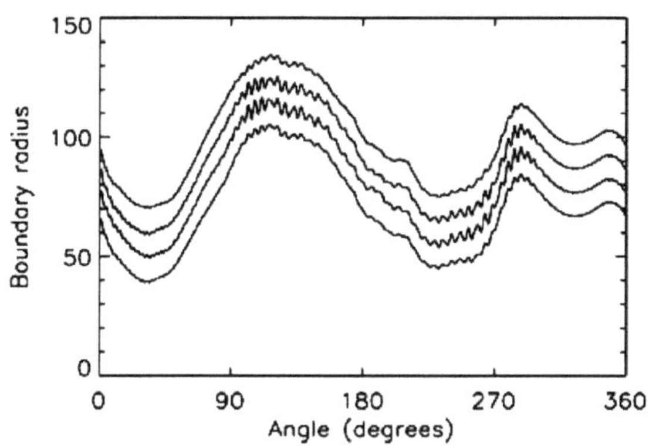

Fig. 8.14. The reconstructed radial contour functions of the segmented structure. From the bottom to the top there are the contours of original raw data, and subsequently, the contours obtained on denoised data clipped with $k = 1$, 3, and 6, respectively. The higher the threshold is, the upper a line is on the plot. Each line is shifted artificially due to the previous one by 10 points, just to enable the reader to compare them. In the real dimensions the lines are overploted

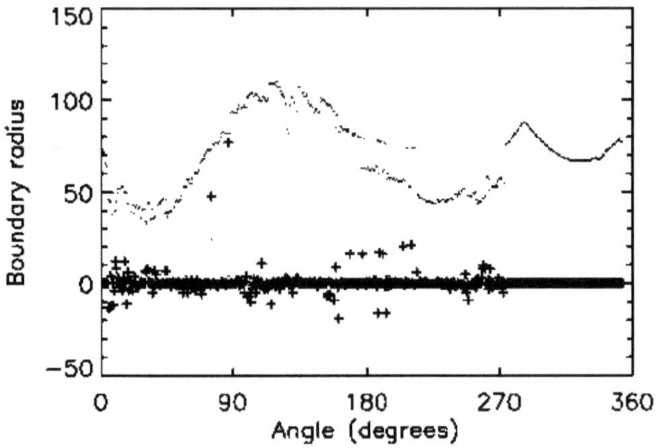

Fig. 8.15. Bayesian inferred edge map of raw data represented by edge point radii ploted in the function of angle, marked by points. The crosses are the residuals obtained by subtraction of the edge map obtained on the data clipped with $k = 6$ from the edge of raw data. These residuals show the imperfection in edge map estimation if the noise is present

8.4 Applications of Bayesian-constrained Spectral Method (BCSM) of Segmentation

Automatic Delineation of Left Ventricle in Ultrasonic Imaging of Cardiac Cycle

Presented method is widely adaptable to many modalities and different problems of segmentation as it is briefly shown through this section. The method provides fast and robust framework to automatically segment the cardiac cycle's ultrasonic images. Following steps were taken:

- Automatic centroid calculation of presegmented contour
- Selection of subsequent frame of the cycle (see figure 8.16 (a) for example)
- Noise reduction by *à trous* wavelet transform and $k = 1$ clipping of wavelet coefficients (figure 8.17).
- Construction of patterns used as a priori knowledge (presegmented contour) – priors.
- Construction of enhanced patterns by application of technic of multiresolution support [45], another method for multiscale image binarization (figure 8.18).
- Bayesian inference on edge position. 6 edge classes were assumed, parameters $\mu = 80$, $s = 20$. Multiple priors were used. Additional limitation was established to automatically correct misclassified edge points. The final edge found in a previous step was used as a limit for the currently investigated edge – if the calculated distance between the edges for the same scanning radius from two subsequent time points

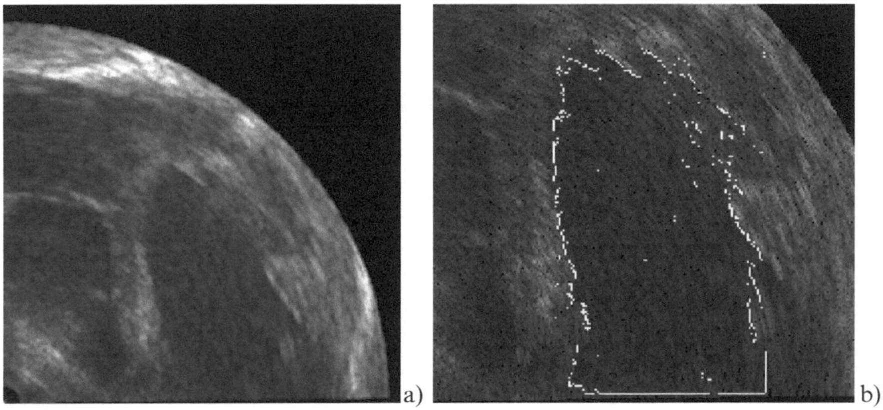

Fig. 8.16. An ultrasonic data sample. A frame before conversion, showing heart's left ventricle **(a)**, as an example of noisy medical imaging. ROI of this frame containing the ventricle only with Bayesian inferred edge map **(b)**

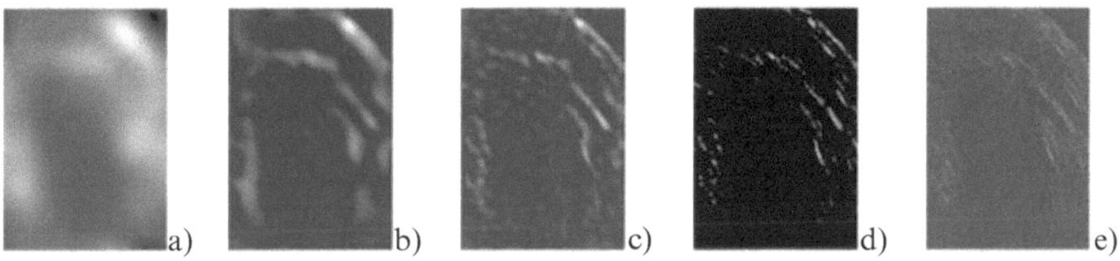

Fig. 8.17. Multiscale *à trous* decomposition of heart's left ventricle ultrasonic image of one frame of cardiac cycle. Scales of decomposition, from grain level **(a)** to finer scales **(b,c,d,e)**

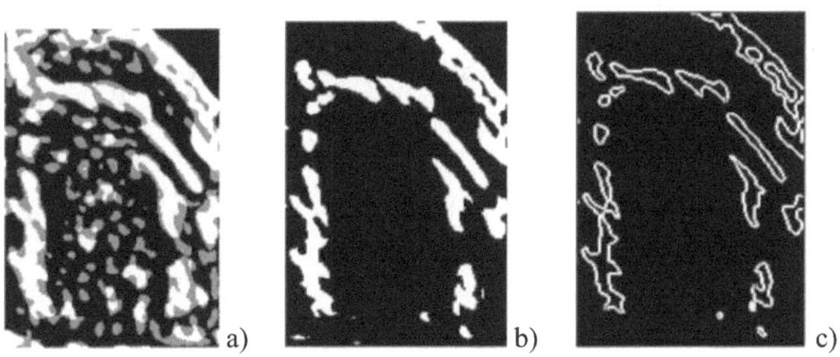

Fig. 8.18. Construction of enhanced prior for improved strategy in Bayesian inference based on multiresolution support (MRS), a technics based on *à trous* multiscale decomposition. Original image of MRS **(a)**, filtered image **(b)** and the same image with edges extracted by Sobel filtration **(c)**, the final prior used in inference

(frames) was greater than certain value the current edge position was corrected by assigning the value found in the previous step. Anatomical knowledge places limits on speed of ventricle walls movement what justify this operation.

- Contour reconstruction from Bayesian edge map by spectral method.
- Next step with another frame.

All subsequent reconstructed contours are shown on figure 8.19.

Fig. 8.19. All the cycle contours are derived in fully automatic manner from raw, ultrasonic image data. The dynamics of mitral valve's region is visible

Bone Shape Reconstruction

Another example of application of the new method is bone shape reconstruction from CT scans. The segmentation has been done with the following steps:

- Selection of scans from 3D data set.
- Initial thresholding
- I step of masking – mask was generated from a summarized image of all subsequent scans containing the tissue of bone of interest
- II step of masking – mask was generated from some predefined masks defining ROI for particular parts of bone. The partial masks were set as ellipses. Their sum, the final mask was conjugated (logical operation AND) with the mask obtained in step I
- The centroid has been calculated
- Bayesian inference with additional prior generated by Sobel filter acting on the thresholded and masked data
- Application of spectral method

The result, compared with the bone segmented with a standard technic of Sobel filtering of thresholded image is shown on figure 8.20. Obtained 3D shapes, combined from 2D radial functions revealed by Bayesian-constrained spectral method and visualised are shown on figure 8.21.

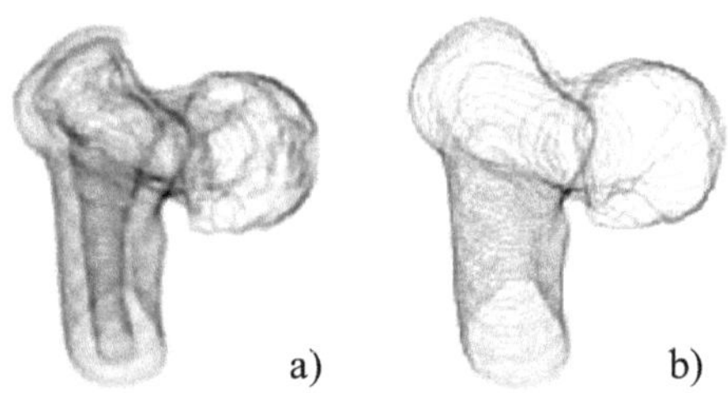

Fig. 8.20. Comparison of contours in 3D structure of a piece of thigh bone obtained by Sobel edge detection **(a)** and proposed method based on Bayesian inference **(b)**

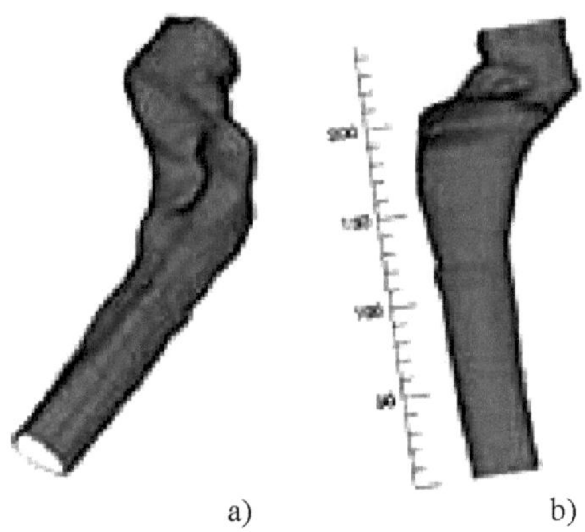

Fig. 8.21. Examples of the bone shown on fig. 8.20 reconstructed by proposed method and visualized in IDL environment

3D PET-CT Imaging of Active Part of the Liver

Diagnostics based on multimodal imaging are important part of clinical practice. The proposed method is applicable to bimodal medical images to support the diagnostics. When the combined functional and structural information is available some diagnostic questions are better addressed if they take both modalities as a source of information into account. For instance, if there is a question what is the PET active part of the liver the answer that we look for are the PET active regions that must belong to the liver even if in some close neighborhood there are some other emitting spots. Hence, to find the useful answer to the question one may need to segment the CT image taking the limitations from other modality, PET in our case. On the other hand CT image of liver is composed of the image of soft tissue that is hardly separable from surrounding soft tissue of spleen or digestive system as their Hounsfield number values are similar or overlapping. Then the information from PET modality is required that limits the tissue selection in CT mode. This self feedback is very well described in terms of probability, Bayesian inference and priors. Using CT mode as a primary source of information, the data and the PET mode data to derive a prior the Bayesian constrained spectral method may be applied. To construct the prior the multiscale decomposition was used together with some morphological operations done on image from each modality as well as on fusion of images from both modalities. The results of such application of the proposed method are shown on figures 8.22 and 8.23. Projecting the data into 3D space and visualization allow us to determine the PET emitting shape, or liver in the presented case, according to the rest of the body, as seen on figure 8.24.

Application to MRI-PET Bimodally Imaged Tumor Morphology

Bayesian constrained spectral method reveals the radial functions describing the most probable representation of a real contour that is hidden in data. This

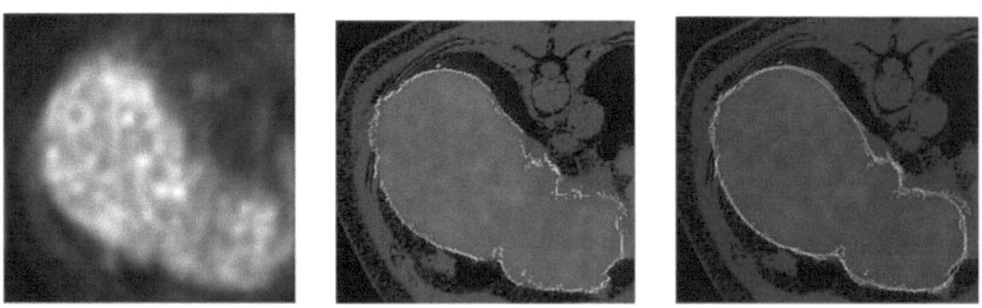

a) b) c)

Fig. 8.22. The prior for Bayesian inference on the region of PET activity in human liver (**a**). Initial edge map revealed by Bayesian inference (**b**) and the resulting contour based on this map, returned by spectral method (**c**)

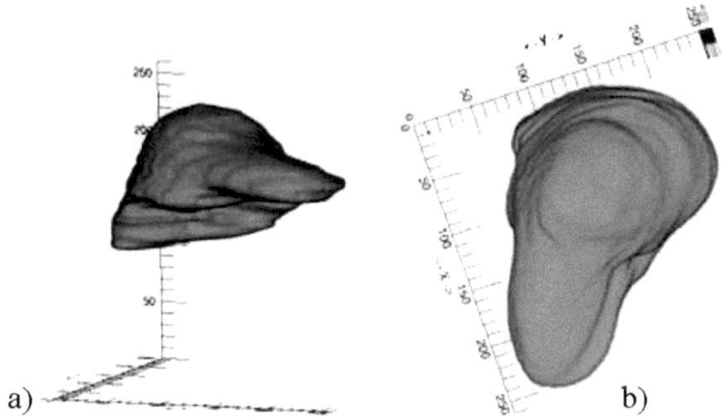

Fig. 8.23. Visualizations of 3D structure PET active region in human liver determined by proposed method

functional form makes it very straightforward to do some morphometry of the organ of interest. If the data is segmented by any means and the 3D representation of organs or objects of interest, like tumors, is available the proposed method may be applied to measure the fraction of the glucose consuming tissue to nonconsuming one in a tumor. This is done by virtual slicing of the object in any direction and application of BCSM to delineate the structure and derive the diameters in particular plane. Example of such object is shown on figure 8.25 where there is a fusion of MRI-imaged and PET-imaged brain tumor.

Application for Morphometry of Cells

Histopathological samples of a tissue contain numerous cells. Any automatic analysis of such samples is done by counting of the cells of interest, usually prepared and coloured differently than the surroundings. Then the measurement of cells properties is done and their total number, area, circumference length, shape, etc. is calculated. BCSM fits very well the requirements for such analysis. Using the method a number of parameters may be derived, the area, the circumference and the diameters of each cell. Example of delineation of a cell extracted by masking from a histopathological sample is shown on figure 8.26. This sample was prepared for angiogenesis research however a numerous different applications of BCSM are possible in the emerging field of molecular imaging [50].

Spleen's Semiautomatic Morphometry in Ultrasonic Imaging

Scanning of internal organs like spleen is often a challenging task. The organ is partially hidden beneath the rib, there may be a lack of echo from some parts of the scanning region, the organ lies beneath the fat layer, etc. However, if some a priori knowledge is available the organ may be reconstructed and its morphometry may be done. This is a crucial point for many

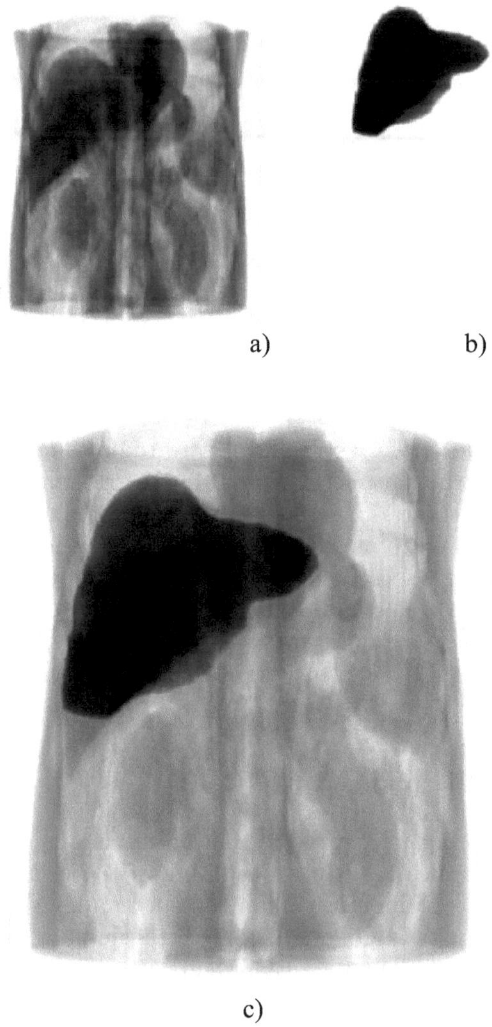

Fig. 8.24. Visualizations of 3D structure PET active region in human liver determined by proposed method. Structural 3D projection based on the CT volume **(a)**, functional 3D projection of PET active region of liver obtained by proposed method **(b)** and the fusion of two projections **(c)**

clinical applications, like estimation of the progress of splenomegaly, etc. The a priori knowledge in the discussed case, which is shown on figure 8.27, was put manually by simple pointing few marks, around 10, in the ROI where the spleen was displayed. Then the initial contour was found used further as a prior, the original data has been decomposed, noise reduced, automatic additional priors constructed and after Bayesian inference the initial edge map

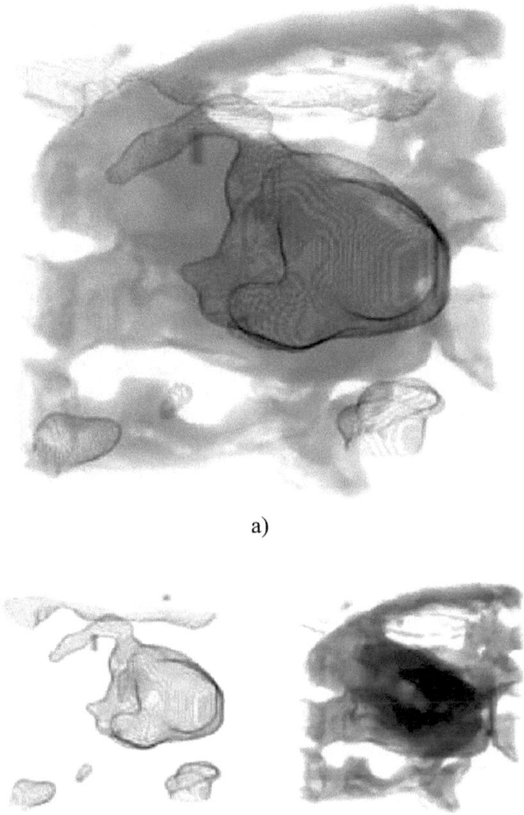

a)

b) c)

Fig. 8.25. Fusion **(a)** of structural MRI **(c)** and functional PET 3D volumes **(b)** limited to the tissue of brain cancer. The data was registered first by a method based on mutual information estimation

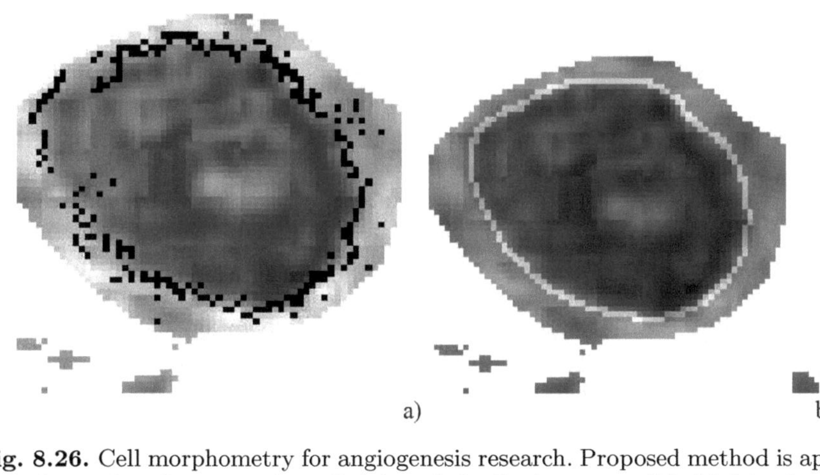

a) b)

Fig. 8.26. Cell morphometry for angiogenesis research. Proposed method is applied to find out the edge map of a cell **(a)** and the final contour **(b)**. Multiscale priors were used

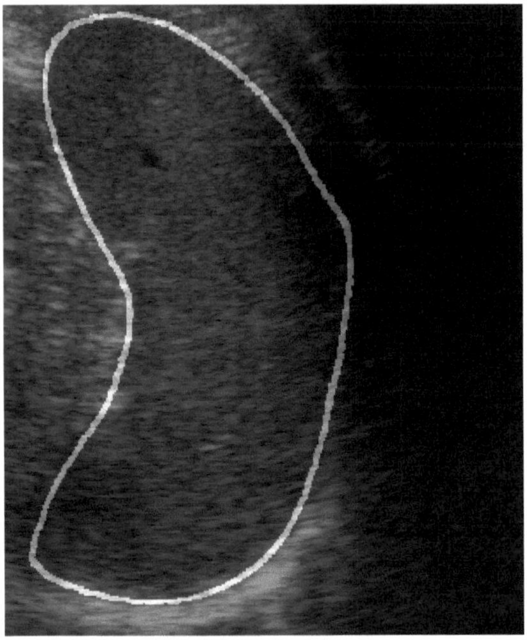

Fig. 8.27. Ultrasonic noisy image of spleen with delineated organ contour. The proposed method has been used

has been converted into the most probable representation of contour by spectral method. The result of delineation is also shown on figure 8.27. Similar applications for different inner organs are straightforward.

8.5 Conclusions and Future Directions

The method has been tested in many scales from cell level through internal organs to whole body. This makes it a universal tool for segmentation of a human tissue and organs of body in hierarchical or dynamical digital models. Another advantage of the method is arbitrary scaling of surface of visualized object and compression of information which is necessary for object's description.

The method is well suited for the analysis of noisy and disturbed data like that obtained by ultrasonography. Applications of the method to ultrasonic data is an alternative for existing methods [48, 49] especially in the case of dynamical modeling. Moreover, it offers a unique opportunity for missing information reconstruction. This is the main advantage of the method in applications to multimodal data as well. High ability of mutual information recovering supports the medical diagnostic process based on human-computer interaction.

Presented method is suitable for supporting the diagnostic process, it helps to manage huge amount of information about human body and its functions, provides tools for virtual reality, academic training and complex digital human modeling. Possible future direction of the method development is its fully 3D version, with spectral method working in 3D space [40] and appropriate novel Bayesian inference strategies and automatic incorporation of standard anatomic atlases. The, most interesting modification or development of the method would be done by applications of different PDE enhanced by additional driving terms and working in complementary to real space of adapted transform, that may be based on different than Fourier bases. Particularly suitable bases for such a purpose are different orthogonal wavelet bases.

Acknowledgments

This scientific work has been funded by resources of Science and High Education Ministry of Poland for years 2006–2007, in the frame of research grant number N518 023 31/1387.

References

1. Rogowska J. "Overview of fundamentals of medical image segmentation", I. N. Bankman ed., Handbook of Medical Imaging, Processing and Analysis, Academic Press, 69–86, 2000.
2. Sahoo P. K., Soltani S., Wong A. K. C. "A survey of thresholding techniques," *Computer Vision, Graphics, and Image Processing*, Vol. 41, 1988, 233–260.
3. Haralick R. M. and Shapiro L. G. *Computer and Robot Vision*, Vol. 1, Addison-Wesley, Reading, MA, 1992.
4. Beucher S. and Lantuejoul C. "Use of watersheds in contour detection" International Workshop on image processing, real-time edge and motion detection/estimation, Rennes, France, Sept. 1979.
5. Vincent L. and Soille P. "Watersheds in digital spaces: an efficient algorithm based on immersion simulations" IEEE Transactions on Pattern Analysis and Machine Recognition, Vol. 13, No. 6, 1991, pp. 583–598.
6. Drop D., Latala Z., Kasperek J., Patury R., Rajda P.J., Sadowski J., Szydlowski L., Wojnar L. "Hardware accelerated watershed based echocardiographic image segmentation" Computers in Cardiology, 2005 Volume, Issue, Sept. 25–28, 2005, page(s): 793–796.
7. Brice, C. R. and Fennema, C. L. "Scene Analysis Using Regions", AI(1), No. 3–4, Fall 1970, pp. 205–226.
8. Droske M., Meyer B., Rumpf M., Schaller C. "An Adaptive Level Set Method for Medical Image Segmentation", Lecture Notes In Computer Science; Vol. 2082 Proceedings of the 17th International Conference on Information Processing in Medical Imaging Pages: 416–422, 2001.
9. Osher S. and Paragios N. "Geometric Level Set Methods in Imaging, Vision, and Graphics", Springer-Verlag, New York, 2003.

10. Sethian J. "Level Set Methods and Fast Marching Methods: Evolving Interfaces in Computational Geometry", Fluid Mechanics, Computer Vision, and Materials Science, Cambridge University Press, Cambridge, UK, 2003.
11. Suri J., Liu L., Singh S., Laxminarayan S., Zeng X., Reden L. "Shape recovery algorithms using levels sets in 2-D/3-D Medical Imagery: A state-of-the-art review", IEEE Transactions on Information Technology in Biomedicine, volume 6, No. 1, 2002.
12. Wismuller A., Vietze F., Dersch D. R. "Segmentation with neural networks". I. N. Bankman, ed., *Handbook of Medical Imaging, Processing and Analysis*, pages 107–126. Academic Press, 2000.
13. Kass M., Witkin A., Terzopoulos D. "Snakes – Active Contour Models" International Journal of Computer Vision, 1(4): 321–331, 1987.
14. Cohen L. D. and Cohen I. "Finite element methods for active contour models and balloons for 2D and 3D images", IEEE-PAMI, Nov. 1993.
15. Osher S. and Sethian J. A. "Fronts propagating with curvature dependent speed: Algorithms based on Hamilton-Jacobi Formulations", Journal of Computational Physics, volume 79, pp. 12–49, 1988.
16. Caselles V., Kimmel R., Sapiro G., Sbert C. "Minimal surfaces: a geometric three-dimesional segmentation approach", Numer. Math., 1997.
17. McInerney T. and Terzopulos D. "Deformable models in medical image analysis: A survey": Med. Img. Analysis, no. 2 1996.
18. Malladi R., Sethian J. A., Vemuri B. C. "Shape modeling with front propagation: A level set approach," IEEE Transactions on Pattern Analysis and Machine Intelligence, 17(2): 158–175, Feburary 1995.
19. Caselles V., Catte F., Coll T., et al., "A Geometric Model for Active Contours in Image Processing," Numerische Mathematik, 66(1): 1–31 October 1993.
20. Cootes T. F., Taylor C. J., Cooper D. H., et al., "Active Shape Models – Their Training and Application", Computer Vision and Image Understanding, 61(1): 38–59, January 1995.
21. Delingette H. "General object reconstruction based on simplex meshes", Int. J. of Computer Vision, 1999.
22. Lachaud J.-O. and Montanvert A. "Deformable meshes with automated topology changes for coarse-to-fine 3-D surface extraction", Med. Img. Analysis, 1998.
23. McInerney T. and Terzopoulos D. "Topology adaptive deformable surfaces for medical image volume segmentation", IEEE-TMI, Oct. 1999.
24. Xu C. and Prince J. L. "Gradient Vector Flow: A New External Force for Snakes", Proc. IEEE Conf. on Comp. Vis. Patt. Recog. (CVPR), Los Alamitos: Comp. Soc. Press, pp. 66–71, June 1997.
25. Xu C. and Prince J. L. "Snakes, Shapes, and Gradient Vector Flow", *IEEE Transactions on Image Processing*, 7(3), pp. 359–369, March 1998.
26. Bard Y., *Nonlinear Parameter Estimation*, Academic, New York, 1974.
27. Bernardo J. M. and A. F. M. Smith, *Bayesian Theory*, John Wiley & Sons, New York, 1994.
28. Berry D. A., *Statistics: A Bayesian Perspective*, Duxbury, Belmont, 1996.
29. Berger J. O., Statistical Decision Theory and Bayesian Analysis, Springer, New York, 1985.
30. Box G. E. P. and Tiao G. C., *Bayesian Inference in Statistical Analysis*, John Wiley & Sons, New York, 1973.

31. de Stefano, A. and White P. R. "Selection of thresholding scheme for image noise reduction on wavelet components using bayesian estimation", *Jour. of Math. Imaging and Vision*, 21:225–233, 2004.
32. Fieguth P. W., Karl W. C., Willsky A. S., Wunsch C. "Multiresolution optimal interpolation and statistical analysis of TOPEX/POSEIDON satellite altimetry" *IEEE Transactions on Geoscience and Remote Sensing*, 33:280–292, 1995.
33. Sharon E., Brandt A., Basri R. "Segmentation and boundary detection using multiscale intensity measurements" *IEEE Computer Society Conference on Computer Vision and Pattern Recognition*, 1:469, 2001.
34. Sharon E., Brandt A., Basri R. "Fast multiscale image segmentation" *IEEE Conference on Computer Vision and Pattern Recognition*, 1:70–77, 2000.
35. Takemura C. M., et al. "Morphometrical data analysis using wavelets", *Realtime imaging*, 10:239–250, 2004.
36. Gefen S., Tretiak O., Bertrand L., Rosen D. G., Nissanov J. "Surface alignment of an elastic body using a multiresolution wavelet representation", *IEEE Transactions on Biomedical Engineering*, 51:1230–1241, 2004.
37. Wang H.-H. "A new multiwavelet-based approach to image fusion", *Journal of Mathematical Imaging and Vision*, 21:177–192, 2004.
38. Sołtysiński T. "Novel algorithm for active surface reconstruction by Bayesian constrained spectral method," Hozman J., Kneppo P., eds. IFMBE Proceedings, Vol. 11. Prague: IFMBE, 4191–4195, 2005.
39. Sołtysiński T., Kałużynski K., Pałko T. "Cardiac ventricle contour reconstruction in ultrasonographic images using Bayesian constrained spectral method", Lecture Notes in Artificial Intelligence Series, Springer-Verlag, 2006, in press.
40. Li J., Hero A. O. "A fast spectral method for active 3D shape reconstruction", Journal of Mathematical Imaging and Vision, 20, 73–87, 2004.
41. Holschneider M., Kronland-Martinet R., Morlet J., Tchamitchian P. "A real time algorithm for signal analysis with the help of the wavelet transform", w Wavelets: Time-Frequency Methods and Phase-Space, Springer-Verlag, 286–297, 1989.
42. Sołtysiński T., Rodatus A., Golnik N., Pałko T. "Comparison of multiscale entropy of healthy and cancer tissue imaged by optical polarimeter", IFMBE Proceedings, vol. 14, 2006.
43. Sołtysiński T. "Speckle Noise Removal By *À Trous* Decomposition And Threshold-limited Synthesis In Ultrasonic Cardiac Images", Proceedings of the conference Biosignal 2006, Brno Technical University, Czech Republic, vol. 18, 2006.
44. Gravel P., Beaudoin G., De Guise J.A. "A method for modeling noise in medical images", IEEE Transactions on medical imaging, vol. 23, no. 10, 1221–1232, 2004
45. Starck J.-L. and Murtagh F., Astronomical image and data analysis, Berlin: Springer, 2002.
46. Cheong, H. "Double Fourier series on a sphere: Applications to elliptic and vorticity equations", Journal of Computational Physics, 157, 1, 327–349, 2000.
47. Sołtysiński T. "Influence of multiscale denoising on Bayesian constrained spectral method in segmentation of noisy medical images", IFMBE Proceedings, vol. 14, 2006.
48. Dydenko I., Friboulet D., Gorce J. M., D'Hooge J., Bijnens B., Magnin I. E., "Towards ultrasound cardiac image segmentation based on the radiofrequency signal", Medical Image Analysis, 7, 353–367, 2003.

49. Hammoude A. "Endocardial border identification in two-dimensional echocardiographic images: review of methods", Computers in Medical Imaging and Graphics 32, 181–193, 1998.
50. Sołtysiński T., "Novel Bayesian constrained spectral method for cell morphometry in multimodal molecular imaging", Proceedings of ESMI, 2007.
51. Handbook of Medical Imaging, Processing and Analysis, I. N. Bankman ed., Academic Press, 2000.

9

Breaking Accessibility Barriers: Computational Intelligence in Music Processing for Blind People

Wladyslaw Homenda

Faculty of Mathematics and Information Science, Warsaw University of Technology, Plac Politechniki 1, 00-660 Warszawa, Poland
homenda@mini.pw.edu.pl

Summary. A discussion on involvement of knowledge based methods in implementation of user friendly computer programs for disabled people is the goal of this paper. The paper presents a concept of a computer program that is aimed to aid blind people dealing with music and music notation. The concept is solely based on computational intelligence methods involved in implementation of the computer program. The program is build around two research fields: information acquisition and knowledge representation and processing which are still research and technology challenges. Information acquisition module is used for recognizing printed music notation and storing acquired information in computer memory. This module is a kind of the paper-to-memory data flow technology. Acquired music information stored in computer memory is then subjected to mining implicit relations between music data, to creating a space of music information and then to manipulating music information. Storing and manipulating music information is firmly based on knowledge processing methods. The program described in this paper involves techniques of pattern recognition and knowledge representation as well as contemporary programming technologies. It is designed for blind people: music teachers, students, hobbyists, musicians.

9.1 Introduction

In this paper we attempt to study application of computational intelligence in a real life computer program. The program is supposed to handle music information and to provide an access for disabled people, for blind people in our case. The term *computational intelligence*, though widely used by computer researchers, has neither a common definition nor it is uniquely understood by the academic community. However, it is not our aim to provoke a discussion on what artificial intelligence is and which methods it does embed. Instead, we rather use the term in a common sense. In this sense intuitively understood knowledge representation and processing is a main feature of it. Enormous development of computer hardware over past decades has enabled

W. Homenda: *Breaking Accessibility Barriers: Computational Intelligence in Music Processing for Blind People*, Studies in Computational Intelligence (SCI) **107**, 207–232 (2008)
www.springerlink.com

bringing computers as tools interacting with human partners in an intelligent way. This required, of course, the use of methods that firmly belong to the domain of computational intelligence and widely apply knowledge processing.

Allowing disabled people to use computer facilities is an important social aspect of software and hardware development. Disabled people are faced problems specific to their infirmities. Such problems have been considered by hardware and software producers. Most important operating systems include integrated accessibility options and technologies. For instance, Microsoft Windows includes Active Accessibility techniques, Apple MacOS has Universal Access tools, Linux brings Gnome Assistive Technology. These technologies support disabled people and, also, provide development tools for programmers. They also stimulate software producers to support accessibility options in created software. Specifically, if a computer program satisfies necessary cooperation criteria with a given accessibility technology, it becomes useful for disabled people.

In the age of information revolution development of software tools for disabled people is far inadequate to necessities. The concept of music processing support with a computer program dedicated to blind people is aimed to fill in a gap between requirements and tools available. Bringing accessibility technology to blind people is usually based on computational intelligence methods such as pattern recognition and knowledge representation and processing. Music processing computer program discussed in this paper, which is intended to contribute in breaking the accessibility barrier, is solely based on both fields. Pattern recognition is applied in music notation recognition. Knowledge representation and processing is used in music information storage and processing.

9.1.1 Notes on Accessibility for Blind People

The population of blind people is estimated to up to 20 millions. Blindness, one of most important disabilities, makes suffering people unable to use ordinary computing facilities. They need dedicated hardware and, what is even more important, dedicated software. In this Section our interest is focused on accessibility options for blind people that are available in programming environments and computer systems.

An important standard of accessibility options for disabled people is provided by IBM Corporation. This standard is common for all kinds of personal computers and operating systems. The fundamental technique, which must be applied in blind people aimed software, relies on assigning all program functions to keyboard. Blind people do not use mouse or other pointing devices, thus mouse functionality must also be assigned to keyboard. This requirement allows blind user to learn keyboard shortcuts which activates any function of the program (moreover, keyboard shortcuts often allow people with good eyesight to master software faster then in case of mouse usage). For instance, Drag and Drop, the typical mouse operation, should be available from keyboard. Of course, keyboard action perhaps will be entirely different then mouse action, but results must be the same in both cases. Concluding, well design computer program must allow launching menus and context menus, must give access to all menu options, toolbars. Such a program must allow launching dialog boxes and give access to all their elements like buttons, static and active text elements, etc. These constraints need careful design of program interface. Ordering of dialog box elements which are switched by keyboard actions is an example of such a requirement.

Another important factor is related to restrictions estimated for non disabled users. For instance, if application limits time of an action, e.g. waiting time for an answer, it should be more tolerant for blind people since they need more time to prepare and input required information.

Application's design must consider accessibility options provided by the operating system in order to avoid conflicts with standard options of the system. It also should follow standards of operating system's accessibility method. An application for blind people should provide conflict free cooperation with screen readers, which are common tools by blind people. It must provide easy-to-learn keyboard interface duplicating operations indicated by pointing devices.

Braille display is the basic hardware element of computer peripherals being a communicator between blind man and computer. It plays roles of usual screen, which is useless for blind people, and of control element allowing for a change of screen focus, i.e. the place of text reading. Braille display also communicates caret placement and text selection.

Braille printer is another hardware tool dedicated to blind people. Since ordinary printing is useless for blind people, Braille printer punches information on special paper sheet in form of the Braille alphabet of six-dots combinations. Punched documents play the same role for blind people as ordinary printed documents for people with good eyesight.

Screen reader is the basic software for blind people. Screen reader is the program which is run in background. Screen reader captures content of an active window or an element of a dialog box and communicates it as synthesized speech. Screen reader also keeps control over Braille display communicating information that is simultaneously spoken.

Braille editors and converters are groups of computer programs giving blind people access to computers. Braille editors allow for editing and control over documents structure and contents. Converters translate ordinary documents to Braille form and oppositely.

9.1.2 Notes on Software Development for Blind People

Computers become widely used by disabled people including blind people. It is very important for blind people to provide individuals with technologies of easy transfer of information from one source to another. Reading a book becomes now as easy for blind human being as for someone with good eyesight.

Blind person can use a kind of scanning equipment with a speech synthesizer and, in this way, may have a book read by a computer or even displayed at a Braille display. Advances in speech processing allow for converting printed text into spoken information. On the other hand, Braille displays range from linear text display to two dimensional Braille graphic windows with a kind of gray scale imaging. Such tools allow for a kind of reading or seeing and also for editing of texts and graphic information.

Text processing technologies for blind people are now available. Text readers, though still very expensive and not perfect yet, becomes slowly a standard tool of blind beings. Optical character recognition, the heart of text readers, is now well developed technology with almost 100% recognition efficiency. This perfect technology allows for construction of well working text readers. Also, current level of development of speech synthesis technology allows for acoustic communicating of a recognized text. Having text's information communicated, it is easy to provide tools for text editing. Such editing tools usually use a standard keyboard as input device.

Text processing technologies are rather exceptions among other types of information processing for blind people. Neither more complicated document analysis, nor other types of information is easily available. Such areas as, for instance, recognition of printed music, of handwritten text and handwritten music, of geographical maps, etc. still raise challenges in theory and practice. Two main reasons make that software and equipment in such areas is not developed for blind people as intensively as for good eyesight ones. The first reason is objective - technologies such as geographical maps recognition, scanning different forms of documents, recognizing music notation are still not well developed. The second reason is more subjective and is obvious in commercial world of software publishers - investment in such areas scarcely brings profit.

9.2 Acquiring Music Information

Any music processing system must be supplied with music information. Manual inputs of music symbols are the easiest and typical source of music processing systems. Such inputs could be split in two categories. One category includes inputs from - roughly speaking - computer keyboard (or similar computer peripheral). Such input is usually linked to music notation editor, so it affects computer representation of music notation. Another category is related to electronic instruments. Such input usually produce MIDI commands which are captured by a computer program and collected as MIDI file representing live performance of music.

Besides manual inputs we can distinguish inputs automatically converted to human readable music formats. The two most important inputs of automatic conversion of captured information are automatic music notation recognition which is known as Optical Music Recognition technology and audio music recognition known as Digital Music Recognition technology. In this paper we discuss basics of automatic music notation recognition as a source of input information feeding music processing computer system.

9.2.1 Optical Music Recognition

Optical Music Recognition is an example of paper-to-computer-memory information transfer technologies. Printed music notation is scanned to get image files in TIFF or similar graphical format of music notation sheets. Then, OMR technology converts music notation to the internal format of computer system of music processing.

Optical music recognition brings difficulties common to general pattern recognition as well as domain specific problems. Scanned music notations subjected to recognition are blurred, noised, fragmented or overlapping printing; rotated and shifted symbol placement; skewed and curved scanning, etc. On the other hand, music symbols appearance is highly irregular: symbols may be densely crowded in one region and sparsely placed in other regions. Instances of the same symbol lay on, above or below staff lines. Thus, copies of the same symbol may be affected by staff lines or may be isolated from staff lines influence. A further difficulty is raised by irregular sizing and shaping of music symbols. Music notation includes symbols of full range of size: starting from small dot (staccato symbol or rhythmic value prolongation of a note or a rest) and ending with page width arc or dynamic hairpin. Sophisticated shaping of music symbols would be illustrated by clefs, rests, articulation markings, etc.

The structure of automated notation recognition process has two distinguishable stages: location of staves and other components of music notation and recognition of music symbols. The first stage is supplemented by detecting score structure, i.e. by detecting staves, barlines and then systems and systems' structure and detecting other components of music notation like title, composer name, etc. The second stage is aimed on finding placement and classifying symbols of music notation. The step of finding placement of music notation symbols, also known as segmentation, must obviously precede the step of classification of music notation symbols. However, both steps segmentation and classification often interlace: finding and classifying satellite symbols often follows classification of main symbols. In this section we briefly discuss the process of music notation recognition.

Staff Lines and Systems Location

Music score is a collection of staves which are printed on sheets of paper, c.f. [8]. Staves are containers to be filled in with music symbols. Stave(s) filled in with music symbols describe a part played by a music instrument. Thus, stave assigned to one instrument is often called a part. A part of one instrument is described by one stave (flute, violin, cello, etc.) or more staves (two staves for piano, three staves for organ).

Staff lines location is the first stage of music notation recognition. Staff lines are the most characteristic elements of music notation. They seem to be easily found on a page of music notation. However, in real images staff lines are distorted raising difficulties in automatic positioning. Scanned image of a sheet of music is often skewed, staff line thickness differs for different lines and different parts of a stave, staff lines are not equidistant and are often curved, especially in both endings of the stave, staves may have different sizes, etc., c.f. [8] and Figure 9.1.

Having staves on page positioned, the task of system detection is performed. Let us recall that the term system (at a page of music notation) is used in the meaning of all staves performed simultaneously and joined together by beginning barline. Inside and ending barlines define system's structure. For instance, in Figure 9.1 we can see two inside and ending barlines connecting two lower staves of piano part and separated upper stave of violin part. Thus, detection of systems and systems' structure relies on finding barlines.

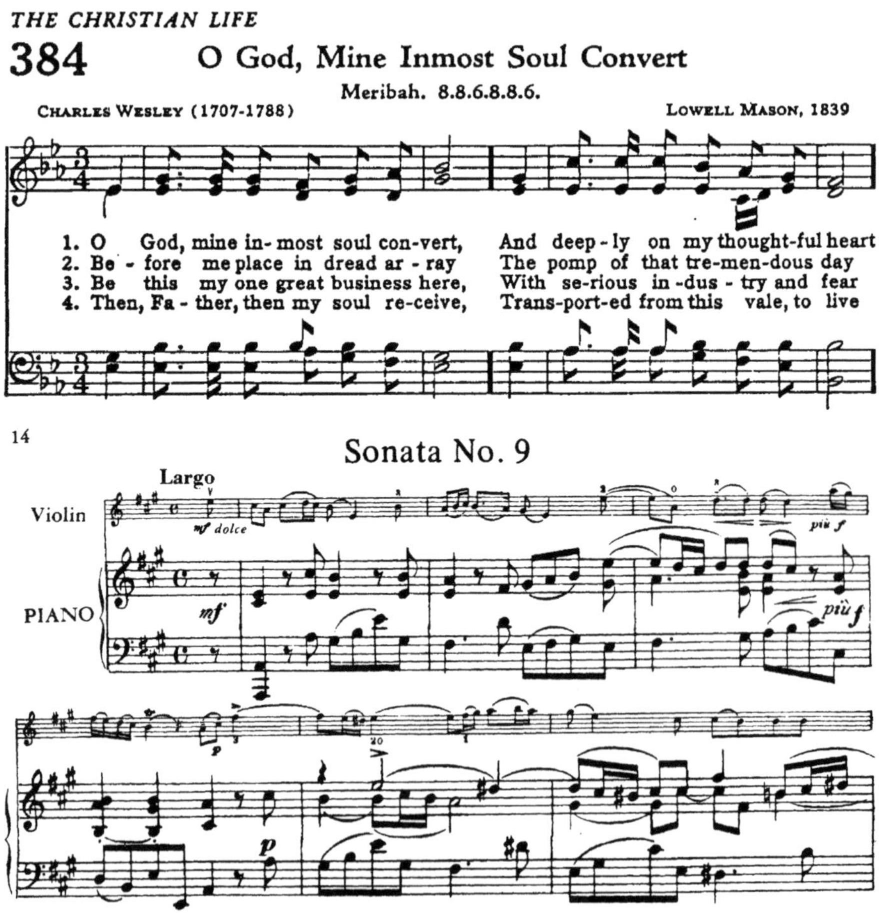

Fig. 9.1. Examples of real notations subjected to recognition

Score Structure Analysis

Sometimes one stave includes parts of two instruments, e.g. simultaneous notation for flute and oboe or soprano and alto as well as tenor and bass. All staves, which include parts played simultaneously, are organized in systems. In real music scores systems are often irregular, parts which not play may be missing.

Each piece of music is split into measures which are rhythmic, (i.e. time) units defined by time signature. Measures are separated each from other by barlines.

The task of score structure analysis is to locate staves, group them into systems and then link respective parts in consecutive systems. Location of barlines depicts measures, their analysis split systems into group of parts and defines repetitions.

Music Symbols' Recognition

Two important problems are raised by symbol recognition task: locating and classifying symbols. Due to irregular structure of music notation, the task of finding symbol placement decides about final symbol recognition result. Symbol classification could not give good results if symbol location is not well done. Thus, both tasks are equally important in music symbols recognition.

Since no universal music font exits, c.f. Figure 9.1, symbols of one class may have different forms. Also size of individual symbols does not keep fixed proportions. Even the same symbols may have different sizes in one score. Besides usual noise (printing defects, careless scanning) extra noise is generated by staff and ledger lines, densely packed symbols, conflicting placement of other symbols, etc.

Music notation is built around staves. The position and size of symbols are restricted and determined by the stave. Having staves and systems located, automated recognition of music is run. Recognition is done for every stave and then, after notation is recognized and analyzed for given stave, the acquired music data pours internal format of music representation.

The first step of music symbols' recognition - symbol location - is aimed at preparing a list of located symbols of music notation and defining bounding boxes embodying symbols of music notation. The process of symbols location is based on analysis of vertical projection. First, vertical projection of the whole region of given stave is analyzed. This analysis is mainly based on processing of derivative of vertical projection and can be interpreted as applyingextended and improved projection methods, c.f. [5]. Derivative processing gives a horizontal approximation of object location. Then, for every roughly located object, horizontal projection of local area is analyzed. This analysis gives vertical location of the object and its improved horizontal location. The most important difficulties are related to objects which cannot be separated by horizontal and vertical projections. Also wide objects as slurs, dynamic 'hairpin' signs, etc. are hardly located.

The next step of recognition process is undertaken on the basis of a list of located objects. This step, in fact, essentially has two permeating tasks: feature extraction and classification of symbols. Both tasks are being done simultaneously and it is not possible to separate them. Feature extraction step starts from extracting the simplest and most obvious features as height and width of the bounding box containing given object. Examining of such simple features allows for classification only in a few cases. In most cases additional features must be extracted and context analysis must be done. The extraction of features is based on filtering of projections in the bounding box, analysis of chosen columns and rows of pixels, etc. Several classification methods are applied for final classification of symbols including context analysis, decision trees, and syntactical methods.

A wide range of methods are applied in music symbol recognition: neural networks, statistical pattern recognition, clustering, classification trees, etc., c.f. [1, 5, 10, 15].

9.2.2 Automatic Conversion of MIDI to Notation

Braille Score program can acquire music information from MIDI files. MIDI file is a container of music information itself. However, music information stored in MIDI file is awkward to be used in music editing. Thus, MIDI file should be converted to more suitable format. Braille Score program converts MIDI file to BSF format. Both MIDI format and BSF format are container for music. Yet, both formats are directed to different tasks. MIDI format is performance and thus time oriented. Its main data inform about beginning and ending time of notes. For instance, in MIDI format division of music to measures does not explicitly exists, such a division could be concluded from other parameters of MIDI format. BSF format is notation oriented. In BSF format measure is a fundamental unit of data. MIDI to BSF conversion should reconstruct missing data necessary to set up BSF format. Before MIDI is converted to BSF, MIDI data must be ordered in order to adjust times (NoteOn, NoteOff, c.f. [20]) to given quantization. This problem is observed for live recorded MIDI files.

MIDI to BSF conversion itself raises interesting algorithmic problems: voice lines detection, flags/beams designation, measures detection, depicting clefs and key signatures, splitting music to staves/systems, identifying of rhythmic groupings, recognizing of articulation and ornamentation figures.

9.3 Representing Music Information

Acquired knowledge has to be represented and stored in a format *understandable* by the computer brain, i.e. by a computer program - this is a fundamental observation and it will be exploited as a subject of discussion in this section. Of course, a computer program cannot work without low level support - it uses a processor, memory, peripherals, etc., but they are nothing more than only primitive electronic tools and so they are not interesting from our point of view. Processing of such an acquired image of the paper document is a clue to the paper-to-memory data transfer and it is successfully solved for selected tasks, c.f. OCR technology. However, documents that are more complicated structurally than linear (printed) texts raise the problem of data aggregation into information units in order to form structured space of information. Such documents raise the problem of acquiring of implicit information/knowledge that could be concluded from the relationships between information units. Documents containing graphics, maps, technical drawings, music notation, mathematical formulas, etc. can illustrate these aspects of difficulties of paper-to-computer-memory data flow or MIDI-to-notation conversions. They are research subjects and still raise a challenge for software producers.

Optical music recognition (OMR) is considered as an example of paper-to-computer-memory data flow. This specific area of interest forces specific methods applied in data processing but, in principle, gives a perspective on the merit of the subject of knowledge processing. Data flow starts from a raster image of music notation and ends with an electronic format representing the information expressed by a scanned document, i.e. by music notation in our case. Several stages of data mining and data aggregation convert the chaotic ocean of raster data into shells of structured information that, in effect, transfer structured data into its abstraction - music knowledge. This process is firmly based on the nature of music notation and music knowledge. The global structure of music notation has to be acquired and the local information fitting this global structure must also be recovered from low level data. The recognition process identifies structural entities like staves, group them into higher level objects like systems, than it links staves of consecutive systems creating instrumental parts. Music notation symbols exist very rarely as standalone objects. They almost exclusively belong to structural entities: staves, systems, parts, etc. So that the mined symbols are poured into these prepared containers - structural objects, cf. [1,4,8,19]. Music notation is a two dimensional language in which the importance of the geometrical and logical relationships between its symbols may be compared to the importance of the symbols alone. This phenomenon requires that the process of music knowledge acquisition must also be aimed at recovering the implicit information represented by the geometrical and logical relationships between the symbols and then at storing the recovered implicit relationships in an appropriate format of knowledge representation.

There are open problems of information gaining and representation like, for instance, performance style, timbre, tone-coloring, feeling, etc. These kinds of information are neither supported by music notation, not could be derived in a reasoning process. Such kinds of information are more subjectively perceived rather than objectively described. The problem of definition, representation and processing of "subjective kinds of information" seems to be very interesting from research and practical perspectives. Similarly, problems like, for instance, human way of reading of music notation may be important from the point of view of music score processing, cf. [6, 7]. Nevertheless, processing of such kinds of information does not fit framework of the paper and is not considered.

The process of paper-to-computer-memory music data flow is presented from the perspective of a paradigm of granular computing, cf. [17]. The low-level digitized data is an example of numeric data representation, operations on low-level data are numeric computing oriented. The transforming of a raster bitmap into compressed form, as e.g. run lengths of black and while pixels, is obviously a kind of numeric computing. Numeric computing transfers data from its basic form to more compressed data. However, the next levels of the data aggregation hierarchy, e.g. finding the handles of horizontal lines, begins the process of data concentration that become embryonic information units, or even knowledge units, rather than more compressed data entities, cf. [8].

9.3.1 Staves, Measures, Systems

Staves, systems, measures are basic concepts of music notation, cf. Figure 9.2. They define the structure of music notation and are considered as information quantities included into the data abstraction level of knowledge hierarchy. The following observations justify such a qualification.

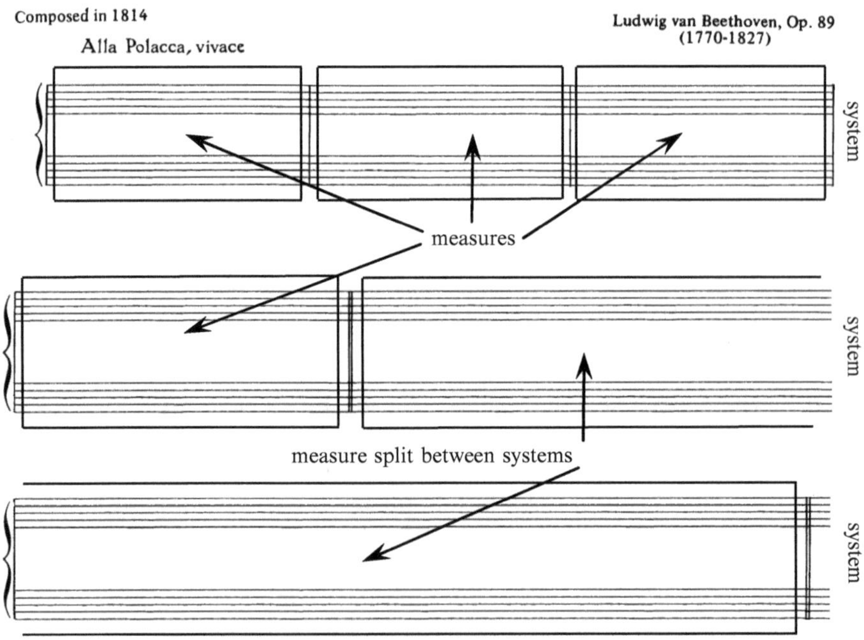

Fig. 9.2. Structuring music notation - systems and measures

A stave is an arrangement of parallel horizontal lines which together with the neighborhood are the locale for displaying musical symbols. It is a sort of vessel within a system into which musical symbols can be "poured". Music symbols, text and graphics that are displayed on it belong to one or more parts. Staves, though directly supported by low-level data, i.e. by a collection of black pixels, are complex geometrical shapes that represent units of abstract data. A knowledge unit describing a stave includes such geometrical information as the placement (vertical and horizontal) of its left and right ends, staff lines thickness, the distance between staff lines, skew factor, curvature, etc. Obviously, this is a complex quantity of data.

A system is a set of staves that are played in parallel; in printed music all of these staves are connected by a barline drawn through from one stave to next on their left end. Braces and/or brackets may be drawn in front of all or some of them. Braces and brackets, if present, define internal system structuring linking staves allocated for one instrument and linking staves of similar instruments. For instance, both staves of piano part are indicated by brace placed in front of their beginning. Similarly, staves of string quintet is grouped with bracket facing beginning of staves.

A measure is usually a part of a system, sometimes a measure covers the whole system or is split between systems, cf. Figure 9.2. A measure is a unit of music identified by the time signature and rhythmic value of the music symbols of the measure. Thus, like in the above cases, a measure is also a concept of data abstraction level.

9.3.2 Notes, Chords, Vertical Events, Time Slices

Such symbols and concepts as notes, chords, vertical events, time slices are basic concepts of music notation, cf. Figure 9.3. They define the local meaning of music notation and are considered as information quantities included in the data abstraction level of the knowledge hierarchy. Below a description of selected music symbols and collections of symbols are described. Such a collection constitutes a unit of information that has common meaning for musician. These descriptions justify classification of symbols to a respective unit of the data abstraction level of the music knowledge hierarchy.

Note - a symbol of music notation - represents basically the tone of given time, pitch and duration. A note may consist of only a notehead (a whole note) or also has a stem and may also have flag(s) or beam(s). The components of a note are information quantities created at the data concentration and the data aggregation stages of data aggregation process [8,13]. This components linked in the concept of a note create an abstract unit of information that is considered as a more complex component of the data abstraction level of the music knowledge hierarchy.

A chord is composed of several notes of the same duration with noteheads linked to the same stem (this description does not extend to whole notes due to the absence of a stem for such notes). Thus, a chord is considered as dataabstraction.

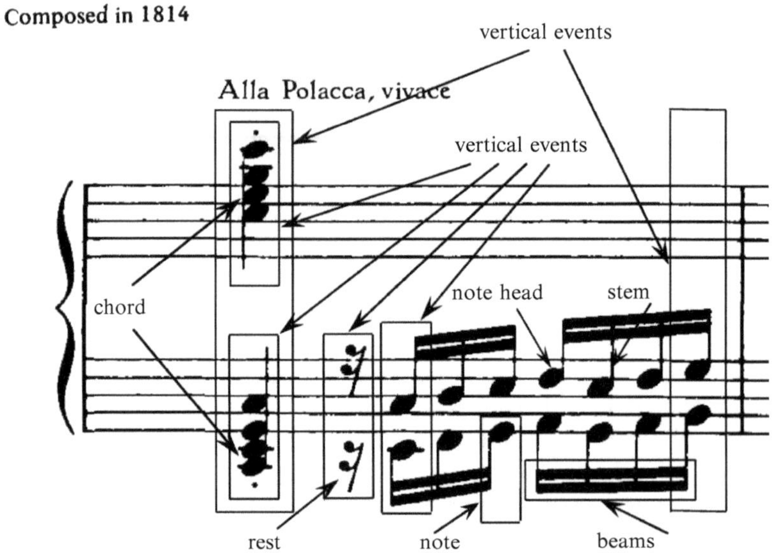

Fig. 9.3. Structuring music notation - symbols, ensembles of symbols

A vertical event is the notion by which a specific point in time is identified in the system. Musical symbols representing simultaneous events of the same system are logically grouped within the same vertical event. Common vertical events are built of notes and/or rests.

A time slice is the notion by which a specific point in time is identified in the score. A time slice is a concept grouping vertical events of the score specified by a given point in time. Music notation symbols in a music representation file are physically grouped by page and staff, so symbols belonging to a common time slice may be physically separated in the file. In most cases time slice is split between separated parts for the scores of part type, i.e. for the scores with parts of each performer separated from others. Since barline can be seen as a time reference point, time slices can be synchronized based on barline time reference points. This fact allows for localizing recognition's timing errors to one measure and might be applied in error checking routine.

9.4 Approximated Data Structuring

The notion of *understanding* is regarded as the main feature of intelligent communication and an important goal of the present paper. We would like to characterize the meaning in which the word *understanding* is used in the paper. Understanding is an ability to identify objects and sets of objects defined by concepts expressed in a given language. The concept's description in a given language is what the syntax is. A mapping which casts the concepts' description on the real world objects is what the semantics is. Ability to recognize the semantics is the meaning of understanding. We reflect meanings of the above notions in music notation seen as a language of natural communication.

9.4.1 Syntax

Syntactic approach is a crucial stage and a crucial problem in the wide spectrum of tasks as, for instance, pattern recognition, translation of programming languages, processing of natural languages, music processing, etc. Syntactic approach is generally based on the context-free methods which have been intensively studied. Context-free methods have also been applied in practice for the processing of artificial languages as, for instance, programming languages, in technical drawings, etc. We can even say that application in this field has been successful.

Unfortunately, natural communication between people, e.g. communication in a natural language or using music notation, is too complex to be formalized in a context-free way, though it is clear that such communication is rule-governed, cf. [2]. Even if there is a definite set of rules defining a language of natural communication, the rules are much more complicated than those describing artificial languages of formal communication. And such rules can often be broken with little impact on communication. Thus, a description of such tools as a natural language or music notation must definitely be highly flexible and deeply tolerant to natural anarchy of its subjects. With all that in mind, the proposed approach to describing languages of natural communication will rely on the sensible application of the proposed context-free methods applied locally in the structured space of a language of natural communication. Moreover, it is assumed that the context-free methods will not be applied unfairly to generate incorrect constructions of them. Those assumptions allow for a raw approximation of languages of natural communication as, for instance, natural language or music notation, which are far more complex than a context-free tools utilized for such an approximation. Of course, such assumptions are real shortcomings in accurate description of a language of natural communication and in its processing. These shortcomings must be solved by employing some other methods, perhaps not context-free.

Below, we present an approximated description of a local area of music notation. This description is given in the form of context free grammar. For more details on context free descriptions of music notation see [11, 13].

<stave> → *<beginning_barline>* *<bl_stave>*
→ *<bl_stave>*
<bl_stave> → *<key_signature>* *<ks_stave>*
→ *<ks_stave>*
<ks_stave> → *<time_signature>* *<ts_stave>*
→ *<ts_stave>*

<ts_stave>	→ *<measure> <barline> <ts_stave>*
	→ *<measure> <barline>*
<measure>	→ *<change_of_k_sign.> <ks_measure>*
	→ *<ks_measure>*
<ks_measure>	→ *<change_of_t_sign.> <ts_measure>*
	→ *<ts_measure>*
<ts_measure>	→ *<vertical event> <ts_measure>*
	→ *<vertical event>*
<vertical event>	→ *<stem> <vertical event>*
	→ *<stem>*
<stem>	→ *<beams> <note_stem>*
	→ *<flags> <note_stem>*
	→ *<note_stem>*
<stem>	→ *<beams> <rhythm_group> <note_stem>*
	→ *<flags> <rhythm_group> <note_stem>*
	→ *<note_stem> <rhythm_group>*
<beams>	→ *left beam <beams>*
	→ *right beam <beams>*
	→ *right beam*
<rhythm_group>	→ *left rh gr <rhythm_group>*
	→ *right rh gr <rhythm_group>*
	→ 3
<flags>	→ *flag <flags>* | *flag*
<note_stem>	→ *note head <note_stem>*
	→ *note head stem*

9.4.2 Semantics

As mentioned above, people use different tools for communication: natural languages, programming languages, artificial languages, language of gesture, drawings, photographs, music notation. All those tools could be seen as tools used for describing a matter of communication and as information carriers. We can observe that different tools can be used for encoding the same communication matter description. Immersing our deliberations into music notation we should be aware that among different tools of natural communication, natural languages are most universal. In general, they cover most parts of information spaces spanned by other tools. Therefore, a natural language can alternatively describe constructions of music notation. Interpreting this observation we can notice that, for instance, a given score can also be described in Braille Music [14], MusicXML [3] or other formats or even, e.g., in the English language. Moreover, all such descriptions carry similar information space.

Likewise, a description of a subject (a thing, a thought, an idea, etc.) may be prepared in different natural languages. Such descriptions approximate the subject bringing its projection onto the language used for description. And such a description could be translated to other natural language without a significant lost of information. This means that the subject being described could be seen as a meaning of a description. So, a study on a subject described in a natural language (or even in any language of natural communication) may supplement the study on descriptions themselves. In other words, syntactic analysis of language descriptions may be supplemented by a semantic analysis of description's subject.

In this study music notation, as a language of natural communication, cast onto a space of communication subjects (i.e. onto musical scores, as texts of the language of natural communication) is understood as the semantic approach to music information processing. Formally, the mapping V describes semantics of the music notation description:

$$V : L \to M$$

where: L is a music notation lexicon, M is music notation.

The mapping V assigns objects of a given musical score M to items stored in the corresponding lexicon L. The lexicon L is a set of local portions of the derivation tree of the score. For details see [11].

9.5 Men-machine Communication as an Intelligent Information Exchange

As mentioned before, communication is understood as a presentation or an exchange of information between two (or more then two) objects of communication. Essential feature communication is understanding information being exchanged. Understanding requires exact description of relations between information entities, what is done in the form of syntactic and semantic structuring integrated in frames of information granulation paradigm.

9.5.1 Syntactic Analysis - a Tool Describing Communicated Information

Syntactic analysis is a tool used for data space structuring. As discussed above, syntactic methods cannot be used for full structuring of complex data spaces as, for instance, for structuring music information. Thus, it is used for approximation of data structuring. Such an approximation is often sufficient for revealing structures of data that could be extracted form the data space and possibly subjected to further processing.

Syntactic analysis is a suitable tool for acquiring user's choice of data. Selection tool is usually used to define user's choice. A selection done by user could either be interpreted at the lowest level of data structures, or may be performed to a part of structured data space. In Figure 9.4 we have two rectangle selections. These selections could be interpreted as numerical data representing raster bitmaps which have nothing common with displayed music

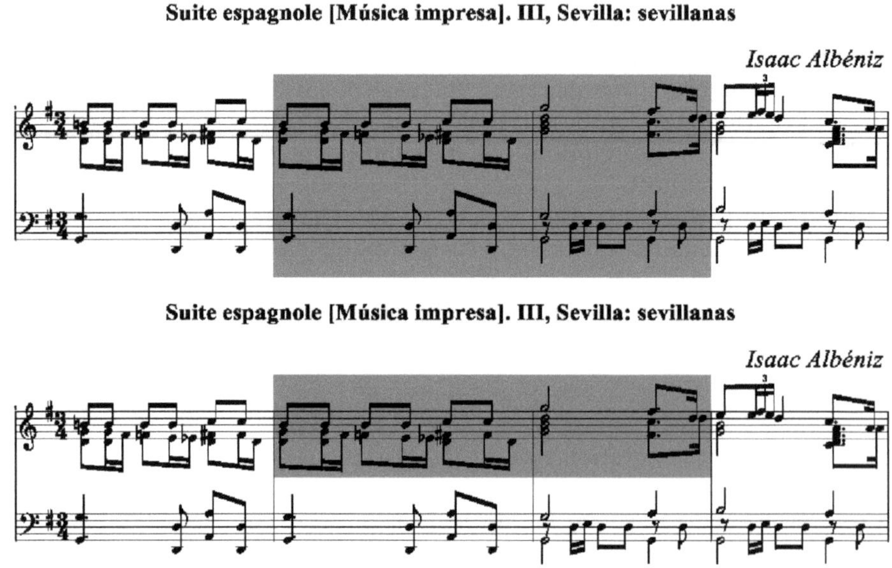

Fig. 9.4. Examples of blocks selections: two measures in a system and two measures in a stave

notation. On the other hand these selections could be understood as a part of music notation, namely: two measures in a system and two measures in a stave. In case of Figure 9.5 selections shown as grayed symbols of music notation cannot be interpreted as a raw numerical data. These selections are parts of the structured data space.

Syntactic analysis allows for immersion of user's selection into structured information space. Syntactic interpretation of user's selection of data gives the first significant raise leading to full identification of information intended to be communicated by men. It needs to be mentioned that, in this discussion, we drop a category of technical details like, for instance, which programming tools are used to point out desired objects at a computer screen and how to indicate options of a selection.

Let us look at the selection of two measures in the stave. It is defined as a part of derivation tree in a grammar generating the score (part of this grammar is outlined in section 9.4.1). This selection corresponds to paths from the root to two indicated vertexes *<measure>* of the part of derivation tree shown in Figure 9.6. The selection of two triplets in lower part of Figure 9.6 is described by the indicated vertex *<ts_measure>*, which is also taken as one vertex path. Description of voice line selection cannot be described as easily as other selections, it requires context analysis.

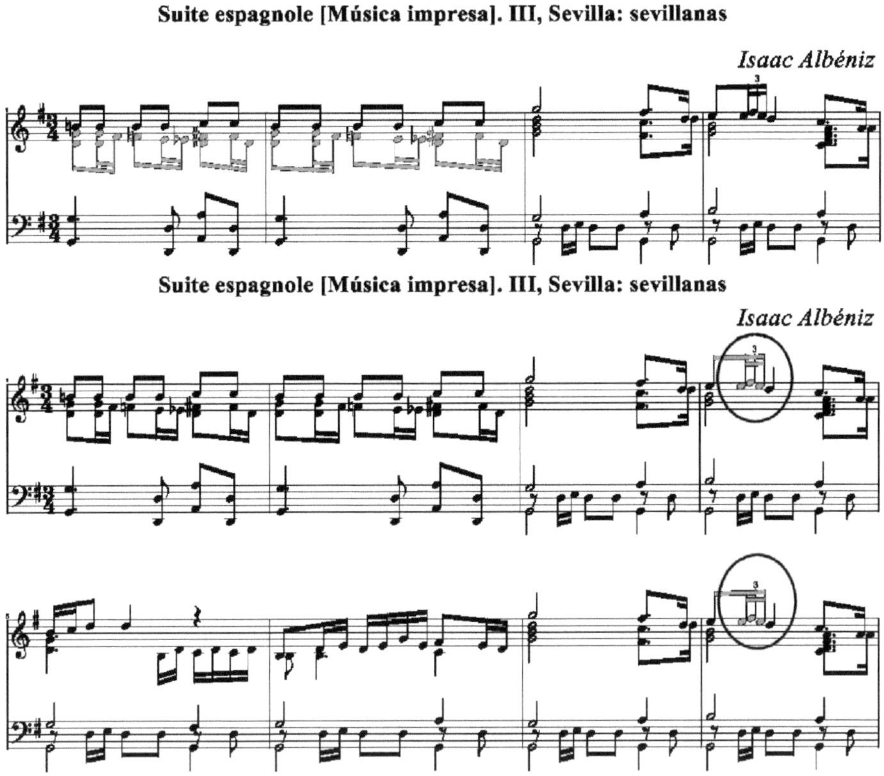

Fig. 9.5. Examples of selections: lower voice line in first two measures and triplets on sixteens

9.5.2 Semantic Mapping as Identification of Communicated Information

Syntactic descriptions of information entities is a basis for identification of relevant area of information space. This identification is done by casting the lexicon of a given score, i.e. the space syntactic granules, onto the space of objects of sematic granules of the score. Semantic granules are subjects of understanding and of possible processing.

The meaning of paths from the root to two indicated vertexes *<measure>* (being syntactic granules) is defined as follow. It is the crop of all subtrees of derivation tree, which include both paths together with subtrees rooted in vertexes ending both paths. The structure of symbols of music notation that are included into selected two measures corresponds to this meaning.

On the other hand, crops of all subtrees of the derivation tree in Figure 9.6, which are equal to the subtree defined by the indicated vertex *<ts_measure>*, is the meaning of syntactic granules (in this case, the subtree has excluded its part denoted by indicated multidots vertex).

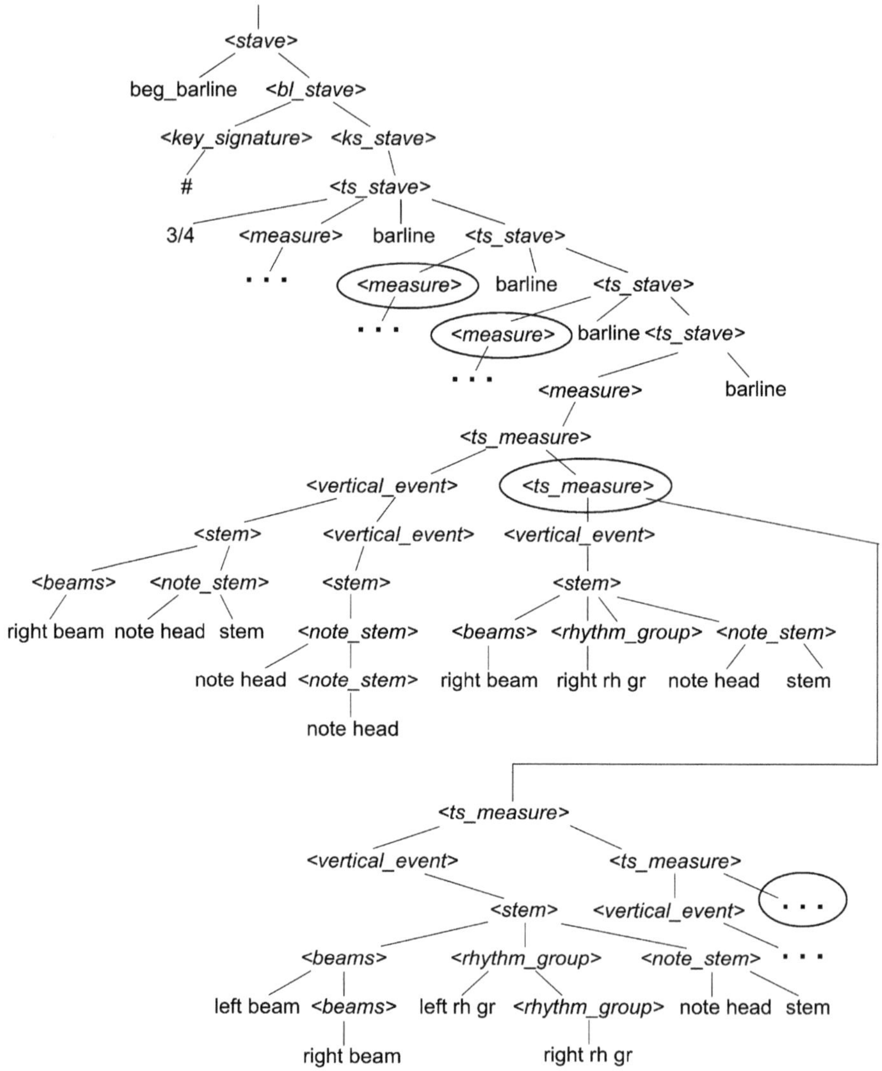

Fig. 9.6. Derivation tree of the first triplet marked at Figure 9.5

It is worth to notice that the description of the first semantic granule is a special case of the the description of the second semantic granule. Having a path, which begins in the root of derivation tree, we can find only one subtree equal this path with subtree rooted in its ending vertex.

Semantic granules define meaning of information being exchanged and allow for responding to requests. Such responses are outlined in Figure 9.7. Its upper part shows original score. two other parts illustrate transposition performed on recognized notation. The middle parts shows three voice lines.

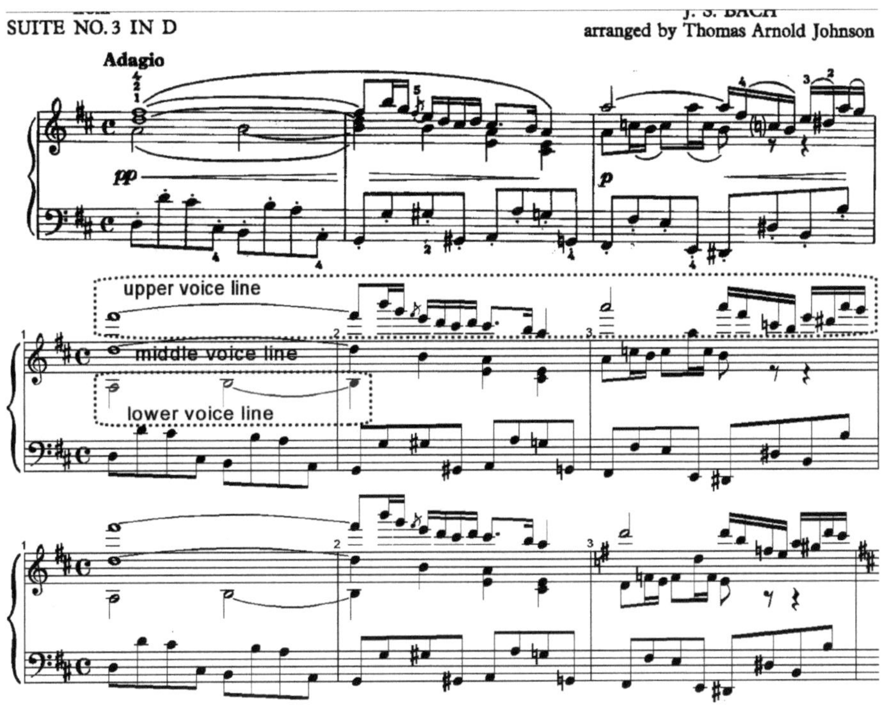

Fig. 9.7. Examples of transpositions: original score, automatic recognition of the original score, upper voice line moved one octave up and lower voice line moved one octave down, third measure transposed from D to G

The upper voice line was subjected to transposition by one octave up. The lower voice line was subjected to transposition by one octave up. The third part of shows transposition of the third measure from D to G.

9.5.3 Granulation as a Form of Understanding

Information exchanged in communication is materialized in the form of texts of a language of natural communication. Thus, the term *text* spans not only over texts of natural languages, but also over constructions like, for instance, musical scores, medical images, etc. (we can also apply this term to constructions of languages of formal communication, e.g. to computer programs). Revealing recent sections let us say that a study on how texts are constructed is what we mean as syntax. A matter described by such a text is what is understood as semantics. Integrating syntax and semantics leads to information granulation and identification of relations between granules of information, c.f. [13, 18]. Discovering relations between both aspects is seen as understanding.

The description of music notation as well as music notation itself could be innately subjected to the paradigm of granular computing elucidation. As stated in [17], granular computing as opposed to numeric computing is knowledge-oriented. Information granules exhibit different levels of knowledge abstraction, what strictly corresponds to different levels of granularity. Depending upon the problem at hand, we usually group granules of similar size (i.e. similar granularity) together into a single layer. If more detailed (and computationally intensive) processing is required, smaller information granules are sought. Then, those granules are arranged in another layer. In total, the arrangement of this nature gives rise to the information pyramid. In the granular processing we encounter a number of conceptual and algorithmic layers indexed by the *size* of information granules. Information granularity implies the usage of various techniques that are relevant for the specific level of granularity.

The meaning of granule size is defined accordingly to real application and should be consistent with common sense and with the knowledge base. Roughly speaking size of syntactic granules is a function of of depth of the syntactic structure. Size of the syntactic granule *<score><score_part><page> <system>* is smaller then size of the syntactic granule *<score><score_part> <page><system><stave>* which, in turn, is smaller then size of the syntactic granule *<score><score_part><page><system><measure>*, c.f. Figure 9.8.

On the other hand, we can define size of semantic granule. It is defined as a quantity of real world objects or a length of continue concept. Size of the semantic granule $V($*<score><score_part><page><system>*$)$ is greater

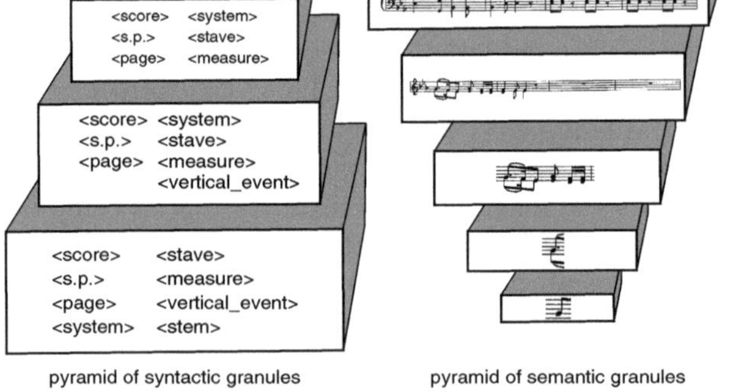

Fig. 9.8. Duality of syntax and semantics for music notation. Relevance of syntactic and semantic granules' pyramids

than size of *V*(<*score*><*score_part*><*page*><*system*><*stave*>), which, in turn, is greater then *V*(<*score*><*score_part*><*page*><*system*><*stave*> <*measure*>). Amazingly, greater size of syntactic granule correspond to smaller size of respective semantic granule. The relevance between syntactic and semantic granules is shown in Figure 9.8. And, as in music notation case, this relevance is a manifestation of duality phenomenon in syntax-semantic related spaces.

9.6 Braille Score

Braille Score is a project developed and aimed on blind people. Building integrated music processing computer program directed to a broad range of blind people is the key aim of Braille Score, c.f. [16]. The program is built around methods of computational intelligence discussed in this paper. The use of computational intelligence tolls improves the program part devoted to recognition and processing of music notation. The attention is focused on user interface with special interest given to communication of the program with blind user.

The program is mastered by a man. Both the man and computer program create an integrated system. The structure of the system is outlined in Figure 9.9.

The system would act in such fields as:

- creating scores from scratch,
- capturing existing music printings and converting them to electronic version,

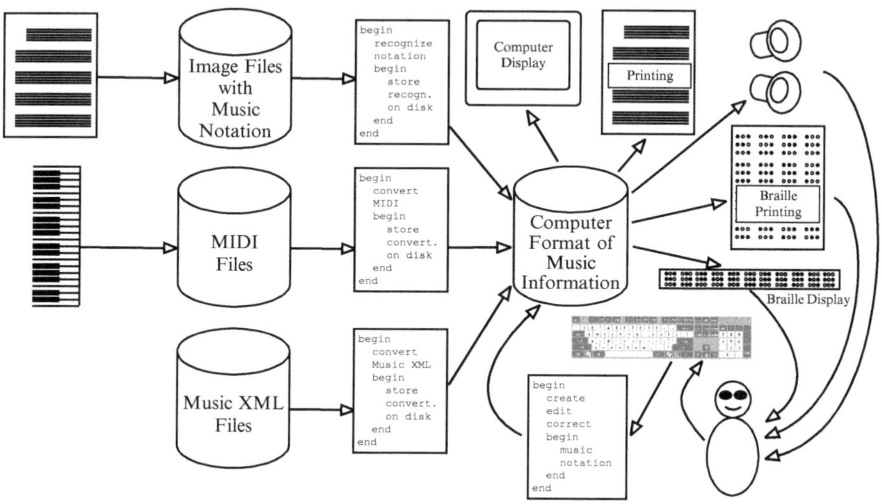

Fig. 9.9. The structure of Braille Score

- converting music to Braille and printing it automatically in this form,
- processing music: transposing music to different keys, extracting parts from given score, creating a score from given parts,
- creating and storing own compositions and instrumentations of musicians,
- a teacher's tool to prepare teaching materials,
- a pupil's tool to create their own music scores from scratch or adapt acquired music,
- a hobby tool.

9.6.1 User Interface Extensions for Blind People

Braille Score is addressed to blind people, c.f [16]. Its user interface extensions allow blind user to master the program and to perform operations on music information. Ability to read, edit and print music information in Braille format is the most important feature of Braille Score. Blind user is provided the following elements of interface: Braille notation editor, keyboard as input tool, sound communicator.

Blind people do not use pointing devices. In consequence, all input functions usually performed with mouse must be mapped to computer keyboard. Massive communication with usage of keyboard requires careful design of interface mapping to keyboard, c.f. [16].

Blind user usually do not know printed music notation. Their perception of music notation is based on Braille music notation format presented at Braille display or punched sheet of paper, c.f. [14]. In such circumstances music information editing must be done on Braille music notation format. Since typical Braille display is only used as output device, such editing is usually done with keyboard as input device. In Braille Score Braille representation of music is converted online to internal representation and displayed in the form of music notation in usual form. This transparency will allow for controlling correctness and consistency of Braille representation, c.f. [16].

Sound information is of height importance for blind user of computer program. Wide spectrum of visual information displayed on a screen for user with good eyesight could be replaced by sound information. Braille Score provides sound information of two types. The first type of sound information collaborates with screen readers, computer programs dedicated to blind people. Screen readers could read contents of a display and communicate it to user in the form of synthesized speech. This type of communication is supported by contemporary programming environments. For this purpose Braille Score uses tools provided by Microsoft .NET programming environment. The second type of sound information is based on own Braille Score tools. Braille Score has embedded mechanism of sound announcements based on its own library of recorded utterances.

9.6.2 Braille Score Output

Interaction between computer and blind user cannot use standard display and visual communication. Use of pointing devices is heavily restricted and must be integrated with other then visual computer feedback to user action. Blind users can fully operate typical keyboard to input data to computer. Of course, a kind of acoustic feedback must be launched to communicate exceptions or alerts. On the other hand, Braille displays are basic computer output for blind users. Unfortunately, usage of Braille display is not effective for massive communication.

Braille Score uses two online methods as its output, c.f. Figure 9.10. The first one is based on Braille display. The second is based on acoustic communication. Braille Score also have two off line outputs: printing music notation and punching its Braille version.

BSF format represents music notation which is a two dimensional language. Printed music notation is direct image of BSF format. For instance, note pitch and time are described by its placement on a stave: vertical placement determines its pitch while horizontal placement - its beginning time.

A unified international Braille system of music notation, respective to classical music notation, was developed, c.f. [14]. Braille system is strictly linear. Thus, representation of music notation must also be linear. This implies that note pitch neither can be determined by its placement on a page, nor by placement relative to other symbols. Anyway, Braille system of music notation uniquely determines features of music symbols and is useful and practical. User of Braille system of music must employ more characters and more rules in order to describe music symbols, c.f. [14].

In Braille Score both types of Braille outputs: online with Braille display and offline with Braille printer are based on the unified system of Braille music notation.

As it was mentioned earlier, acoustic output is very important for blind people. This type of communication is faster then the one based on Braille

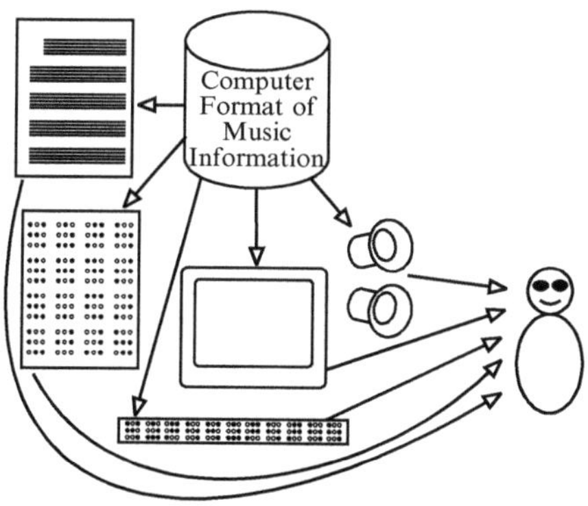

Fig. 9.10. Braille Score output

display. Acoustic output integrated with keyboard shortcuts used for navigation and editing provides very efficient tool for mastering Braille Score Format.

And, finally, Braille Score is able to display music notation on computer screen and to print it. These two outputs, though cannot be directly used by blind people, are necessary in computer program even as a development tool. Yet, these outputs help in mastering Braille Score by good eyesight users as, for instance, music teachers to prepare class materials or to work together with blind students.

9.7 Conclusions

The aim of this paper is a discussion on involvement of computational intelligence methods in implementation of user friendly computer programs focused on disabled people.

Optical music recognition has been intensively developed for last two decades gaining promising results. However, practical realizations in this field are still far from perfection. The field of music notation recognition is still open for research and further improvements of OMR technology are still sought. In Sections 2 and 3 of the paper a brief overview of OMR technology from the perspective of pattern recognition paradigm is presented. Optical music recognition (OMR) is considered as an example of paper-to-computer-memory data flow. This specific area of interest forces specific methods to be applied in data processing, but in principle, gives a perspective on the merit of the subject of data aggregation. The process of paper-to-computer-memory music data flow is presented from the perspective of the process of acquiring information from plain low-level data. Three important aspects of recognition process are distinguished: structure of music notation analysis, music symbol recognition and context knowledge acquisition. The discussion outlines an interpretation of this process as a metaphor of granular computing.

The new framework on men-machine intelligent communication is presented in the Sections 4 and 5. The term intelligent communication is understood as information exchange with identified structure of information, which is presented by a side of communication to his/its partner(s) or is exchanged between sides of communication. Of course, identification of information structure is a natural feature of human's side of such communication. An effort is focused on automatic identification of information structure based on syntax and semantics of information description. Syntactic and semantic descriptions have dual structure revealing granular character of represented information. Complementary character of both attempts allow for automation of information structuring and - in consequence - intelligent information maintenance and processing, what is the basis of intelligent communication in men-machine intelligent communication. In this paper the problem of men-machine intelligent communication is reflected in the area of music notation treated as a language of natural communication. However, reflection of this problem in natural language as a language of natural communication give similar conclusions, c.f. [9]. Thus, we can expect that integrated syntactic and semantic data structuring guides to rational interpretation of men-machine communication in many areas of human activity. This framework permits for better understanding of communication process as well as leads to practical solutions.

In the paper we describe a concept of Braille Score the specialized computer program which should help blind people to deal with music and music notation. The program is built around methods of computational intelligence discussed in this paper. The use of computational intelligence tolls improves the program part devoted to recognition and processing of music notation. The attention is focused on user interface with special interest given to communication of the program with blind user.

References

1. Bainbridge D., Bell T., The challenge of optical music recognition, Computers and the Humanities 35 (2001) 95-121.
2. Bargiela A., Homenda W., Information structuring in natural language communication: Syntactical approach, Journal of Intelligent & Fuzzy Systems, 17 (2006) 6, 575-581
3. Castan G., Good M., Roland P., Extensible Markup Language (XML) for Music Applications: An Introduction. in: Walter B. Hewlett and Eleanor Selfridge-Field (Eds.) The Virtual Score: Representation, Retrieval, Restoration, Cambridge, MA: MIT Press, pp. 95-102.
4. Dannenberg R., Music Representation Issues, Techniques, and Systems, Computer Music Journal (17:3) (1993) 20-30.
5. Fujinaga I., Adaptive optical music recognition, 16th Inter. Congress of the Inter. Musicological Society, Oxford, Oxford University Press, 2001.
6. Goolsby T. W., Eye movement in music reading: Effects of reading ability, notational complexity, and encounters, Music Perception, 12,1(1994) 77-96.
7. Goolsby T. W., EProfiles of processing: Eye movements during sightreading, Music Perception, 12,1(1994) 97-123.
8. Homenda W., Granular Computing as an Abstraction of Data Aggregation - a View on Optical Music Recognition, Archives of Control Sciences, Vol. 12 (XLVIII) (2002) No. 4, pp 433-455.
9. Homenda W., Information Structuring in Natural Language Communication: Syntax versus Semantic, in: Rutkowski L. et al (Eds.), Artificial Intelligence and Soft Computing - ICAISS, Lecture Notes in Artificial Intelligence, pp. 872-878, Springer, 2004.
10. Homenda W., Optical Music Recognition: the Case Study of Pattern Recognition, in: Computer Recognition Systems, Kurzyski et al (Eds.), pp. 835-842, Springer Verlag, 2005.

11. Homenda W., Automatic understanding of images: integrated syntax and sematic analysis of music notation, IEEE World Congress on Computational Intelligence, July 16-21, 2006, Sheraton Vancouver Wall Centre, Vancouver, BC, Canada
12. Homenda W., Breaking Accessibility Barriers: Computational Intelligence in Music Processing for Blind People, ICINCO 2007 - Fourth International Conference on Informatics in Control, Automation and Robotics, 32-39, Angers, France; 9-12 May, 2007
13. Homenda W., Towards automation of data understanding: integration of syntax and semantics into granular structures of data, Fourth International Conference on Modeling Decisions for Artificial Intelligence MDAI 2007, Kitakyushu, Fukuoka, Japan, 16-18 August, 2007
14. Krolick B., How to Read Braille Music, 2nd Edition, Opus Technologies, 1998.
15. McPherson J. R., Introducing feedback into an optical music recognition system, Third Internat. Conf. on Music Information Retrieval, Paris, France, 2002.
16. Moniuszko T., Design and implementation of music processing computer program for blind people (in Polish), Master Thesis, Warsaw University of Technology, Warsaw, 2006.
17. Pedrycz W., Granular Computing: An Introduction, in: Joint 9th IFSA World Congress and 20th NAFIPS International Conference, Vancouver, pp. 1349-1354, 2001.
18. Pedrycz W., Bargiela A., Granular mappings, IEEE Transactions on Systems, Man, and Cybernetics-part A, 35(2005)2, 292-297.
19. Taube H., Stella: Persistent Score Representation and Score Editing in Common Music, Computer Music Journal, 17,3(1993) 38-50.
20. MIDI 1.0, Detailed Specification, Document version 4.1.1, February 1990.

10

Ethical Healthcare Agents

Michael Anderson[1] and Susan Leigh Anderson[2]

[1] Department of Computer Science, University of Hartford 200 Bloomfield Avenue, West Hartford, CT 06776
anderson@hartford.edu

[2] Department of Philosophy, University of Connecticut One University Place, Stamford, CT 06901
susan.anderson@uconn.edu

Summary. We have combined a bottom-up casuistry approach with a top-down implementation of an ethical theory to develop a system that uses machine-learning to abstract relationships between *prima facie* ethical duties from cases of particular types of ethical dilemmas where ethicists are in agreement as to the correct action. This system has discovered a novel ethical principle that governs decisions in a particular type of dilemma that involves three potentially conflicting *prima facie* duties. We describe two prototype systems in the domain of healthcare that use this principle, one that advises human beings as to the ethically correct action in specific cases of this type of dilemma and the other that uses this principle to guide its own behavior, making it what we believe may be the first explicit ethical agent.

10.1 Introduction

A pressing need for personnel in the area of healthcare, caused in no small part by the aging "baby boomer" population, has fueled interest in possible technological solutions, including developing intelligent healthcare agents. Before such agents can be deployed, however, ethical concerns pertaining to their use need to be addressed. Unfortunately, at the present time, there is no consensus among ethicists as to the ideal ethical theory and few of the proposed candidates obviously lend themselves to machine implementation. Although more agreement exists among ethicists as to the correct action in biomedical ethical dilemmas than in other areas of applied ethics, this agreement has yet to be fully codified in such a way that it can be incorporated into a machine. The new interdisciplinary research area of "Machine Ethics" is concerned with solving this problem not only for dilemmas that an artificial agent might face in healthcare, but in other areas as well.

The ultimate goal of machine ethics, we believe, is to create a machine that itself follows an ideal ethical principle or set of principles, that is to say, it is guided by this principle or these principles in decisions it makes about

M. Anderson and S.L. Anderson: *Ethical Healthcare Agents*, Studies in Computational Intelligence (SCI) **107**, 233–257 (2008)
www.springerlink.com

possible courses of actions it could take. To accomplish this goal, the machine ethics research agenda will involve testing the feasibility of a variety of approaches to capturing ethical reasoning, with differing ethical bases and implementation formalisms, and applying this reasoning in intelligent agents engaged in ethically sensitive activities, such as healthcare. Machine ethics researchers must investigate how to determine and represent ethically relevant features of ethical dilemmas, discover and implement ethical principles, incorporate ethical principles into an intelligent agent's decision procedure, make ethical decisions with incomplete and uncertain knowledge, provide explanations for decisions made using ethical principles, and evaluate intelligent agents that act upon ethical principles.

It might seem impossible to "compute" ideas that humans feel most passionately about and have such difficulty codifying: their ethical beliefs. Despite this, our interdisciplinary team of an ethicist and computer scientist believe that it is essential that we try, since there will be benefits not only in the domain of healthcare, but for the fields of Artificial Intelligence and Ethics as well. We've been attempting to make ethics computable for three reasons: First, to avert possible harmful behavior from increasingly autonomous machines, we want to determine whether one can add an ethical dimension to them. Second, we want to advance the study of ethical theory by making it more precise. Finally, we want to solve a particular problem in ethical theory—namely, to develop a decision procedure for an ethical theory that involves multiple, potentially competing, duties.

Our research in machine ethics has been concerned with leveraging machine learning techniques to facilitate the codification of ethics, biomedical ethics in particular, and developing ethical healthcare agents whose actions are guided by the principles resulting from this codification. In our work to date in machine ethics [3,4] we have, at a proof of concept level, developed a representation of ethically relevant features of ethical dilemmas that is needed to implement a *prima facie* duty approach to ethical theory, discovered an ethical principle that governs decisions made in a particular type of ethical dilemma involving three *prima facie* duties, and implemented this principle in prototype intelligent agent systems. In the following, we summarize this work and present two proof-of-concept systems in the domain of healthcare: MedEthEx [4], a system that uses a machine-discovered ethical principle to resolve particular cases of a general type of biomedical ethical dilemma, and EthEl, a prototype eldercare system that uses the same principle to provide guidance for its actions. We believe that MedEthEx and EthEl demonstrate the feasibility of developing systems governed by ethical principles and lend credence to the view that intelligent agents can play an important role in the domain of healthcare and do so in an ethically sensitive manner.

10.2 One Approach to Computing Ethics

In our research, we've adopted the action-based approach to ethical theory, where the theory tells us how we should act in ethical dilemmas. This approach lends itself to machine implementation by giving the agent either a single principle or several principles to guide its actions, unlike other approaches (e.g. virtue-based ethics that emphasizes virtues that an ethical agent should possess) that don't clearly specify the correct action in an ethical dilemma. A good action-based ethical theory should satisfy these criteria [2]:

- *Consistency.* The theory shouldn't contradict itself by saying that a single action in a given set of circumstances is simultaneously right and wrong.
- *Completeness.* It should tell us how to act in any ethical dilemma in which we might find ourselves.
- *Practicality.* We should be able to follow it.
- *Agreement with intuition.* The actions it requires and forbids should agree with expert ethicists' intuition.

We started our project by programming the one action-based ethical theory that clearly attempts to make ethics computable: Hedonistic Act Utilitarianism (HAU). According to one of its creators, Jeremy Bentham, HAU simply involves doing "moral arithmetic." [7] HAU maintains that an action is right when, of all the possible actions open to the agent, it will likely result in the greatest net pleasure, or happiness, taking all those affected by the action equally into account. HAU involves first calculating the units of pleasure and displeasure that each person affected will likely receive from each possible action. It then subtracts the total units of displeasure from the total units of pleasure for each of those actions to get the total net pleasure. The action likely to produce the greatest net pleasure is the correct one. If the calculations end in a tie, where two or more actions are likely to result in the same greatest net pleasure, the theory considers these actions equally correct.

The program JEREMY [5] is our implementation of HAU with simplified input requirements. JEREMY (fig. 10.1) presents the user with an input screen that prompts for an action's description and the name of a person that action affects. It also requests a rough estimate of the amount (very pleasurable, somewhat pleasurable, not pleasurable or displeasurable, somewhat displeasurable, or very displeasurable) and likelihood (very likely, somewhat likely, or not very likely) of pleasure or displeasure that the person would experience from this action. The user enters this data for each person affected by the action and for each action under consideration. When data entry is complete, JEREMY calculates the amount of net pleasure each action achieves. (It assigns 2, 1, 0, -1, or -2 to pleasure estimates and 0.8, 0.5, or 0.2 to likelihood estimates, and sums their product for each individual affected by each action.) It then presents the user with the action or actions achieving the greatest net pleasure.

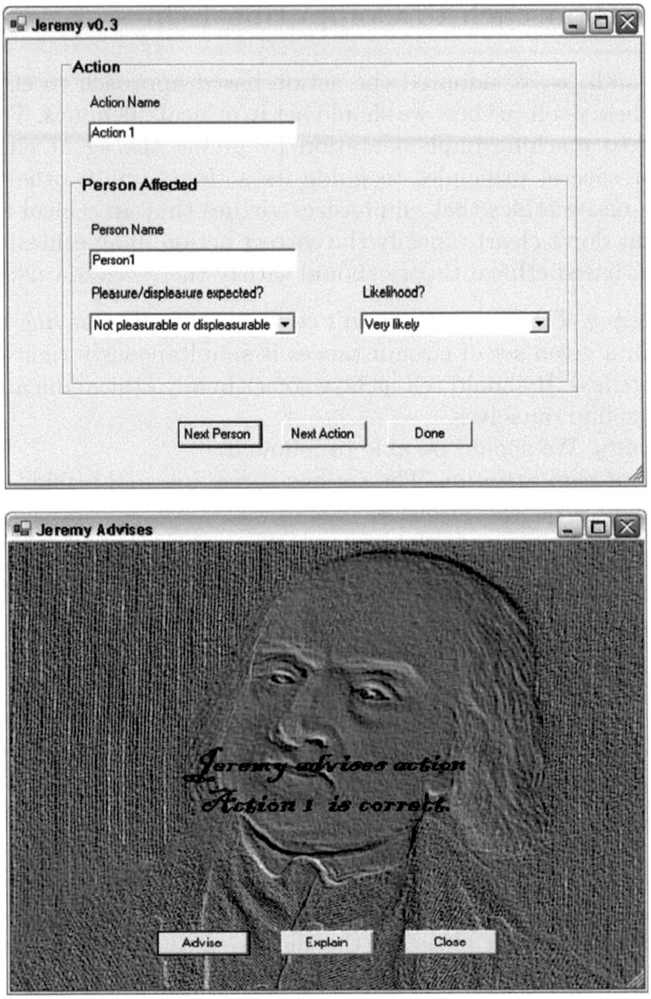

Fig. 10.1. JEREMY, a hedonistic act utilitarian advisor system

An ideal version of a system such as JEREMY might well have an advantage over a human being in following HAU because you can program it to do the arithmetic strictly (rather than simply estimate), be impartial, and consider all possible actions. We conclude, therefore, that machines can follow HAU at least as well as human beings and perhaps even better, given the same data that human beings would need to follow the theory.

Even though HAU is consistent, complete, and can be made practical, most ethicists believe that it fails the test of agreement with intuition. Despite John Stuart Mill's heroic attempt in chapter five of *Utilitarianism* to show that considerations of justice can be subsumed under the utilitarian principle [16], ethicists generally believe that HAU can allow for the violation of individual rights if this will likely result in the greatest net good consequences, taking everyone affected into account. One could, for instance, construct a case to show that HAU permits killing one unimportant person to save the lives of five important persons. This violates the intuition that it's wrong to kill one person to save several persons.

We have, however, adopted one aspect of HAU in our current approach to ethical decision-making. When applying an ethical duty to a particular dilemma, we consider such factors as the duty's intensity and duration and the number of persons affected—which we have initially combined as the level of satisfaction or violation of the duty involved.

10.3 A More Comprehensive Ethical Theory

In agreement with W.D. Ross [20], we believe that all single-principle, absolute duty ethical theories (such as HAU and Kant's Categorical Imperative, a principle that requires you to act in a way that can be universalized) are unacceptable because they don't appreciate the complexity of ethical decision making and the tensions that arise from different ethical obligations pulling us in different directions.

Ross's theory consists of seven *prima facie* duties. A *prima facie* duty is an obligation that we should try to satisfy but that can be overridden on occasion by another, currently stronger duty. Ross's suggested list of *prima facie* duties (which he says can be altered) captures the best of several single-principle ethical theories, while eliminating defects by allowing for exceptions. His suggested duties are those of

- *fidelity*—you should honor promises and live up to agreements that you've voluntarily made,
- *reparation*—you should make amends for wrongs you've done,
- *gratitude*—you should return favors,
- *justice*—you should treat people as they deserve to be treated, in light of their past behavior and rights they might have,
- *beneficence*—you should act so as to bring about the most amount of good,
- *nonmaleficence*—you should act so as to cause the least harm, and
- *self-improvement*—you should develop your talents and abilities to the fullest.

The first four duties are Kantian in spirit. The next two duties—beneficence and nonmaleficence—derive from the single utilitarian principle. Ross maintains that one must separate the likely harm that can be caused from the possible good consequences, rather than simply subtract the one from the other, because the duty of nonmaleficence is generally stronger than that of beneficence. This accounts for our intuition that it's wrong to kill one person to save five. Finally, the last duty, that of self-improvement, captures the best of "ethical egoism" by acknowledging that we have a special duty to ourselves that we don't have to others.

Ross's *prima facie* duty approach to ethical theory incorporates the good aspects of the rival teleological and deontological approaches to ethics (emphasizing consequences vs. principles), while allowing for needed exceptions to adopting one or the other approach exclusively. It also has the advantage of being better able to adapt to the specific concerns of ethical dilemmas in different domains. There may be slightly different sets of *prima facie* duties for legal ethics, business ethics, journalistic ethics and eldercare ethics, for example.

While everyone agrees that Ross's duties seem intuitively plausible, he doesn't tell us how to determine the ethically correct action when the duties give conflicting advice, beyond saying that one should use one's intuition to resolve the conflict. Unfortunately, this would allow someone to rationalize doing whatever he or she feels like doing, by maintaining that a duty that supported that action is the most important one in the dilemma.

Without an objective decision procedure, furthermore, the theory can fail all the requirements of an acceptable action-based ethical theory. In a given ethical dilemma, one of Ross's duties could tell us that a particular action is right, while another could tell us that the same action is wrong, making the theory inconsistent. By not giving us a single correct action in that dilemma, we don't know what we ought to do, so the theory could also be considered incomplete and impractical. Finally, because you could rationalize doing an action that an ethical expert, and most of us, would consider wrong, the theory could fail the test of agreement with intuition.

We've concluded that the ideal ethical theory incorporates multiple *prima facie* duties, like Ross's theory, with some sort of a decision procedure to determine the ethically correct action in cases where the duties give conflicting advice.

10.4 A Decision Procedure for Competing Duties

We've formulated a method that could help make a multiple *prima facie* duty theory, like Ross's, workable. Our method essentially adopts John Rawls' *reflective equilibrium* approach to creating and refining ethical principles, which goes back and forth between particular cases and principles, generalizing from particular cases and testing those generalizations on further cases [19]. First, we find or create ethical dilemmas where tension exists between the *prima facie* duties involved and where ethicists have reached a consensus as to the correct action. We then use machine learning to abstract a general decision principle from those cases. Finally, we test this principle on further cases and refine it as needed to reflect ethicists' intuitions about the correct action in these other cases. (The system can learn a decision principle only to the extent that ethical experts agree on the answers to particular dilemmas.)

Our method uses a trainer (fig. 10.2) to develop the decision principle. It prompts an expert ethicist for an action's description and an estimate of each

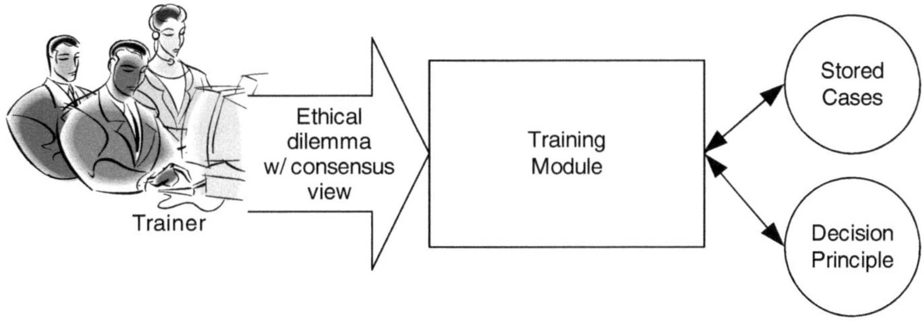

Fig. 10.2. Developing a decision principle

of the affected duties' satisfaction or violation level (very satisfied, somewhat satisfied, not involved, somewhat violated, or very violated). The expert enters this data for each action under consideration. When data entry is complete, the trainer seeks the intuitively correct action from the expert. It combines this information with the input case to form a new training example that it stores and uses to refine the decision principle. After such training, the decision principle can be used to provide the correct action for this case, should it arise in the future, as well as for all previous cases encountered. Furthermore, because the decision principle learned is the least-specific one required to satisfy cases seen so far, it might be general enough to be used to determine correct actions in previously unseen cases as well.

To capture expert ethical opinion, we use *inductive-logic programming* (ILP) [14] to learn the relationships between the duties involved in a particular dilemma. ILP is a machine learning technique that inductively learns relations represented as first-order Horn clauses (i.e. universally quantified conjunctions of positive literals L_i implying a positive literal $H : H \leftarrow (L_1 \wedge \cdots \wedge L_n)$), classifying positive and negative examples of a relation. To train a system using ILP, one presents it with examples of the target relation, indicating whether they're positive (true) or negative (false). The object of training is for the system to learn a new hypothesis that, in relation to all input cases, is complete (covers all positive cases) and consistent (covers no negative cases).

We chose this machine learning technique for a number of reasons. First, the properties of set of *prima facie* duties aren't clear. For instance, do they form a partial order? Are they transitive? Do subsets of duties have different properties than other subsets? We have shown, previously, that simply assigning linear weights to the duties isn't sufficiently expressive to capture the relationships between those duties [5]. ILP provides a rich representation language that's more likely to express potentially nonclassical relationships. Furthermore, representing the relationships as Horn clauses lets us automatically confirm a decision principle's consistency regarding the relationships between duties across all cases. Finally, ILP's declarative representation language lets us more readily express, consult, and update commonsense background knowledge regarding duty relationships.

The decision principle learned is based on a predicate, *supersedes(Action1, Action2)*, that's true when the first of the two actions that it is given is ethically preferable to the second. We represent each action as an ordered list of values specifying the level of satisfaction or violation for each duty involved. The selection of the range of possible satisfaction or violation levels of a particular duty should, ideally, depend upon how many gradations are needed to distinguish between cases that are ethically distinguishable. We have chosen, initially, the following range of values: -2 represents a serious violation, -1 represents a less serious violation, 0 indicates that the duty is neither satisfied nor violated, $+1$ indicates minimal satisfaction, and $+2$ indicates maximal satisfaction. Clauses in the *supersedes* predicate are represented as disjunctions of lower bounds for differentials of these values between actions.

We believe it is likely that new duties will need to be added, as other ethical dilemmas are considered, in order to make distinctions between ethically distinguishable cases that would otherwise have the same representation. There is a clear advantage to an approach to ethical decision-making that can accommodate changes to the range of satisfaction or violation of duties, as well as the addition of duties, as needed.

We chose to develop a decision principle based upon Beauchamp's and Childress' Principles of Biomedical Ethics (PBE) [6], a *prima facie* duty theory having only four duties which include: The *Principle of Respect for Autonomy* that states that the health care professional should not interfere with the effective exercise of patient autonomy (reflecting the recent shift from a paternalistic model of the healthcare worker-patient relationship to one giving the patient a more active role). For a decision by a patient concerning his/her care to be considered fully autonomous, it must be intentional, based on sufficient understanding of his/her medical situation and the likely consequences of foregoing treatment, sufficiently free of external constraints (e.g. pressure by others or external circumstances, such as a lack of funds) and sufficiently free of internal constraints (e.g. pain/discomfort, the effects of medication, irrational fears or values that are likely to change over time) [15]. The *Principle of Nonmaleficence* requires that the health care professional not harm the patient, while the *Principle of Beneficence* states that the health care professional should promote patient welfare. Finally, the *Principle of Justice* states that health care services and burdens should be distributed in a just fashion.

We chose PBE and biomedical ethical dilemmas for five reasons: First, PBE uses a more manageable total of four duties, instead of Ross' seven. Second, one member of our research team has a biomedical ethics background. Third, healthcare workers will likely have the information needed to judge whether a particular duty is involved in an ethical dilemma and to judge that duty's intensity. Fourth, there's a pressing need for ethical advice in this area, as biomedical research introduces new, challenging ethical dilemmas and as baby boomers begin to age (many ethical dilemmas involve end-of-life care). Finally, more agreement exists among biomedical ethicists as to the ethically preferable action than in other areas of applied ethics.

The field of Biomedical Ethics has arisen out of a need to resolve pressing problems faced by health care workers, insurers, hospital ethics boards, and biomedical researchers. As a result of there having been more discussion of actual cases in this field, a consensus is beginning to emerge as to how to evaluate ethical dilemmas in this domain, leading to the ethically correct action in many dilemmas. A further reason why there might be more of a consensus in this domain than in others is because in the area of biomedical ethics there is an ethically defensible goal (the best possible health of the patient), whereas in other areas (e.g. business, law) the goal may not be ethically defensible (make as much money as possible, serve the client's interest even if she is guilty of an offense or doesn't deserve a settlement) and ethics enters the picture as a limiting factor (the goal must be achieved within certain ethical boundaries).

To begin to apply PBE, we chose a representative type of ethical dilemma that health care workers often face that involves three of the four Principles of Biomedical Ethics (Respect for Autonomy, Nonmaleficence and Beneficence): A health care worker has recommended a particular treatment for her competent adult patient and the patient has rejected that treatment option. Should the health care worker try again to change the patient's mind or accept the patient's decision as final? The dilemma arises because, on the one hand, the healthcare professional should not challenge the patient's autonomy unnecessarily; on the other hand, the health care worker may have concerns about why the patient is refusing the treatment, i.e. whether it is a fully autonomous decision.

This dilemma is constrained to three of the four duties of PBE (nonmaleficence, beneficence, and respect for autonomy) and involves only two possible actions in each case. We've drawn on the intuitions of Allen Buchanan and Dan Brock [9] and our project's ethicist (whose views reflect a general consensus) to determine the correct actions in particular cases of this type of dilemma.

In the type of dilemma we consider, we can assign specific meanings to each duty's possible values. For nonmaleficence,

- -2 means that this action will likely cause severe harm to the patient that could have been prevented,
- -1 means that this action will likely cause some harm to the patient that could have been prevented,
- 0 means that this action isn't likely to cause or prevent harm to the patient,
- $+1$ means that this action will likely prevent harm to the patient to some degree, and
- $+2$ means that this action will likely prevent severe harm to the patient.

For beneficence,

- -2 means that the other action would likely have improved the patient's quality of life significantly,

- -1 means that the other action would likely have improved the patient's quality of life somewhat,
- 0 means that neither action is likely to improve the patient's quality of life,
- $+1$ means that this action will likely improve the patient's quality of life somewhat, and
- $+2$ means that this action will likely improve the patient's quality of life significantly.

For respect for autonomy,

- -1 means not immediately acquiescing to the patient's wishes but trying again to change the patient's mind,
- $+1$ means that the healthcare worker acts according to the patient's wishes but believes that the patient's decision isn't fully autonomous, and
- $+2$ means that the healthcare worker acts according to the patient's wishes and believes that the patient's decision is fully autonomous.

(Because this dilemma always involves autonomy, but never to the extent of forcing a treatment on the patient, 0 and -2 aren't options.)

As an example, consider a specific case of the type of dilemma we're considering. A patient refuses to take an antibiotic that's almost certain to cure an infection that would otherwise likely lead to his death. He decides this on the grounds of long-standing religious beliefs that forbid him to take medications. The correct action in this case is for the healthcare worker to accept the patient's decision as final because, although severe harm (his death) will likely result, his decision can be seen as being fully autonomous. The healthcare worker must respect a fully autonomous decision of a competent adult patient, even if he or she disagrees with it, because the decision concerns the patient's body and a patient should have control over what is done to his or her body. This case appears as training case 1 in Table 10.1. In this case, the predicate *supersedes*(Accept, Try Again) would be true and *supersedes*(Try Again, Accept) would be false.

The chosen type of dilemma has only 18 possible cases where, given the two possible actions, the first action supersedes the second (i.e. is ethically preferable). Four of these were provided to the system as examples of when the target predicate (supersedes) is true. Four examples of when the target predicate is false (obtained by inverting the order of the actions where the target predicate is true) were also provided. Positive training case 1 was just described in the previous paragraph.

In training case 2, a patient won't consider taking medication that could only help alleviate some symptoms of a virus that must run its course. He refuses the medication because he has heard untrue rumors that the medication is unsafe. Even though the decision is less than fully autonomous, because it's based on false information, the little good that could come from taking the medication doesn't justify trying to change his mind. So, the doctor should accept his decision.

Table 10.1. The levels of duty satisfaction or violation for the two possible actions in four MedEthEx training cases. A check mark indicates the ethically correct action in each case.

Case no. & action	*Nonmaleficence value*	*Beneficence value*	*Autonomy value*
Case 1			
Try Again	+2	+2	−1
√ Accept	−2	−2	+2
Case 2			
Try Again	0	+1	−1
√ Accept	0	−1	+1
Case 3			
√ Try Again	+1	+1	−1
Accept	−1	−1	+1
Case 4			
√ Try Again	0	+2	−1
Accept	0	−2	+1

In training case 3, a patient with incurable cancer refuses further chemotherapy that will let him live a few months longer, relatively pain free. He refuses the treatment because, ignoring the clear evidence to the contrary, he's convinced himself that he's cancer-free and doesn't need chemotherapy. The ethically preferable answer is to try again. The patient's less than fully autonomous decision will lead to some harm (dying sooner) and deny him the chance of a somewhat longer life (a violation of the duty of beneficence), which he might later regret.

In training case 4, a patient, who has suffered repeated rejection from others due to a very large non-cancerous abnormal growth on his face, refuses to have simple and safe cosmetic surgery to remove the growth. Even though this has negatively affected his career and social life, he's resigned himself to being an outcast, convinced that this is his lot in life. The doctor is convinced that his rejection of the surgery stems from depression due to his abnormality and that having the surgery could vastly improve his entire life and outlook. The doctor should try again to convince him because so much of an improvement is at stake and his decision is less than fully autonomous.

Table 10.1 summarizes the levels of duty satisfaction or violation for both of the possible actions in all four training cases and indicates the correct action in each case.

We can more succinctly characterize the cases using the difference between the values for duties in the ethically preferable action and the values for corresponding duties in the less preferable action. For example, in training case 1, the differences between the duties of the Accept and the Try Again actions are −4, −4, 3. Positive differences signify duties that are favored in the ethically preferable action (respect for autonomy in this example); negative differences signify duties that are favored in the less preferable action (nonmaleficence and beneficence in this example).

$$\Delta nonmaleficence \geq -4 \wedge \Delta beneficence \geq -4 \wedge \Delta autonomy \geq 3$$
$$\vee$$
$$\Delta nonmaleficence \geq -1 \wedge \Delta beneficence \geq -3 \wedge \Delta autonomy \geq -1$$
$$\vee$$
$$\Delta nonmaleficence \geq 1 \wedge \Delta beneficence \geq -4 \wedge \Delta autonomy \geq -2$$
$$\vee$$
$$\Delta nonmaleficence \geq -4 \wedge \Delta beneficence \geq 3 \wedge \Delta autonomy \geq -2$$

Fig. 10.3. The set of clauses defining the discovered supersedes predicate

The learning task is to find a set of clauses that covers all the positive training examples while not covering any negative training examples. Figure 10.3 illustrates the set of clauses defining the *supersedes*(*Action1*, *Action2*) predicate discovered by the system, where Δ <*duty*> denotes the difference between *Action1*'s <*duty*> value and *Action2*'s <*duty*> value.

Each clause specifies a lower bound for each of the three duty differentials that must hold for that clause to be true. As each clause is joined to the others disjunctively, any one true clause will cause the *supersedes* predicate to be true. For example, the third clause states that in order for it to consider *Action1* ethically preferable to *Action2*,

- the value for nonmaleficence must be 1 or more in favor of *Action1*,
- the value for beneficence can be any value (as −4 is the lowest possible bound), and
- the value for respect for autonomy can be in favor of *Action2* by no more than 2.

The system discovered a principle that provided the correct answer for the remaining 14 positive cases, as verified by the consensus of ethicists abstracted from a discussion of similar types of cases given by Buchanan and Brock [9]. The complete and consistent decision principle that the system discovered can be stated as follows: A healthcare worker should challenge a patient's decision if it is not fully autonomous and there is either any violation of the duty of nonmaleficence or a severe violation of the duty of beneficence. Although, clearly, this rule is implicit in the judgments of the consensus of ethicists, we believe that this principle has never before been stated explicitly. This philosophically interesting result lends credence to Rawls' "reflective equilibrium" approach — the system has, through abstracting and refining a principle from intuitions about particular cases, discovered a plausible principle that tells us which action is correct when specific duties pull in different directions in a particular type of ethical dilemma. Furthermore, the discovered principle supports an insight of Ross' [19] that violations of the duty of nonmaleficence should carry more weight than violations of the duty of beneficence. We offer this principle as evidence that making ethics more precise will permit machine-learning techniques to discover philosophically novel and interesting principles in ethics. It should also be noted that the learning system that discovered this principle is an instantiation of a general architecture.

With appropriate content, it can be used to discover relationships between any set of *prima facie* duties where there is a consensus among ethicists as to the correct answer in particular cases.

Once the decision principle is discovered, the needed decision procedure can be fashioned. Given two actions, each represented by the satisfaction/violation levels of the duties involved, values of corresponding duties are subtracted (those of the second action from those of the first). The principle is then consulted to see if the resulting differentials satisfy any of its clauses. If so, the first action is considered to be ethically preferable to the second.

10.5 An Ethical Advisor System

A good first step toward the eventual goal of developing machines that can follow ethical principles is creating programs that enable machines to act as ethical advisors to human beings [5]. We begin this way for four pragmatic reasons:

First, one could start by designing an advisor that gives guidance to a select group of persons in a finite number of circumstances, thus reducing the assignment's scope.

Second, the general public will probably more easily accept machines that just advise human beings than machines that try to behave ethically themselves. In the first case, it's human beings who will make ethical decisions by deciding whether to follow the machine's recommendations, preserving the idea that only human beings will be moral agents. The next step in the Machine Ethics project is likely to be more contentious: creating machines that are autonomous moral agents.

Third, a problem for AI in general, and so for this project too, is how to get needed data—in this case, the information from which to make ethical judgments. With an ethical advisor, human beings can be prompted to supply the needed data.

Finally, ethical theory hasn't advanced to the point where there's agreement, even by ethical experts, on the correct answer for all ethical dilemmas. An advisor can recognize this fact, passing difficult decisions that must be made in order to act onto the human user.

Figure 10.4 depicts a general architecture for an ethical advisor system. With appropriate data, it can be used to permit a user access to any decision procedure, using any discovered principle. A user inputs details of a particular case into the system and is presented with the ethically preferable action in accordance with the decision principle. In order to permit a user unfamiliar with the representation details required by the decision procedure, a *knowledge-based interface* provides guidance in determining satisfaction or violation levels of duties in particular cases. It 1) asks ethically relevant questions of the user, determining the ethically relevant features of the particular

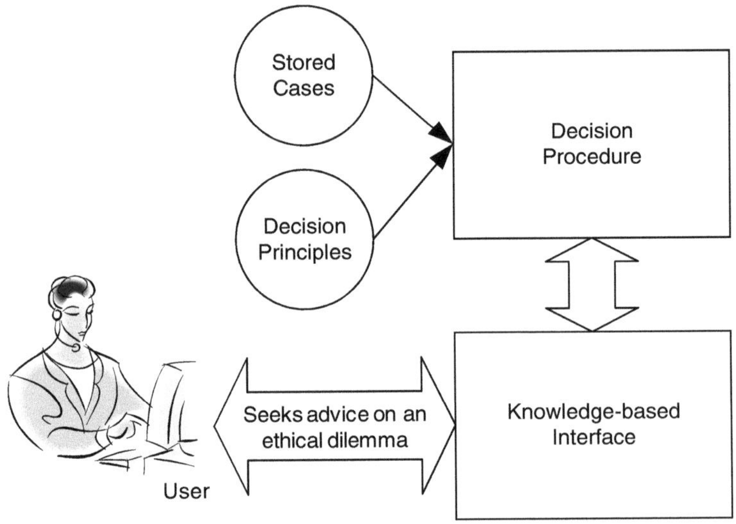

Fig. 10.4. An ethical advisor system architecture

case at hand, 2) transforms the answers to these questions into the appropriate representations (in terms of the level of satisfaction/violation of the *prima facie* duties for each action), 3) sends these representations to the decision procedure, and 4) presents the answer provided by the decision procedure, i.e. the action that is considered to be correct (consistent with the system's training), as well as an explanation of this answer to the user. The interface uses knowledge derived from ethicists concerning the dimensions and duties of the particular ethical dilemma. Knowledge is represented as finite-state automata (FSA) for each duty entailed. Questions pertinent to the dilemma serve as start and intermediate states, and intensities of duty satisfaction or violation levels (as well as requests for more information) are final states. The input to the interface is the user's responses to the questions posed; the output is a case with duty satisfaction or violation levels corresponding to these responses.

Given the details of the case from the knowledge-based interface, the decision procedure consults the decision principle and determines whether one action supersedes all others in the current case. If it discovers such an action, it outputs that action as the ethically correct action in this case—that is, the action that's consistent with the system's training.

MedEthEx[1] [4], an instantiation of the general ethical advisor architecture, uses the discovered principle to give advice to a user faced with a case of the dilemma type previously described. To illustrate this system, consider the following dilemma: A patient refuses to take an antibiotic that is likely to

[1] For further exploration, the MedEthEx prototype can be accessed online at http://www.machineethics.com.

prevent complications from his illness, complications that are not likely to be severe, because of long-standing religious beliefs that don't allow him to take medications.

When the system is consulted, it first seeks information to determine the satisfaction/violation level of the duty of autonomy for each action. To do so, it presents questions as required. The system first asks whether or not the patient understands the consequences of his decision. If the health care worker is not sure, she may need to seek more information from the patient or, depending upon her answers to later questions, the system may determine that this is not a fully autonomous decision. If we assume that the health care worker believes that the patient does indeed know the consequences of his action, the system then asks questions to determine if the patient is externally constrained. The healthcare worker answers "no" because the reason why the patient is refusing to take the antibiotic has nothing to do with outside forces. Finally, it asks questions to determine if the patient is internally constrained. Since the patient is not constrained by pain/discomfort, the effects of medication, irrational fears or values that are likely to change over time, the answer is "no." This is because the belief that has led to his refusing the antibiotic is a *long-standing* belief of his. The answers provided to these questions have the system conclude that the patient's decision is fully autonomous, giving the value +2 to the duty of autonomy for accepting the patient's decision. The value for challenging the patient's decision is −1 because questioning the patient's decision, which challenges his autonomy, is not as strong as acting against the patient's wishes, which would have been a −2.

The system then seeks information to determine the satisfaction/violation level of the duty of nonmaleficence for each action. To do so, it presents questions concerning the possibility and severity of harm that may come to the patient given his decision. As harm will likely result from the patient's decision, but it will not be severe, the system gives the value of −1 to the duty of nonmaleficence for accepting the patient's decision. Challenging the patient's decision could avoid this moderate harm, so a +1 to the duty of nonmaleficence is assigned to this action.

The system then seeks information to determine the satisfaction/violation level of the duty of beneficence for each action. To do so, it presents questions concerning the possibility and level of improvement of quality of the patient's life that may result from accepting/challenging his decision. As the quality of the patient's life would worsen somewhat if the patient's decision were accepted and improve somewhat if not, the system gives the value of −1 to the duty of beneficence for accepting the patient's decision and a +1 for challenging it. The test case, then, is generated as:

Test Case	Autonomy	Nonmaleficence	Beneficence
Try Again	−1	+1	+1
Accept	+2	−1	−1

The system then consults the principle for both *supersedes(try again, accept)* and *supersedes(accept, try again)*. It finds that the first is not covered by the principle but the second is covered. As action 1 in this case is *accept*, the system advises the user to accept the patient's decision. This answer is consistent with ethicists' intuition. The healthcare worker should accept the patient's decision, since, as in Training Case 2, the decision appears to be a fully autonomous one and with even less possible harm at stake.

10.6 An Ethical Eldercare System

Eldercare is a domain where we believe that, with proper ethical considerations incorporated, robots can be harnessed to aid an increasingly aging human population, with an expectation of a shortage of human caretakers in the future. We believe, further, that this domain is rich enough in which to explore most issues involved in general ethical decision-making for both machines and human beings.

EthEl (ETHical ELdercare system) (fig. 10.5) is a prototype system in the domain of eldercare that takes ethical concerns into consideration when reminding a patient to take his/her medication. EthEl must decide how often to remind a patient to take a prescribed medication, when to accept a patient's refusal to take the medication that might prevent harm and/or provide benefit to the patient, and when to notify the overseer, if he/she continues to refuse to take the medication. Whether to accept a patient's refusal to take the medication or notify an overseer is an ethical dilemma analogous to the dilemma originally used to discover the previously stated decision principle in that the same duties are involved (nonmaleficence, beneficence, and respect for autonomy) and "notifying the overseer" in the new dilemma corresponds

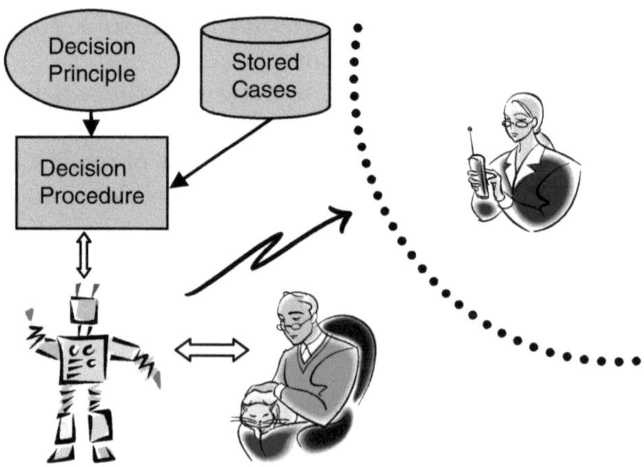

Fig. 10.5. EthEl, an ethical eldercare system prototype

to "trying again" in the original. There is a further ethical dimension that is implicitly addressed by the system: In not notifying the overseer – most likely a doctor – until absolutely necessary, the doctor will be able to spend more time with other patients who could be benefited, or avoid harm, as a result of the doctor's attending to their medical needs. Finally, we believe that there is an ethical dimension to the scheduling of reminders itself, since too many reminders is a challenge to patient autonomy and too few could lead to the patient being harmed or losing a benefit from not taking the medication soon enough.

Machines are currently in use that face this dilemma.[2] The state of the art in these reminder systems entails providing "context-awareness" (i.e. a characterization of the current situation of a person) to make reminders more efficient and natural. Unfortunately, this awareness does not extend to consideration of ethical duties that such a system should observe regarding its patient. In an ethically sensitive eldercare system, both the timing of reminders and responses to a patient's disregard of them should be tied to ethical duties involved. The system should challenge patient autonomy only when necessary, as well as minimize harm and loss of benefit to the patient. The decision principle discovered from the MEDETHEX dilemma can be used to achieve these goals by directing the system to remind the patient only at ethically justifiable times and notifying the overseer only when the harm or loss of benefit reaches a critical level. In the following, we describe ETHEL, a reminder system that follows this principle, in detail. To facilitate prototype implementation, reasonable and liftable assumptions have been made regarding numeric values and calculations.

ETHEL receives initial input from an overseer (most likely a doctor) including: what time to take a medication, the maximum amount of harm that could occur if this medication is not taken (e.g. none, some or considerable), the number of hours it would take for this maximum harm to occur, the maximum amount of expected good to be derived from taking this medication, and the number of hours it would take for this benefit to be lost. The system then determines from this input the change in duty satisfaction/violation levels over time, a function of the maximum amount of harm/good and the number of hours for this effect to take place.

The change in nonmaleficence equals the maximum harm that could occur divided by the number of hours it would take for this harm to occur. The change in beneficence equals the maximum good that could be gained divided by the number of hours it would take for this benefit to be lost. The change in respect for autonomy, if the maximum possible harm is greater than the maximum possible good, is the same as the change in nonmaleficence. (The principle states that it is twice as bad to ignore harm than to ignore benefit, so suspected loss of autonomy should be keyed to change in harm when this is greater than the amount of good involved.) Otherwise, the change in

[2] For an example, see http://www.ot.utoronto.ca/iatsl/projects/medication.htm

respect for autonomy equals the average of the changes in nonmaleficence and beneficence, since both could be factors in satisfying the decision principle. These values are used to increment, over time, duty satisfaction/violation levels for the *remind* action and, when a patient disregards a reminder, the *notify* action. They are used to decrement duty satisfaction/violation levels for the *don't remind* and *don't notify* actions as well.

The starting values for the *remind* action duties are $0, 0, -1$ (for nonmaleficence, beneficence, and respect for autonomy respectively) because as yet there is no harm or loss of benefit and there is somewhat of a challenge to the patient's autonomy in giving a reminder. Nonmaleficence and/or beneficence values (at least one of these duties will be involved because the medication must prevent harm and/or provide a benefit or it would not be prescribed) will be incremented over time because reminding will increasingly satisfy the duties not to harm and/or benefit the patient as time goes by. Respect for autonomy will not increase over time because reminding is consistently a minimal challenge to patient autonomy (unlike notifying the overseer which would be a serious violation of respect for patient autonomy).

For the *don't remind* action, the starting values are 0, 0, 2 because as yet there is no harm or loss of benefit and patient autonomy is being fully respected in not reminding. Nonmaleficence and/or beneficence are gradually decremented over time because there is more harm and/or loss of benefit (negative effects) for the patient as time goes by. Autonomy decreases as well over time because as more and more harm is caused and/or benefit is lost, the fact that the patient has chosen to bring this harm upon his or herself and/or forgo the benefits, in not taking the medication, raises increasing concern over whether the patient is acting in a fully autonomous manner.

For the *notify* action, the starting values are $0, 0, -2$ because as yet there is no harm or loss of benefit and there is a serious challenge to the patient's autonomy in notifying the overseer immediately. Nonmaleficence and/or beneficence will be gradually incremented because the duties not to harm and/or benefit the patient will become stronger since, as time goes by, there is increasing harm and/or loss of benefit. Autonomy will increase from -2 (the worst it could be) because, as time goes by and the harm increases and/or more and more benefits are being lost, the suspicion that the patient is not making a fully autonomous decision in not taking the medication increases, so there is less of a violation of the duty to respect patient autonomy.

For the *accept* action, the starting values are 0, 0, 2 because as yet there is no harm or loss of benefit and full patient autonomy is being respected in accepting the patient's decision. Nonmaleficence and/or beneficence are gradually decremented because, as time goes by, there is more harm and/or loss of benefit (negative effects) for the patient. Autonomy decreases as well, as time goes by, because as more and more harm is caused and/or benefit is lost, the fact that the patient has chosen to bring this harm upon his or her self and/or forgo the benefits, in not taking the medication, raises increasing concern over whether the patient is acting in a fully autonomous manner.

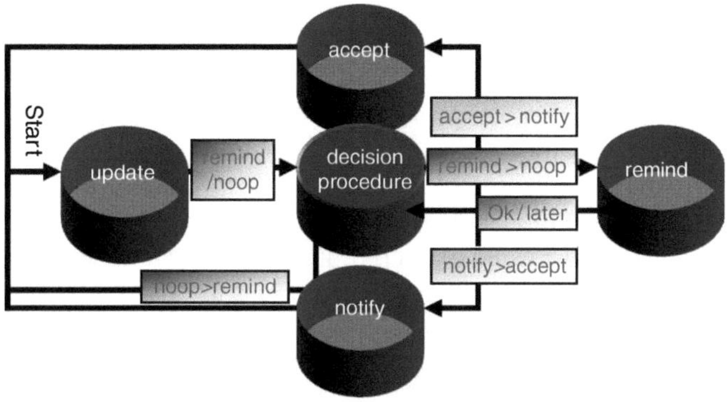

Fig. 10.6. EthEl flow of control

Beginning with the time that the patient is supposed to take the medication, EthEl (fig. 10.6) follows the overseer's orders and reminds the patient to take the medication. If the patient refuses to take the medication, and it is ethically preferable to accept this refusal rather than notify the overseer at that point, EthEl considers whether to remind again or not in five minute intervals. Another reminder is issued when, according to the principle, the differentials between duty satisfaction/violation levels of the *remind/don't remind* actions have reached the point where reminding is ethically preferable to not reminding. Similarly, the overseer is notified when a patient has disregarded reminders to take medication and the differentials between the duty satisfaction/violation levels of the *notify/don't notify* actions have reached the point where notifying the overseer is ethically preferable to not notifying the overseer.

The number of reminders, when they should be offered, and when to contact the overseer are all keyed to possible harm and/or loss of benefit for the patient, as well as violation of the duty to respect patient autonomy. There are three categories of cases for determining number of reminders:

1. When neither the amount of harm nor loss of benefit is expected to reach the threshold required to overrule autonomy. (According to the principle discovered, the threshold is reached only when some harm results or maximum benefit is lost.) Since notifying the overseer would never be triggered, the number of reminders should be minimal.
2. When either the harm caused or loss of benefit is expected to reach the threshold necessary to overrule autonomy. Since either value would be sufficient to trigger notifying the overseer, reminders should occur more often.
3. When there is maximum harm to the patient at stake, if the patient does not take the medication. Since the amount of possible harm to the patient is twice what would trigger notifying the overseer, assuming the autonomy condition is satisfied (that is, the patient's decision to forgo taking the

medication is considered to be less than fully autonomous), reminders are critical and should be given often to prevent harm and avoid notifying overseer.

Given current possible satisfaction/violation values, the following seems to be a reasonable first pass at capturing the relationship between the above categories: if there is no harm to be expected from not taking the medication, give the amount of good to be expected +1 reminders; else give the amount of harm to be expected +2 reminders. These values are used to scale the changes in duty satisfaction/violation values of the *remind/don't remind* actions over time in such a way that they move toward their critical thresholds at a faster rate than these values in the *notify/accept* actions. Such scaling permits the principle to adjudicate between actions of differing ethical relevance.

Given, as an example, a starting time of 12:00 p.m. and six hours for both maximum harm and maximum loss of benefit to occur, figure 10.7 illustrates the behavior of the system when the patient repeatedly refuses to take his/her medication under a variety of values for nonmaleficence (harm) and beneficence (benefit). Given maximum possible harm and benefit, the system responds by frequently reminding the patient and finally contacting the overseer well before the maximum harm occurs. When there is some harm, not the maximum, at stake and maximum possible benefit, fewer, more widely spaced reminders are given. The overseer is notified later than in the previous case, but still in advance of the attainment of maximal harm and maximal loss of benefit. When there is both some (less than maximum) harm and benefit at stake, the same number of reminders given in the previous case are spread further apart and notification of the overseer only occurs when the maximum for either one has been reached. Lastly, when there is no possible harm and only some (less than maximum) benefit at stake, a reminder is given only when the benefit from taking this medication will be lost. Since in this case there is no harm involved, the overseer is never contacted.

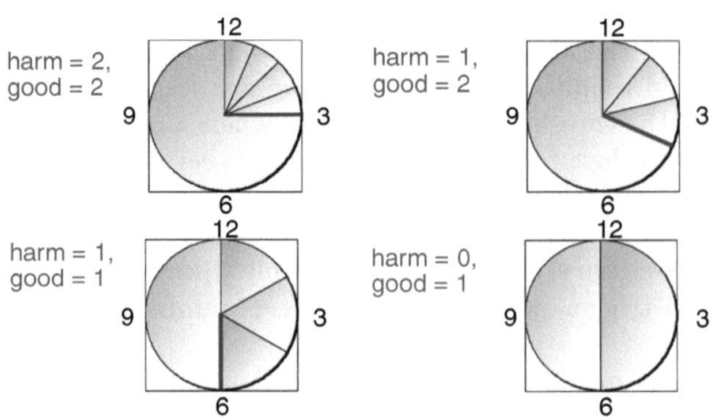

Fig. 10.7. EthEl system behavior with a start time of 12:00 and 6 hours for maximum harm and loss of benefit, both

In designing a reminding system for taking medications, there is a continuum of possibilities ranging from those that simply contact the overseer upon the first refusal to take medication by the patient to a system such as EthEl that takes into account ethical considerations. Clearly, systems that do not take ethical considerations into account are less likely to meet ethical obligations to their charges (and, implicitly, to the overseer as well). Systems that choose a less ethically sensitive reminder/notification schedule for medications are likely to not remind the patient often enough or notify the overseer soon enough, in some cases, and remind the patient too often or notify the overseer too soon in other cases.

EthEl uses an ethical principle learned by a machine to determine reminders and notifications in a way that is proportional to the amount of maximum harm to be avoided and/or benefit to be achieved by taking a particular medication, while not unnecessarily challenging a patient's autonomy. EthEl is an explicit ethical agent (in a constrained domain), according to Jim Moor's [18] definition of the term: A machine that is able to calculate the best action in ethical dilemmas using an ethical principle, as opposed to having been programmed to behave ethically, where the programmer is following an ethical principle. We believe that EthEl is the first system to use an ethical principle to determine its actions.

10.7 Related Research

Although many have voiced concern over the impending need for machine ethics (e.g. [10, 13, 23]), there have been few research efforts towards accomplishing this goal. Of these, a few explore the feasibility of using a particular ethical theory as a foundation for machine ethics without actually attempting implementation: Christopher Grau [11] considers whether the ethical theory that most obviously lends itself to implementation in a machine, Utilitarianism, should be used as the basis of machine ethics; and Tom Powers [19] assesses the viability of using deontic and default logics to implement Kant's categorical imperative.

Efforts by others that do attempt implementation have been based, to greater or lesser degree, upon *casuistry*—the branch of applied ethics that, eschewing principle-based approaches to ethics, attempts to determine correct responses to new ethical dilemmas by drawing conclusions based on parallels with previous cases in which there is agreement concerning the correct response. Rafal Rzepka and Kenji Araki [22], at what might be considered the most extreme degree of casuistry, are exploring how statistics learned from examples of ethical intuition drawn from the full spectrum of the World Wide Web might be useful in furthering machine ethics in the domain of safety assurance for household robots. Marcello Guarini [12], at a less extreme degree of casuistry, is investigating a neural network approach where particular actions concerning killing and allowing to die are classified as acceptable or unacceptable depending upon different motives and consequences. Bruce McLaren [16], in the spirit of a more pure form of casuistry, uses a case-based reasoning approach to develop a system that leverages information concerning a new ethical dilemma to predict which previously stored principles and cases are relevant to it in the domain of professional engineering ethics.

Other research of note investigates how an ethical dimension might be incorporated into the decision procedure of autonomous systems and how such systems might be evaluated. Selmer Bringsjord, Konstantine Arkoudas, and Paul Bello [8] are investigating how formal logics of action, obligation, and permissibility might be used to incorporate a given set of ethical principles into the decision procedure of an autonomous system, contending that such logics would allow for proofs establishing that such systems will only take permissible actions and perform all obligatory actions. Colin Allen, Gary Varner, and Jason Zinser [1] have suggested that a "moral Turing test" might be used to evaluate systems that incorporate an ethical dimension.

10.8 Future Directions

We plan to investigate the learned decision principle further to see if it can be applied to other dilemmas involving the same three duties. Also, it will be interesting to add the fourth duty from the PBM, justice, to see to what extent there's a consensus among bioethicists in cases where this duty is involved from which we can abstract a decision principle. There's disagreement about what is just among those working in ethics in other domains, but there might not be disagreement among bioethicists. Furthermore, we would like to see if our approach to learning decision principles will prove viable for other sets of duties, including sets of higher cardinality, and in other domains. It's reasonable to believe that each specific applied ethics domain (legal ethics, business ethics, journalistic ethics, and so on) involves juggling a set of *prima facie* duties that's specific to that domain. In each case, there will be the problem of abstracting a decision principle to determine the correct action when the duties conflict. We plan, therefore, to look at other domains to see whether our approach to creating an ethical-advisor system might be helpful in solving ethical dilemmas for those who work in those domains.

We further plan to investigate systems that follow ethical principles themselves. We believe, though, that the first step in the development of machine ethics must be to work on making ethics computable. If that task can't be accomplished, at least to the extent to which ethics experts are in agreement as to what's ethically right, then creating a machine that behaves ethically will be impossible. Creating ethical-advisor systems lets us explore the extent to which ethics can be computed in specific domains. Once ethics experts are comfortable with the results, then an ethical dimension can, at least in principle, be incorporated into machines, like EthEl, that function in those domains. This should not only avert unethical behavior on the part of machines, but also allow them to do tasks that we would have previously thought only human beings should do.

The process of making an ethical theory precise enough to be computed will likely lead to a sharpening and revision of the theory itself. This research provides an opportunity for applying AI techniques in a new domain, developing new areas of applied ethics, as well as making a contribution to ethical theory itself.

Our results demonstrate that a problem in ethical theory—devising a decision procedure for an ethical theory involving multiple *prima facie* duties—can be solved at least in a constrained domain and that AI techniques can help solve it. So, we believe that not only is it possible to train a machine to make ethical decisions, but also that machines can help human beings codify the principles that should guide them in ethical decision making.

In our preliminary research, we committed to a specific number of particular *prima facie* duties, a particular range of duty satisfaction/violation values, and a particular analysis of corresponding duty relations into differentials. To minimize bias in the constructed representation scheme, we propose to lift these assumptions and make a minimum epistemological commitment: Ethically relevant features of dilemmas will initially be represented as the degree of satisfaction or violation of at least one duty that the agent must take into account in determining the ethical status of the actions that are possible in that dilemma. A commitment to at least one duty can be viewed as simply a commitment to ethics – that there is at least one obligation incumbent upon the agent in dilemmas that are classified as ethical. If it turns out that there is only one duty, then there is a single, absolute ethical duty that the agent ought to follow. If it turns out that there are two or more, potentially competing, duties (as we suspect and have assumed heretofore) then it will have been established that there are a number of *prima facie* duties that must be weighed in ethical dilemmas, giving rise to the need for an ethical decision principle to resolve the conflict.

We envision a general system that will incrementally construct, through an interactive exchange with experts in ethics, the representation scheme needed to handle the dilemmas with which it is presented and, further, discover principles consistent with its training that lead to their resolution. Such a dynamic representation scheme is particularly suited to the domain of ethical decision-making, where there has been little codification of the details of dilemmas and principle representation. It allows for changes in duties and the range of their satisfaction/violation values over time, as ethicists become clearer about ethical obligations and discover that in different domains there may be different duties and possible satisfaction/violation values. Most importantly, it accommodates the reality that completeness in an ethical theory, and its representation, is a goal for which to strive, rather than expect at this time. The understanding of ethical duties, and their relationships, evolves over time.

Acknowledgment

This material is based upon work supported in part by the National Science Foundation grant number IIS-0500133.

References

1. Allen, C., Varner, G. and Zinser, J. 2000. Prolegomena to Any Future Artificial Moral Agent. Journal of Experimental and Theoretical Artificial Intelligence 12, pp. 251–61.
2. Anderson, S. 1999. "We Are Our Values," *Questioning Matters*, D. Kolak, ed., Mayfield, p. 599.
3. Anderson, M. and Anderson, S.L. 2006a. An Approach to Computing Ethics. IEEE Intelligent Systems, vol. 21, no. 4, pp. 22–28, July/August.
4. Anderson, M. and Anderson, S.L. 2006b. MedEthEx: A Prototype Medical Ethics Advisor. Proceedings of the Eighteenth Conference on Innovative Applications of Artificial Intelligence, Boston, Massachusetts, August.
5. Anderson, M., Anderson, S. and Armen, C. 2005. "Toward Machine Ethics: Implementing Two Action-Based Ethical Theories," *Proc. AAAI 2005 Fall Symp. Machine Ethics*, AAAI Press, pp. 1–16.
6. Beauchamp, T.L. and Childress, J.F. 1979. Principles of Biomedical Ethics, Oxford University Press.
7. Bentham, J. 1799. *An Introduction to the Principles and Morals of Legislation*, Oxford Univ. Press.
8. Bringsjord, S., Arkoudas, K. and Bello, P. 2006. Toward a General Logicist Methodology for Engineering Ethically Correct Robots. IEEE Intelligent Systems, vol. 21, no. 4, pp. 38–44, July/August.
9. Buchanan, A.E. and Brock, D.W. 1989. Deciding for Others: The Ethics of Surrogate Decision Making, pp. 48–57, Cambridge University Press.
10. Gips, J. 1995. Towards the Ethical Robot. Android Epistemology, Cambridge MA: MIT Press, pp. 243–252.
11. Grau, C. 2006. There Is No "I" in "Robot": Robots and Utilitarianism. IEEE Intelligent Systems, vol. 21, no. 4, pp. 52–55, July/August.
12. Guarini, M. 2006, Particularism and the Classification and Reclassification of Moral Cases. IEEE Intelligent Systems, vol. 21, no. 4, pp. 22–28, July/August.
13. Khan, A.F.U. 1995. The Ethics of Autonomous Learning Systems. Android Epistemology, Cambridge MA: MIT Press, pp. 253–265.
14. Lavrač, N. and Džeroski, S. 1997. Inductive Logic Programming: Techniques and Applications. Ellis Harwood.
15. Mappes, T.A. and DeGrazia, D. 2001. *Biomedical Ethics*, 5th ed., McGraw-Hill, pp. 39–42.
16. McLaren, B.M. 2003. Extensionally Defining Principles and Cases in Ethics: an AI Model. Artificial Intelligence Journal, Volume 150, November, pp. 145–181.
17. Mill, J.S. 1899. *Utilitarianism*, Boston, MA: Willard Small.
18. Moor, J.H. 2006. The Nature, Importance, and Difficulty of Machine Ethics. IEEE Intelligent Systems, vol. 21, no. 4, pp. 18–21, July/August.
19. Powers, T.M. 2006. Prospects for a Kantian Machine. IEEE Intelligent Systems, vol. 21, no. 4, pp. 46–51, July/August.

20. Rawls, J. 1951. Outline for a Decision Procedure for Ethics. Philosophical Review, 60.
21. Ross, W.D. 1930. The Right and the Good. Clarendon Press, Oxford.
22. Rzepka, R. and Araki, K. 2005. What Could Statistics Do for Ethics? The Idea of Common Sense Processing Based Safety Valve. Proceedings of the AAAI Fall Symposium on Machine Ethics, pp. 85–87, AAAI Press.
23. Waldrop, M.M. 1987. A Question of Responsibility. Chap. 11 in Man Made Minds: The Promise of Artificial Intelligence. NY: Walker and Company, 1987. (Reprinted in R. Dejoie et al., eds. Ethical Issues in Information Systems. Boston, MA: Boyd and Fraser, 1991, pp. 260–277.)

MIX
Papier aus verantwortungsvollen Quellen
Paper from responsible sources
FSC® C105338

If you have any concerns about our products,
you can contact us on
ProductSafety@springernature.com

In case Publisher is established outside the EU,
the EU authorized representative is:
Springer Nature Customer Service Center GmbH
Europaplatz 3, 69115 Heidelberg, Germany

Printed by Libri Plureos GmbH
in Hamburg, Germany